Inborn Errors of Metabolism in Humans

Previous Symposia of the Society for the
Study of Inborn Errors of Metabolism*

1. Neurometabolic Disorders in Childhood. Ed. K. S. Holt and J. Milner 1963
2. Biochemical Approaches to Mental Handicap in Children. Ed. J. D. Allan and K. S. Holt 1964
3. Basic Concepts of Inborn Errors and Defects of Steroid Biosynthesis. Ed. K. S. Holt and D. N. Raine 1965
4. Some Recent Advances in Inborn Errors of Metabolism. Ed. K. S. Holt and V. P. Coffey 1966
5. Some Inherited Disorders of Brain and Muscle. Ed. J. D. Allan and D. N. Raine 1969
6. Enzymopenic Anaemias, Lysosomes and other papers. Ed. J. D. Allan, K. S. Holt, J. T. Ireland and R. J. Pollitt 1969
7. Errors of Phenylalanine Thyroxine and Testosterone Metabolism. Ed. W. Hamilton and F. P. Hudson 1970
8. Inherited Disorders of Sulphur Metabolism. Ed. N. A. J. Carson and D. N. Raine 1971
9. Organic Acidurias. Ed. J. Stern and C. Toothill 1972
10. Treatment of Inborn Errors of Metabolism. Ed. J. W. T. Seakins, R. A. Saunders and C. Toothill 1973
11. Inborn Errors of Skin, Hair and Connective Tissue. Ed. J. B. Holton and J. T. Ireland 1975
12. Inborn Errors of Calcium and Bone Metabolism. Ed. H. Bickel and J. Stern 1976
13. Medico-Social Management of Inherited Metabolic Disease. Ed. D. N. Raine 1977
14. The Cultured Cell and Inherited Metabolic Disease. Ed. R. A. Harkness and F. Cockburn 1977
15. Inborn Errors of Immunity and Phagocytosis. Ed. F. Güttler, J. W. T. Seakins and R. A. Harkness 1979
16. Inherited Disorders of Carbohydrate Metabolism. Ed. D. Burman, J. B. Holton and C. A. Pennock 1980
17. Transport and Inherited Disease. Ed. N. R. Belton and C. Toothill 1981

The Society exists to promote exchanges of ideas between workers in different disciplines who are interested in any aspect of inborn metabolic disorders. Particulars of the Society can be obtained from the Editors of this Symposium.

* Symposia 1 10 published by E. & S. Livingstone

Inborn Errors of Metabolism in Humans

Monograph based upon Proceedings
of the International Symposium
held in Interlaken, Switzerland, September 2–5, 1980.

Edited by
Forrester Cockburn
and
Richard Gitzelmann

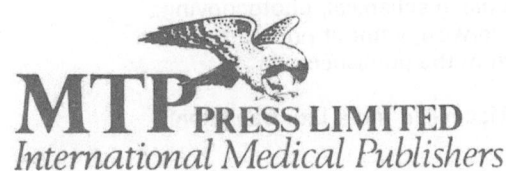

MTP PRESS LIMITED
International Medical Publishers

Published in the UK and Europe by
MTP Press Limited
Falcon House
Lancaster, England

British Library Cataloguing in Publication Data

Inborn errors of metabolism in humans.—(Symposium of the
   Society for the Study of Inborn Errors of Metabolism; 18)
   1. Metabolism, Inborn errors of—Congresses
   I. Cockburn, Forrester   II. Gitzelmann, R.
   III. Series
   616.3'9042   RC627.8
ISBN-13: 978-94-009-7327-5   e-ISBN-13: 978-94-009-7325-1
DOI: 10.1007 / 978-94-009-7325-1

Typeset by Macmillan India Ltd, Bangalore

by McCorquodale (Scotland) Ltd.

Contents

List of contributors   ix

Opening remarks   xiii

Dedication   xv

SECTION ONE

**Pathogenic Mechanisms of Inborn Errors:
Clinical Implications of Biochemical
Diversity**

1   Molecular aspects of genetic heterogeneity
    H. Harris   3

2   Inborn errors of purine metabolism – The
    Milner Lecture
    W. L. Nyhan   13

3   Vitamin-responsive inherited metabolic
    disorders: propionic acidaemia and
    methylmalonic acidaemia
    L. E. Rosenberg   37

4   Homocystinuria: clinical and biochemical
    heterogeneity
    N. A. J. Carson   53

5   Hereditary defects of steroid biosynthesis
    A. Prader and M. Zachmann   69

6   Blood–brain barrier amino-acid transport:
    clinical implications
    W. M. Pardridge   87

SECTION TWO

Treatment: New Aspects and Limits,
Transplantation, Replacement Therapy,
Genetic Engineering

7   Recent studies on the maturation of
    lysosomal enzymes
    E. F. Neufeld   103

8   Enzyme substitution by fibroblast
    transplantation
    *M. F. Dean, H. Muir, P. F. Benson and
    L. R. Button*   111

9   Artificial cell-encapsulated enzymes and
    adsorbents in congenital metabolic
    disorders
    T. M. S. Chang   131

10 Prospects for enzyme replacement therapy
    in heritable metabolic disorders
    *R. O. Brady, J. A. Barranger, P. G. Pentchev,
    F. S. Furbish and A. E. Gal*   139

SECTION THREE

Inborn Errors of Metabolism affecting Brain
Development (Animal Models)

11   Inborn errors of metabolism affecting
     brain development – Introduction
     N. Herschkowitz   157

12   Mutations in mice affecting brain
     development and their correlations
     with human diseases
     N. Baumann, F. Lachapelle and J.-C. Turpin   161

13   Murine mutations affecting myelination:
     models to study myelin diseases in the
     human
     J.-M. Matthieu   173

14   The effect of phenylalanine on myelin
     metabolism in adolescent rats
     F. A. Hommes, A. G. Eller and E. H. Taylor   193

15   Abnormal oligodendrocyte differentiation
     in a mouse mutant with defect in
     myelination
     *L. Bologa-Sandru, H.-P. Siegrist, A. Z'graggen,
     U. Wiesmann and N. Herschkowitz*   201

SECTION FOUR

Consequences of Inborn Errors of
Metabolism for the Individual, the Family
and Society

16   Inborn errors of metabolism – consequences
      of long-term treatment for the individual, as
      derived from observations in phenylketonuria
      H. Bickel and S. Grubel-Kaiser   211

17   Social aspects of the handicapped person
      Y. Posternak   225

18   Psychological and educational aspects of
      handicap
      C. C. Cunningham   237

19   Repercussions of screening
      B. E. Clayton   255

20   Some principles in the management of
      inherited metabolic disease
      D. N. Raine   267

      Index   287

List of contributors

J. A. BARRANGER
Developmental and Metabolic Neurology Branch, National Institute of Neurological and Communicative Disorders and Stroke, NIH, Bethesda, MD 20205, USA

N. BAUMANN
Laboratoire de Neurochimie, Inserm U. 134, Hôpital de la Salpétrière, 47 Boulevard de l'Hôpital, 75651 Paris Cedex 13, France

P. F. BENSON
Paediatric Research Unit, Department of Surgery, Guy's Hospital Medical School, London SE1 9RT, UK

H. BICKEL
Universitäts Kinderklinik, Im Neuenheimer Feld 150, D-6903 Heidelberg, West Germany

L. BOLOGA-SANDRU
Department of Pediatrics, University of Berne, 3010 Berne, Switzerland

R. O. BRADY
Developmental and Metabolic Neurology Branch, National Institute of Neurological and Communicative Disorders and Stroke, NIH, Bethesda, MD 20205, USA

L. R. BUTTON
Paediatric Research Unit, Department of Surgery, Guy's Hospital Medical School, London, SEI 9RT, UK

N. A. J. CARSON
Department of Child Health, The Queens University, Belfast 7, N. Ireland

T. M. S. CHANG
Artificial Cells and Organs Research Centre, McGill University, 3655 Drummond Street, Montreal, P.Q., Canada H3G 1Y6

B. E. CLAYTON
Department of Chemical Pathology and Human Metabolism, University of Southampton, Southampton General Hospital, Tremona Road, Southampton, Hants S09 4XY, UK

F. COCKBURN
University Department of Child Health, Royal Hospital for Sick Children, Yorkhill, Glasgow G3 8SJ, UK

C. C. CUNNINGHAM
Hester Adrian Research Centre, The University of Manchester, Manchester, M13 9PL, UK

M. F. DEAN
Department of Biochemistry, Kennedy Institute of Rheumatology, 6 Bute Gardens, Hammersmith, London W6 7DW, UK

A. G. ELLER
Department of Cell and Molecular Biology, Medical College of Georgia, Augusta, GA 30912, USA

F. S. FURBISH
Developmental and Metabolic Neurology Branch, National Institute of Neurological and Communicative Disorders and Stroke, NIH, Bethesda, MD 20205, USA

A. E. GAL
Developmental and Metabolic Neurology Branch, National Institute of Neurological and Communicative Disorders and Stroke, NIH, Bethesda, MD 20205, USA

R. GITZELMANN
Division of Metabolism, University Paediatric Department, Kinderspital, 8032 Zurich, Switzerland

S. GRUBEL-KAISER
Universitäts Kinderklinik, Im Neuenheimer Feld 150, D-6903 Heidelberg, West Germany

H. HARRIS
Department of Human Genetics, University of Pennsylvania Medical School, Philadelphia, PA 19104, USA

N. HERSCHKOWITZ
Department of Pediatrics, University of Berne, 3010 Berne, Switzerland

F. A. HOMMES
Department of Cell and Molecular Biology, Medical College of Georgia, Augusta, GA 30912, USA

F. LACHAPELLE
Laboratoire de Neurochimie, Inserm U. 134, Hôpital de la Salpétrière, 47 Boulevard de l'Hôpital, 75651 Paris Cedex 13, France

R.-S. MACH
4 rue de l'Athénée, 1205 Genève, Switzerland

J.-M. MATTHIEU
Neurochemistry Laboratory, Department of Pediatrics, University

Medical Center of Lausanne, CHUV, CH-1011 Lausanne, Switzerland

H. MUIR
Department of Biochemistry, Kennedy Institute of Rheumatology, 6 Bute Gardens, Hammersmith, London, W6 7DW, UK

E. F. NEUFELD
Genetics and Biochemistry Branch, National Institute of Arthritis, Diabetes, Digestive and Kidney Diseases, NIH, Bethesda, MD 20205, USA

W. L. NYHAN
Pediatrics Department, University of California, San Diego School of Medicine, La Jolla, CA 92093, USA

W. M. PARDRIDGE
Department of Medicine, Division of Endocrinology, UCLA School of Medicine, Los Angeles, CA 90024, USA

P. G. PENTCHEV
Developmental and Metabolic Neurology Branch, National Institute of Neurological and Communicative Disorders and Stroke, NIH, Bethesda, MD 20205, USA

Y. POSTERNAK
University of Geneva, 36 B route du Vallor, 1224 Chêne-Bougeries, Geneva, Switzerland

A. PRADER
Department of Paediatrics, University of Zurich, Kinderspital, Steinwiesstrasse 75, 8032 Zurich, Switzerland

D. N. RAINE (deceased)
Department of Clinical Chemistry, The Children's Hospital, Ladywood, Birmingham B16 8ET, UK

L. E. ROSENBERG
Department of Human Genetics, Yale University School of Medicine, 333 Cedar Street, New Haven, CT 06510, USA

H.-P. SIEGRIST
Department of Pediatrics, University of Berne, 3010 Berne, Switzerland

E. H. TAYLOR
Department of Cell and Molecular Biology, Medical College of Georgia, Augusta, GA 30912, USA

J.-C. TURPIN
Laboratoire de Neurochimie, Inserm U. 134, Hôpital de la Salpêtrière, 47 Boulevard de l'Hôpital, 75651 Paris Cedex 13, France

U. WIESMANN
Department of Pediatrics, University of Berne, 3010 Berne, Switzerland

M. ZACHMANN
Department of Paediatrics, University of Zurich, Kinderspital, Steinwiesstrasse 75, 8032 Zurich, Switzerland

A. Z'GRAGGEN
Department of Pediatrics, University of Berne, 3010 Berne, Switzerland

Opening Remarks

In the name of the Swiss Academy of Medical Sciences it is my pleasure to welcome you all, speakers and participants, to Interlaken.

My first remark goes to Hugo Aebi, to congratulate him for having set up and organized this meeting.

It is not quite by chance that this meeting on the biochemistry of genetic disorders is held in Switzerland; there are two reasons for that: firstly, the presence in Switzerland of good biochemists, and secondly, it is relevant to recall that Switzerland could be considered the birthplace of the DNA period of genetic research. It was Friedrich Miescher, who in 1869 in Basel (stimulated by his uncle, the embryologist His), isolated DNA for the first time. "That viscous substance", as Miescher referred to the DNA he had isolated from salmon, did not make headlines at the time, however, and Miescher would probably have been very surprised if he could have learned from Avery, more than 80 years later, that this DNA was indeed the chemical support of genetic information.

In the history of the relationship between medical research and inherited metabolic diseases, one can distinguish three overlapping periods. First, the description of the particular signs and symptoms which constitute a particular disease. Then, the elucidation of the biochemical defects involved. And finally, the understanding that these biochemical defects are themselves only the consequence of alterations at the level of DNA, which must be studied and explained in the light of the rapid progress of molecular genetics.

During the 50 years which elapsed between the formulation by Archibald Garrod of the concept of 'Inborn error of metabolism' in 1908 and the first printing of Stanbury's classical book on the biochemistry of inherited diseases, phenomenal progress has been made in the biochemistry of inherited metabolic disorders. The precise understanding of the biochemical defects must be completed by a study of the ultimate genetic origin of the diseases. And here the work of the biochemists and of the clinicians has been complemented by the progress of molecular biology during the last 30 years. An understanding of the origin of inherited diseases in molecular terms indeed draws heavily on that new science, from the concept of 'one gene – one enzyme' of Beadle and Tatum to the more recent discovery that most genes are indeed discontinuous or fragmented along our chromosomes.

Because of the rapid progress of the various areas which have made the field of inborn errors of metabolism what it is today, there is an inherent danger or risk for medical sciences and medicine. This danger is the gap between the professional scientists and medicine. More than ever we need people capable of conducting a dialogue between what sometimes appear to be different worlds. This meeting is a remarkable example of such a dialogue for the ultimate benefit of medicine. In the name of the Swiss Academy of Medical Sciences I am grateful for your contribution.

May your symposium be a great success. Thank you.

RENE-S. MACH

Dedication

Dedication

SECTION ONE

Pathogenic mechanisms of inborn errors: clinical implications of biochemical diversity

1

Molecular aspects of genetic heterogeneity

H. Harris

INTRODUCTION

A student of the literature of the inborn errors of metabolism, and indeed of other inherited diseases, could not fail to have noticed in recent years the increasing use of the term 'genetic heterogeneity'. It is usually meant to imply that what appears to be the same clinical syndrome may be the consequence of a number of quite different gene mutations. That this could indeed occur has, of course, been recognized for a long time[1,2]. But whereas in the past it was considered by most workers, at least implicitly, to be an unusual and somewhat infrequent phenomenon, it is now increasingly apparent that it is a common and widespread feature of inherited disease[3-5]. In other words, one can now say that 'genetic heterogeneity' is the rule rather than the exception, and its possible implications must be considered in the analysis of any inherited clinical disorder.

As different examples of the phenomenon have been analysed, it has become clear that such heterogeneity can arise in several ways. In introducing this book, in which the molecular basis of many different types of inborn error of metabolism will be discussed, I thought it would be useful to consider in general terms the basic types of cause which can give rise to the phenomenon and to propose a simple classification of these causes. This will, perhaps, provide a convenient framework on which to base the analysis of heterogeneity in any particular case.

3

The classification of causes is given in Table 1.1. Although I will consider each of these causes separately, it is important to stress that for any particular disorder more than one of these different types of cause may be operating, so that the heterogeneity may be very complex indeed.

TABLE 1.1   Causes of genetic heterogeneity of inborn errors of metabolism

1. Multiple allelism

2. Multiple loci
    (a) encoding different polypeptide chains in the same enzyme protein
    (b) encoding polypeptide chains in different enzyme proteins

3. Other causes
    (a) genetic background
    (b) gene–environment interactions

Detailed accounts of the various conditions mentioned in this chapter can be found in references 4 and 5.

MULTIPLE ALLELISM

It is now known that the base sequence in the DNA of a so-called 'structural' gene which determines the amino-acid structure of a polypeptide chain of an enzyme or protein includes several distinct regions. These are: the coding sequence regions which are eventually, via mRNA, translated into the amino-acid sequence of the polypeptide; the 5' and 3' sequence regions which are transcribed into RNA, present in the mRNA strand, but not translated into protein; intervening sequence regions which interrupt the coding sequences in the DNA, are transcribed into RNA but removed by processing in the nucleus so that they are not represented in the mRNA strand, and are not translated into protein. The precise functions of the non-translated regions (i.e. the 5' and 3' sequences, and the intervening sequences) are not known, but one must presume that they are necessary in some way for the normal production of the polypeptide and quite possibly are involved in the regulation of its rate of synthesis. A very large number of different mutations can occur within the confines of the gene. These may involve single base substitutions, deletions, or additions of one or a sequence of many bases. Their functional consequences will depend on the regions in which they occur, as well as on the specific character of the alteration in the DNA.

Most inborn errors of metabolism are diseases in which the various pathological manifestations are secondary to a metabolic disturbance resulting from a gross deficiency of a specific enzyme, which in turn is the consequence of a single gene mutation. Many different mutations within a gene can produce a profound loss of activity of the corresponding enzyme, and this loss of activity can arise in a number of different ways. It may, for example, arise because of the synthesis of a structurally altered enzyme protein which has lost its catalytic activity because of a change at the catalytic site. It may also arise because the altered enzyme protein is structurally unstable and so decays much more rapidly than its normal counterpart. Quite a number of examples of both of these types of defect have now been well documented in different conditions, and they can be attributed to mutations which have occurred at one or another site in the coding regions of the gene.

The different mutants can often be differentiated by immunochemical methods and also by enzyme kinetic studies in those cases, which are not uncommon, where the loss of enzyme activity is profound but not complete. This is exemplified by the differentiation of the multiplicity of allelic mutants which give rise to the various hypoxanthine–phos-phoribosyl transferase deficiences which determine the Lesch–Nyhan and other forms of hyperuricaemia and glucose-6 phosphate dehydrogenase deficiencies which determine various forms of chronic haemolytic disease. These examples bear witness to the remarkable number of different mutant alleles which may result in the deficiency of a single enzyme. Nevertheless, the immunochemical and enzyme kinetic methods presently available are probably relatively insensitive in their capacity to discriminate between many of the allelic differences that occur among patients with particular enzyme deficiencies. However, one may expect that the new DNA technology which is currently being developed very rapidly will make it possible before not too long to study many inborn errors at the DNA, rather than at the protein, level. One can anticipate that this will reveal even further heterogeneity among mutations which occur in the coding region of the gene and give rise to enzyme deficiencies. It should also enable us to find out whether, and to what extent, mutations in the untranslated regions of structural genes result in defects in enzyme synthesis and in consequent inborn errors of metabolism. If inborn errors attributable to such mutations can be identified, they should also prove to be extremely informative about the normal function of the particular region of the gene where the mutation is located.

If, as I have argued, many different mutant alleles may in different patients be the cause of a particular inborn error, a rather important inference can be made which undermines one of the standard dogmas of human genetics still expressed, or at least implied, in many text-books. This is, that in the case of disorder which segregates in families in the manner of a typical Mendelian autosomal recessive characteristic, the affected patients are *ipso facto* homozygous for a single mutant gene. If, however, numerous though individually very rare mutant alleles each resulting in the deficiency of the particular enzyme exist in the population, this conclusion will often and perhaps usually be incorrect. Although a condition segregates in families as an autosomal recessive, it will in many cases be due to heterozygosity for two different alleles, each producing a functionally defective enzyme but in different ways. Such heterozygous individuals would have received one of the mutant alleles from one parent and one from the other, each of whom would usually be carrying the normal allele and be clinically unaffected. So typical recessive segregation patterns with one-quarter ratios (after allowing for proband selection) would be obtained. The practical importance of this is that in attempting to characterize the nature of the enzyme deficiency, one has to keep in mind the strong possibility that there may be a mixture of two different variant enzyme proteins rather than just one. A number of well documented examples of the phenomenon have been reported, e.g. in certain cases of pyruvate kinase deficiency and glucose phosphate isomerase deficiency. However, the matter is, in general, very difficult to investigate because of the inevitably low levels of enzyme activity in the patients.

The important exception to the generalization that most individuals with rare autosomal recessive conditions are likely to be compound heterozygotes will occur in situations where there is inbreeding. Patients whose parents are first or second cousins will, for example, usually have received the same mutant allele from each parent and so be homozygotes. Also, in those cases where a particular inborn error has a relatively high incidence in a relatively small population but is rare elsewhere, it is probable that virtually all the affected individuals of that particular population are homozygous. Examples are tyrosinosis among the Quebecois of French origin and Tay–Sachs disease among Ashkenazi Jews. In each of these cases it seems probable that only a single mutation is involved and the two abnormal alleles in a given patient are ultimately derived from a common ancestor.

MULTIPLE LOCI

Mutations at quite separate loci coding for different polypeptide chains can result in the same or very similar clinical syndromes.

In some cases this is because a particular enzyme protein may contain two non-identical polypeptide chains encoded by different loci. Tay–Sachs and Sandhoff disease are examples of this. The two loci encode different polypeptides, both of which are present in the enzyme hexosaminidase A. Mutations at either locus can produce essentially the same clinical consequences because either can result in a loss of hexosaminidase A activity.

More often, however, genetic heterogeneity arises from mutants at gene loci which determine quite distinct enzymes. That this is so is not very surprising. Loss of function of one or another of the enzymes involved in a sequential series of reactions in a metabolic pathway or which are associated together in a complex of metabolic relationships, can well result in the same or very similar consequences at the clinical level.

A rather obvious example is provided by the complex network of metabolic reactions which occurs in the red cell and is necessary for maintaining its functional and structural integrity. Disruption of the normal metabolism of the red cell, with its consequent premature disruption and hence chronic haemolytic disease, can clearly occur as a result of defects of quite of a number of different enzymes. And indeed, a series of clinically not very dissimilar forms of chronic haemolytic anaemia have already been differentiated and shown to be due to deficiencies of different enzymes determined by different loci. These various haemolytic diseases may vary in clinical severity, but in practice it seems that they are rather difficult to differentiate from one another in the absence of information provided by enzyme studies. This difficulty is further enhanced by the fact that at any one of these loci, multiple alleles which differ in the degree of enzyme deficit they produce, and hence in clinical severity, may also occur. So superimposed on the variation due to mutations at separate loci affecting different enzymes is the added variation due to multiple allelism at single loci. Storage diseases such as the Hunter, Hurler and Scheie syndromes, the Sanfilippo syndromes A, B and C, and various glycogen diseases provide further examples of the same general phenomenon.

Enzyme studies provide the most direct approach to such problems. Where, for a variety of technical reasons this may be difficult, other approaches may be of considerable value in unravelling the matter. Complementation analysis in cell culture has, for example, emerged in recent years as a particularly powerful tool. One elegant illustration of this is provided by the complementation analysis of the methylmalonic acidurias carried out by Rosenberg and his colleagues, where five distinct complementation groups were identified among cell lines derived from 21 patients[6].

It is perhaps important to point out here the possible therapeutic implications of genetic heterogeneity. Again the methylmalonic acidurias provide an apt example. Deficient activity of methylmalonyl-CoA mutase is found in many cases. But this enzyme requires 5'-deoxy-adenosylcobalamin as cofactor and the severe syndrome of a critically ill infant with profound ketoacidosis and methylmalonic aciduria can arise either because of a mutation affecting the methylmalonyl-CoA mutase apoenzyme or because of a mutation affecting one or another of the enzymes involved in the biosynthesis of 5'-adenosylcobalamin from cobalamin or vitamin B_{12}, which is a necessary ingredient of a normal diet. Many of the patients with a defect in the 5'-adenosylcobalamin pathway respond dramatically to large doses of vitamin B_{12}, whereas most of those with the defective apoenzyme do not and succumb rapidly.

Inborn errors of metabolism are, as a rule, very rare diseases irregularly distributed in different populations. In view of the high degree of genetic heterogeneity which makes it likely that very often different mutants cause the disease in different families, particularly if they come from different populations, it is clearly unwise to assume that if a particular syndrome has been reported to have failed to respond to a specific line of therapy in some cases, it will necessarily fail to respond in others.

OTHER CAUSES OF HETEROGENEITY

It is implicit in the concept of genetic heterogeneity that different mutants may vary to some degree in the clinical effects they produce, because of subtle differences in the degree and character of the enzyme deficiency. Thus the clinical syndromes under consideration may exhibit a spectrum of variation. However, clinical variation from patient to patient may arise even when the same mutant allele (in the case of homozygotes) or the same mutant alleles (in the case of compound heterozygotes) are the basic cause of the disease in question.

Genetic background

One possible source of such variations is the rest of the genetic constitution of the individuals in which the particular mutant gene or genes occur. There is now an extensive body of data[5] which indicates that, with the exception of monozygotic twins, no two individuals are exactly alike in their enzyme makeup, because of the common allelic differences (so-called polymorphisms) which occur at many gene loci. Such so-called 'normal variations' in genetic background, because they must define many of the details of the biochemical milieu against which the effects of particular abnormal genes are expressed, may well result in subtle differences in the manifestation of a particular disorder in different affected patients. Some combinations of particular genes at other loci might minimize the pathological consequences and others accentuate them. Since such different combinations of genes will often not result in obvious metabolic differences between normal individuals, the detailed manner in which they may contribute to variation in manifestation of particular inborn errors of metabolism is generally very difficult to define.

Gene–environment interactions

The clinical manifestations of an enzyme deficiency determined by a mutant gene may also depend, to some degree, on variations in the environmental circumstances to which individuals with the abnormality are exposed. Often the expression of a particular abnormality appears to be hardly influenced by such environmental variations, but in other cases the effects may be important and give rise to quite unexpected clinical differences.

A striking illustration is provided by the work of Blass and Gibson on the Wernicke–Korsakoff syndrome in chronic alcoholics[7]. The reasons why some people and not others become severe chronic alcoholics are complex and poorly understood. A variety of social factors are no doubt involved, and there may be biological factors as well. One consequence of chronic alcoholism is severe and prolonged malnutrition, including an inadequate vitamin intake. Among such chronically malnourished alcoholics a small minority develop the Wernicke–Korsakoff syndrome, which is a severe confusional state associated with a variety of neurological abnormalities. There is often rapid clinical improvement if large doses of thiamine are administered. Blass and Gibson showed that in patients with the Wernicke–Korsakoff syndrome there is a mutant form of the enzyme transketolase, with a markedly reduced affinity for its essential cofactor, thiamine pyrophosphate. It appears that under normal circumstances, where there is an adequate supply of thiamine in the diet, the concentration of thiamine pyrophosphate in the cells of individuals with this abnormal enzyme is sufficient to allow normal functioning. However, in the profoundly malnourished state that develops in chronic alcoholics, the concentration of thiamine pyrophosphate falls to levels which cause a marked reduction in transketolase activity, and this in turn evidently gives rise to the characteristic neurological abnormalities of the Wernicke–Korsakoff syndrome. Thus the syndrome only occurs in individuals with the abnormal enzyme and who are severely malnourished. Other alcoholics with the same degree of malnutrition do not develop the syndrome, nor presumably do individuals on a normal diet who happen to have the abnormal enzyme.

CONCLUDING REMARKS

In conclusion I would like to emphasize the remarkable degree of genetic heterogeneity that can occur in quite rare disorders. A good illustration is provided by the syndrome of congenital methaemoglobinaemia. This may arise from mutations affecting the structure of haemoglobin, or from mutations causing deficient activity of the enzyme NADH diaphorase, which in the normal individual is concerned with maintaining the iron of haemoglobin in the ferrous state. The abnormality is generally apparent in infancy and persists throughout life with little variation, and because of the marked cyanosis it is readily recognized. Congenital methaemoglobinaemia is extremely rare and probably in most populations occurs with an incidence of less than one in 100 000 births. Nevertheless, at least ten different mutant genes causing it have already been identified, two at one or other of the α-haemoglobin loci, three at the β-haemoglobin locus and at least five at the locus which determines NADH diaphorase. The syndromes they separately produce are very similar clinically.

There is no reason to believe that congenital methaemoglobinaemia is unusual in this respect, and one may anticipate that a similar degree of genetic heterogeneity will be found in many other conditions.

Acknowledgements

This work was supported by grant GM27018 from the National Institutes of Health.

References

1. Harris, H. (1953). *An Introduction to Human Biochemical Genetics*. Eugenics Laboratory Memoirs, XXXVII. (Cambridge: Cambridge University Press)
2. Harris, H. (1974). Genetic heterogeneity in inherited disease. *J. Clin. Pathol.* 27 (Suppl.) (R. Coll. Pathol.), **8**, 32

3. McKusick, V. A. (1973). Phenotypic diversity of human diseases resulting from allelic series. *Am. J. Hum. Genet.,* **25,** 446
4. Stanbury, J. B., Wyngaarden, J. B. and Fredrickson, D. S. (1978). *The Metabolic Basis of Inherited Disease.* 4th Ed. (New York: McGraw-Hill)
5. Harris, H. (1980). *The Principles of Human Biochemical Genetics.* 3rd Ed. (Amsterdam: North Holland)
6. Willard, H. F., Mellman, I. F. and Rosenberg, L. E. (1978). Genetic complementation among inherited deficiencies of methylmalonyl CoA mutase activity: evidence for a new class of human cobalamin variant. *Am. J. Hum. Genet.,* **30,** 1
7. Blass, J. B. and Gibson, G. E. (1977). Abnormality in thiamine-requiring enzyme in patients with Wernicke–Korsakoff syndrome. *N. Engl. J. Med.,* **297,** 1367

2

Inborn errors
of purine metabolism
W. L. Nyhan

INTRODUCTION

The inborn errors of metabolism have played a special role in the development of human genetics as a scientific discipline. The study of these disorders, each of them individually uncommon, has pointed out the ways in which molecular expression of gene action takes place in man. It has given us new understanding of mechanisms of human variation. It has pioneered in the field of prenatal diagnosis and has permitted new approaches to questions of population genetics by permitting the detection of recessive genes in heterozygotes. Each of these aspects of modern biochemical genetics is exemplified by the inborn errors of purine metabolism, an area in which there have been exciting new developments.

Although gout was recognized by Hippocrates, scientific progress in this field was slow until recent years, but now a number of disorders of purine metabolism have been characterized at a molecular level. In addition to the understanding this has brought to the hyperuricaemias, new interrelations have been uncovered between the metabolism of purines and immune function. This chapter will focus on these disorders of purine metabolism, which present with accumulation of uric acid in body fluids.

13

THE LESCH–NYHAN SYNDROME

The modern era of the inborn errors of purine metabolism was ushered in with the discovery of the Lesch–Nyhan syndrome in 1964[1]. The gene responsible for this condition is on the X chromosome and the phenotype is a fully recessive X-linked characteristic. The molecular expression of the abnormal gene is in the defective activity of the enzyme hypoxanthine guanine phosphoribosyl transferase (HGPRT; EC. 2.4.2.8)[2,3]. In this disorder there are far-reaching biological effects.

The cardinal clinical characteristics of the syndrome are mental retardation, spastic cerebral palsy, choreoathetosis and self-multilative behaviour[1,3]. These patients also have hyperuricaemia and may have any of the renal or other consequences of hyperuricaemia seen in populations of patients with gout. They usually develop normally for the first six to eight months, but crystalluria, haematuria or renal-tract stone disease may occur even during these early months of life.

The onset of cerebral manifestations is with athetoid cerebral palsy. Infants who have been sitting and holding their heads up begin to lose these abilities. Intially, they may be hypotonic or hypertonic, but deep tendon reflexes are increased. Later they are all markedly hypertonic. In the established disease, the motor defect is of such severity that the patient can neither stand nor sit unassisted. None of our patients with the Lesch–Nyhan syndrome has walked. I believe that a patient thought to have this syndrome who does walk should be carefully studied with the hypothesis that he has some other disease. Most patients are mentally retarded; their IQs have usually been below 50. Nevertheless, there is a spectrum of intelligence, and a few patients who appear to have had the classic enzyme variant have had normal intelligence.

Involuntary movements of both choreic form and athetoid type are prominent. The movements may appear dystonic. The patients are prone to sudden opisthotonic or extensor spasms of the trunk, and scissoring of the lower extremities is seen regularly. Deep tendon reflexes are increased. The Babinski sign may be present, and many patients have ankle clonus.

The speech is characterized by athetoid dysarthria. Athetoid dysphagia is another problem; these patients have so much difficulty in swallowing that they are difficult to feed. They all vomit frequently. Rarely, a patient may present in the first few days of life with severe vomiting[4]. Because of feeding difficulty and persistent vomiting a patient in a busy, crowded institution for the retarded may die of inanition. Most of the patients are markedly underweight and many are quite short. The bone age may be retarded. These features are probably nutritional. Endocrinological investigation has not revealed abnormalities[5], and a number of patients, particularly those reared at home, have had normal rates of physical growth and normal bone ages. Patients aspirate frequently and may develop pneumonia. Convulsions are not a regular feature of the syndrome but have been observed in a number of patients.

Aggressive, self-multilating behaviour is possibly the most striking aspect of the syndrome[1, 6,7]. Self-multilation may begin as early as the eruption of the teeth. Its onset is seldom delayed long thereafter, but a few children may go for some years before the onset of the characteristic behaviour. Most patients bite both their lips and fingers destructively. Every patient we have seen has bitten his lips unless the primary teeth have been removed early, and in most patients the hallmark of the syndrome is loss of tissue about the lips (Figure 2.1). There may be partial amputations of the fingers.

Sensation is intact in children with the Lesch–Nyhan syndrome. They scream in pain when they bite themselves, and it is clear that they really do not want to do what they are doing. They are really happy only when

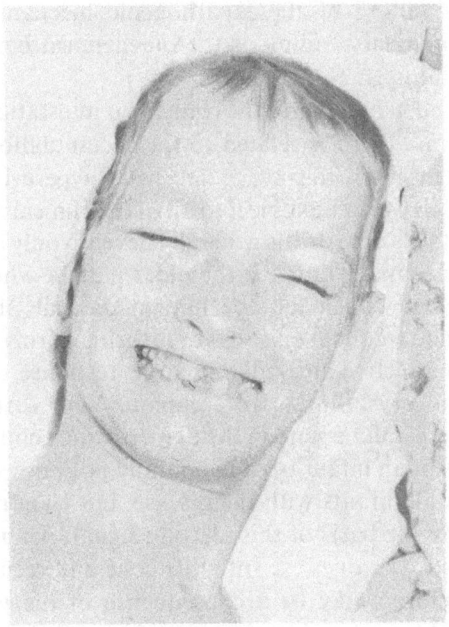

Figure 2.1 A patient with the Lesch–Nyhan syndrome. The loss of tissue about the lip is characteristic of the syndrome

securely protected from themselves[7]. Many of these children scream all night until their parents or guardians are taught how to restrain them securely in bed. As they grow older these children learn to call for help. The cry of the young child with the syndrome carries the same message. Mutilation in this syndrome is caused by a form of compulsive behaviour disorder and does not take the form of biting alone. These children are generally self-destructive, but they will also direct their aggressions against others and bite them. As they learn to speak they become verbally aggressive. Vomiting may be incorporated into this pattern of behaviour, and even the opisthotonic rearward thrust of the head which is so characteristic may be at least semi-voluntary, and effectively agressive against anyone close behind.

The behaviour of these patients is an integral element of the syndrome. I believe that a patient with features of the syndrome including an abnormality in HGPRT who does not mutilate is likely to have a variant protein other than the classic Lesch–Nyhan variant. The pathogenesis of the behaviour is scientifically provocative and not well understood. The syndrome is the first instance in which a stereotyped pattern of human behaviour has been associated with a distinct biochemical abnormality. Improved understanding of these pathogenic mechanisms might contribute to a better understanding of the biochemical basis of behaviour, both normal and abnormal.

On the other hand, a number of the clinical manifestations of the Lesch–Nyhan syndrome are directly related to the accumulation of uric acid in body fluids. Patients with this syndrome have hyperuricaemia from the neonatal period. They may be subject to all of the clinical manifestations of gout, but acute attacks of arthritis generally develop only after a number of years of hyperuricaemia. Thus it is the older patient who develops acute arthritis. An affected cousin of one patient died at 21 years and was reported to have had frequent episodes of arthritis during his last year. We have observed an effective anti-inflammatory response to colchicine.

Haematuria and crystalluria are common. Very early there may be masses of orange crystalline sand in the diapers which could readily lead to an early diagnosis in an infant born in a family not known to be at risk. It seems to occur in all infants with the disease, but I am not aware of any cases diagnosed on the basis of this alerting signal. A number of patients have had urinary tract stones[8, 9]. Infantile colic and recurrent abdominal pains in older children may be a consequence of the presence of large amounts of insoluble material in the urine. Urinary tract infections have been common only in those with stones. Many of these patients develop a renal concentration defect in which there is polyuria and polydipsia[10, 11].

This may protect against the development of stones, but patients may have great difficulty satisfying their thirst in a large, busy institution. Urate nephropathy may lead to renal failure, and this has been the most common cause of early death.

Tophi may also develop, but these take years to form and to become evident. We have observed tophi in three cases, but none recently, as patients are being diagnosed earlier and treated with allopurinol. One patient had a tophus on his ear that was as large as a golf ball. Another had tophi which broke down and drained solid white urate.

Anaemia is observed with some frequency. Sometimes it is macrocytic and megaloblastic[12, 13]. The anaemia often regresses spontaneously. We have observed an associated eosinophilia in one patient, and so has Michel[14].

Autopsies have been carried out in four patients, three of which have been reported. In the first of these[15] some cerebral pathology was observed. There were granules which took the de Galantha stain for urate and there was axonal swelling and demyelination of the white matter. Changes like this have been seen in other patients with uraemia and are generally thought not to be specific for the Lesch–Nyhan syndrome. The patients described by Crussi et al.[16] did not have these lesions in the brain, nor did our second patient. The myelin displayed remarkable integrity, and there were no microscopically discernible lesions in the basal ganglia.

In most patients, the first biochemical evidence of metabolic abnormality is an increased concentration of uric acid in the blood, usually in the range of 10 mg/dl. Occasionally, normal blood concentrations of uric acid have been observed in children and rarely a patient might have consistently normal serum concentrations.

The urinary excretion of uric acid is always increased. Children with this syndrome excrete three to four times as much uric acid (> 600 mg/day) as do control children. Among adult patients with gout those who have excreted this much uric acid have been classified as hyper-excretors. Patients with the Lesch–Nyhan syndrome excrete 40–60 mg/kg body weight per day. Expressed in terms of creatinine excretion, these patients usually excrete 2–4 mg of uric acid/mg of creatinine, while control individuals excrete less than 1 mg uric acid/mg creatinine.

The metabolism of purines has been studied by determining the rate at which uric acid is synthesized from glycine. This has been done by administering isotopically labelled glycine. In our original studies[1, 8, 17], the tracer glycine was labelled with [14]C. More recently, we have explored the utility of the non-radioactive isotope of carbon, ^{13}C, for this purpose[18]. In either case, the uric acid must be isolated from the urine, purified, and its isotope content determined. Isolated uric acid labelled with ^{14}C may be added to a scintillation solution and counted directly. For ^{13}C-labelled uric acid measurements, tetramethyluric acid is made from trimethylalanine hydroxide and purified on a Sephadex G10 column. It is then analysed by gas chromatography and mass spectrometry.

In patients there is a rapid peak of specific activity in the first 24 h; at the peak it is easy to distinguish patients from controls. In studies of this sort in adults, it has not been possible to distinguish the specific activities of patients with gout from those of control individuals. Therefore, it has become conventional to express the data as the cumulative percentage of the isotope of administered glycine that has been converted to uric acid. Adults with overproduction gout convert about twice as much glycine to uric acid as do controls. In children with the Lesch–Nyhan syndrome, about 2 % of the glycine administered has regularly been recovered in uric acid[1, 8, 17, 18]. This is about 20 times the control value[19]. These are the highest rates of purine production ever reported.

In our studies using ^{13}C-labelled glycine, patients with the Lesch–Nyhan syndrome had curves of specific activity as well as cumulative percentage incorporation rates that were virtually identical to those obtained using ^{14}C-labelled glycine. Initially, we studied the simultaneous incorporation of both tracers in the same patient. The high purity obtained by derivatization and the extra column purification leads to smoother specific activity curves for ^{13}C than for ^{14}C. Furthermore, the isotope enrichment obtained with the non-radioactive tracer permits the assay of very small samples. This methodology should have many important applications in the *in vivo* study of metabolism in man.

It would be expected that compounds other than uric acid might accumulate in the presence of overproduction of purine of this magnitude. Patients excrete normal quantities of xanthine. However, the amounts of hypoxanthine excreted are markedly increased[20, 21]. In most normal individuals, the molar ratio of hypoxanthine to xanthine is less than one. In Lesch–Nyhan patients the ratio is greater than one and may be as high as 8. When the patient is treated with allopurinol, which inhibits xanthine oxidase, the excretion of uric acid decreases and the other oxypurines become the major products of overproduction. The hypoxanthine to xanthine ratio decreases with small doses of allopurinol, but as the degree of the block is increased, more and more purine ends up as hypoxanthine. In controls treated with allopurinol, most of the oxypurine excreted is xanthine. These observations indicate that in normal individuals most urinary urate is formed from xanthine which does not come from hypoxanthine. This is consistent with the fact that patients with a congenital absence of xanthine oxidase have xanthinuria. On the other hand, in the Lesch–Nyhan syndrome most of the purine usually seen as urinary urate was previously hypoxanthine.

Uric acid is not formed in the brain. Other oxypurines are the end-products of purine metabolism in the central nervous system. In the cerebrospinal fluid of patients with the Lesch–Nyhan syndrome[22], xanthine concentrations are identical to those of controls but concentrations of hypoxanthine are four times greater than in controls. Treatment with allopurinol increases even further the concentration of hypoxanthine in the cerebrospinal fluid of these patients.

The primary site for the expression of the abnormal gene in the Lesch–Nyhan syndrome is the enzyme hypoxanthine guanine phosphoribosyl transferase (HGPRT) (Figure 2.2). This enzyme converts the purine bases, hypoxanthine and guanine, to their respective nucleotides, inosinic and guanylic acids (IMP and GMP). The purine analogues, 6-mercaptopurine, 6-thioguanine and 8-azaguanine, require the presence of this enzyme and conversion to their respective nucleotides before they can become active chemotherapeutic or cytotoxic agents. Deficiency in the activity of HGPRT in the Lesch–Nyhan syndrome was first reported by Seegmiller et al.[2]. This important observation has been confirmed by a number of investigators[3, 23, 24]. The enzyme is normally present in all tissues of the body. In affected patients, activity is deficient in every tissue.

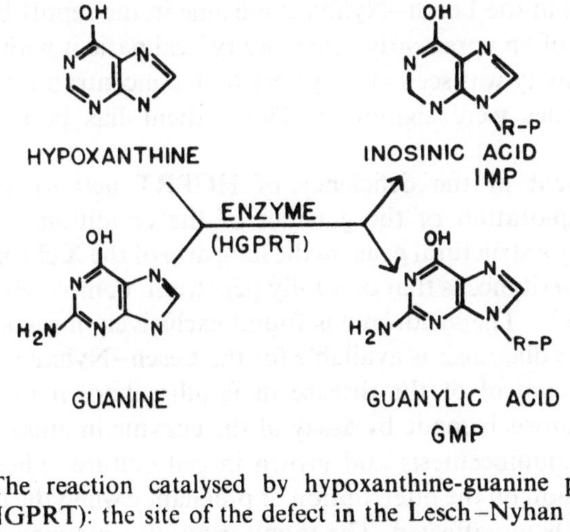

Figure 2.2 The reaction catalysed by hypoxanthine-guanine phosphoribosyl transferase (HGPRT): the site of the defect in the Lesch–Nyhan syndrome

HGPRT is most conveniently measured in the erythrocyte. Quantitative assay of the enzyme in the erythrocyte has regularly revealed no activity. The more precisely quantitative the determination, the more it is clear that the values obtained in Lesch–Nyhan patients cannot be distinguished from zero.

HGPRT may be studied by electrophoresis on polyacrylamide disc gels. The pattern for HGPRT is reproducible, and one in which there is a broad area of activity with four sub-bands[25, 26]. Erythrocyte haemolysates from patients with the Lesch–Nyhan syndrome regularly yield an area compatible with the presence of enzyme in this system[26]. Its mobility is faster than that of the normal enzyme but activity is very low. These observations indicate that the mutation which produces this syndrome is in a structural gene which specifies a protein with an altered primary structure. This conclusion is also supported by the observation that it is possible to activate the variant enzyme with small amounts of normal enzyme[27]. This cannot be done by simply mixing the two together, but occurs when they are subjected together to electrophoresis; two bands of activity appear – one in the variant area, or when they are passed together through a Sephadex column.

Abnormal HGPRT does not exhibit cross-reactivity (CRM) with antibody prepared against purified normal erythrocyte HGPRT[28]. This issue is not completely clear, even in recent literature. It is generally agreed that patients with the classic Lesch–Nyhan syndrome are CRM$^-$ and that early reports to the contrary[29 – 31] resulted from antibodies to impurities. A source of some confusion is the fact that genetic heterogeneity has been demonstrated in the Lesch–Nyhan syndrome in the report by McDonald and Kelley[32] of an apparently otherwise typical patient with a K_m variant HGPRT. Activity was seen at only very high concentrations of substrates and the kinetics were sigmoidal. This patient has been found to be CRM$^+$[33 34].

Establishment of the deficiency of HGPRT activity permitted the molecular exploration of the genetics of the condition. The disease is transmitted by a structural gene on the long arm of the X chromosome. The pattern of inheritance is that of a fully penetrant, completely recessive, X-linked disease[17]. The syndrome is found exclusively in males.

Intrauterine diagnosis is available for the Lesch–Nyhan syndrome, and this permits control of the disease in families known to be at risk[35]. Prenatal diagnosis is made by assay of the enzyme in amniotic fluid cells obtained by amniocentesis and grown in cell culture. These techniques permit a decision on the interruption of pregnancy when the fetus has been diagnosed as being affected. The monitoring of a pregnancy in this way permits a known carrier of the gene to have normal children, since those monitored pregnancies brought to term should have established HGPRT activity.

In an X-linked recessive condition, the fathers should and do have normal activity of the enzyme. The Lyon hypothesis specifies that the mothers, as heterozygotes, should be mosaics in which there are two populations of cells, one completely normal and the other completely deficient. This has been demonstrated by experiments in which fibroblasts in cell culture were cloned[36, 37].

However, assessment of the activity of HGPRT in erythrocytes or leukocytes of obligate heterozygotes for this condition has always revealed normal HGPRT activity. Information on this subject has been obtained through the study of key kindreds in which two types of glucose-6-phosphate dehydrogenase (G6PD) were segregating, as well as two types of HGPRT[38, 39]. In these families women heterozygous for HGPRT and for the G6PD types A and B were studied by cloning fibroblasts cultured from skin, and two populations of cells were proven to be present. However, repeated assay of their erythocytes and leukocytes revealed only one G6PD type, as well as normal activity for HGPRT. These observations indicate a clonal origin of the haematopoietic system. The data could be explained by non-random inactivation of the X chromosome containing the information for G6PD and for HGPRT. A more likely explanation is that there is random inactivation very early in fetal life, but that it is followed by selection against the HGPRT⁻ cell. We have called this phenomenon hemizygous expression. It complicates the detection of heterozygotes in this condition. A molecular diagnosis is essential for precise genetic counselling, but it is clear that heterozygosity cannot be detected using blood.

The presence of both cell types in cultures derived from heterozygote skin has permitted the use of fibroblasts in culture for diagnosis. Heterozygosity can, of course, be demonstrated by cloning[36, 37]. However, the time, expense and attention involved preclude the use of cloning as a routine method for the diagnosis of the gene carrier. Pharmacological methods of cell selection [40, 41] provide the cell culture method of choice for heterozygote detection, as long as enzyme assay is carried out on the populations of cells selected. The principles of selection take advantage of the unique properties of these cells. HGPRT is required for the activation of 6-mercaptopurine (6-MP) and related analogue inhibitors of purine metabolism. These include 6-thioguanine (6-TG) and 8-azaguanine (8-AG). Normal cells containing HGPRT are killed by these compounds, while HGPRT⁻ cells are unaffected. Thus, in the mixed population of cells cultured from a heterozygote, this type of selective medium will permit the growth only of the HGPRT⁻ cells. Selection of a population of HGPRT⁺ cells can be made by growth in hypoxanthine–aminopterin–thymidine

(HAT) medium, but this is not required for diagnosis of heterozygosity. The difficulty with any cell-culture method of heterozygote detection is that sometimes only one cell type grows from the primary explant. There is no problem if this is the HGPRT$^-$ population, but if it is the HGPRT$^+$ population, misdiagnosis would result.

The assay of the enzyme in single hair follicles provides the most reliable, rapid, simple, and the least expensive method of heterozygote detection[42-44]. It is the best method and has supplanted other methods requiring cell culture. It obviates the problem of selection *in vitro*. It also obviates the problem which we have observed of changes in enzyme content and activity during cultivation *in vitro*. On the other hand it is not always possible to obtain follicles. Cell culture methods may, therefore, be required.

For validity, the hair-follicle methods are dependent on the viability of cells and enzymes in each tiny follicle. Gartler and colleagues[42] have controlled this by splitting the extract obtained from each follicle and running both adenine phosphoribosyl transferase (APRT) and HGPRT. We do this electrophoretically and, therefore, can simultaneously assay both HGPRT and APRT on each single follicle. We believe it is preferable to assay 20–30 hairs for diagnosis.

Treatment in the Lesch–Nyhan syndrome is effective only for the complications of the hyperuricaemia. The renal complications, as well as arthritis and tophi, are effectively prevented using allopurinol. The oral administration of allopurinol, in a dose of 200–400 mg/day, causes a reduction of plasma and urinary concentrations of uric acid and a concomitant increase in the oxypurines, hypoxanthine and xanthine[20, 21]. In controls and in adults with gout who have normal HGPRT activity, the total excretion of oxypurines, i.e. the sum of uric acid, xanthine and hypoxanthine, decreases after treatment with allopurinol. In patients with Lesch–Nyhan syndrome, this decrease in oxypurine excretion is not seen[20]. Probenecid and other uricosuric agents are contra-indicated in patients with HGPRT deficiency. The kidneys of these individuals already process enormous amounts of uric acid, and administration of a uricosuric agent could lead to a renal shutdown and death. Alkali therapy with sodium citrate or sodium bicarbonate is effective in the prevention of crystalluria and stones, and the maintenance of a normal level of urea nitrogen in the blood in patients who drink sufficient water. However, this form of management is much more difficult than with allopurinol therapy, particularly at times of intercurrent illness.

Interrelations among the oxypurines are relevant to treatment with allopurinol (Figure 2.3). In normal individuals an increasingly effective

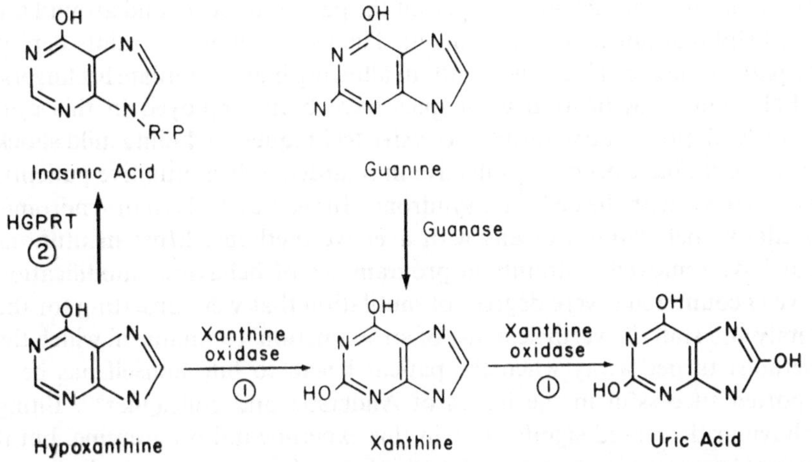

Figure 2.3   Interrelations among the oxypurines. Xanthine oxidase (1) the site of the inhibitory action of allopurinol catalyses the two separate conversions shown. HGPRT (2) is the site of the defect in the Lesch–Nyhan disease, in which hypoxanthine cannot be reutilized and accumulates

blockade of xanthine oxidase with allopurinol results in the excretion of a greater proportion of the purine formed as xanthine. This is consistent with the fact that patients with inherited defects in xanthine oxidase have xanthinuria. Patients with normal HGPRT simply reutilize hypoxanthine accumulating behind a block in xanthine oxidase. This can be a problem, for xanthine is even more insoluble than uric acid and with inappropriate treatment one could convert uric-acid stone disease to xanthine stone disease. On the other hand, in the HGPRT⁻ patient, increasing the degree of inhibition of xanthine oxidase makes him increasingly hypoxanthinuric. Hypoxanthine is quite soluble and does not cause urinary-tract stones. In the management of a patient with very large quantities of uric acid in the urine, adjustment of the ratios of uric acid, xanthine and hypoxanthine through regulation of the dosage of allopurinol may require quantitative measurement of the amounts of these oxypurines in the urine. Xanthine stones have been reported in this syndrome[45] and we have observed them in some of our patients.

The cornerstone of the day-to-day management of the Lesch–Nyhan syndrome is physical restraint aimed at the protection of the patient against himself. We have learned a number of practical procedures that facilitate the care of these patients[7]. Patients do learn some control with age, so it is often possible to prevent disfigurement by the removal of primary teeth.

Individualized wheelchairs that permit the patient to be up and around are very helpful adjuncts to management. The use of elbow restraints permit the patient the use of his hands without allowing him to mutilate his fingers.

Behaviour modification techniques have been employed in this syndrome with provocative results. Aversive techniques, including mild shock with a prod, have been very effective in retarded, self-multilative patients, such as those with the de Lange syndrome. In the Lesch–Nyhan syndrome, mutilative behaviour worsens with aversive methods. Most institutions that have removed restraints in programmes of behaviour modification have encountered severe degrees of mutilation that were upsetting for the family and staff. Nevertheless, use of an 'extinction' technique in which the therapist turned away when the patient began to bite himself has been reported successful in the hands of Anderson and colleagues[46]. Biting behaviour decreased significantly in this experimental programme, but it has not been possible to extrapolate this form of management to the home. Behaviour in this syndrome, like all behaviour, is capable of some modification, but this is clearly not a therapy. A similar comment could be made about pharmacological approaches, using 5-hydroxytryptophan[47]. When 5-hydroxytryptophan is combined with a peripheral decarboxylase inhibitor such as carbidopa, it is possible to modify behaviour[48]. However, tolerance develops very rapidly. These results suggest that biogenic amines may be important in the control of behaviour. Furthermore, the urinary excretion of 5-hydroxyindoleacetic acid is greater in patients with the Lesch–Nyhan syndrome than in controls, which also suggests biogenic amine imbalance[49].

HYPERURICAEMIC DISORDERS IN WHICH THERE ARE OTHER VARIANTS OF HGPRT

In increasing numbers of patients, abnormalities of HGPRT are being recognized in which the phenotype is different from that of the Lesch–Nyhan syndrome. These mutant genes are also on the X chromosome[50-52]. Male patients with these enzyme variants reproduce, and an absence of male to male transmission has been documented[52]. In some families some expression has been observed in the female heterozygote[53]. In view of the number of mutations at the HGPRT locus that have so far been recognized, it appears likely that a considerable molecular heterogeneity is present.

Patients with variants of HGPRT were first found among adult male patients with clinical gout. These patients excrete large amounts of uric acid in the urine and may present in childhood with renal stone disease. They may develop urate nephropathy, and this too may occur in childhood. One of our patients[54] presented with a syndrome of transient haematuria and oliguria following anaesthesia in a pattern that suggested glomerulonephritis. Acute attacks of gouty arthritis and deposits of urate generally appear first in adult life. Many years of hyperuricaemia are required before the onset of the arthritic manifestations that are ultimately the hallmark of gout. Thus we have come to recognize two distinct phenotypes (Table 2.1) of deficiency of HGPRT – the Lesch–Nyhan syndrome and a phenotype in which the manifestations are simply those of hyperuricaemia.

TABLE 2.1   Populations of patients with HPRT deficiency

Defect	HPRT activity	Clinical features
Lesch–Nyhan syndrome	0	Mental retardation, spasticity, choreoathetosis, self-mutilation, hyperuricaemia, nephropathy, stones, arthritis, tophi
Partial defects	1–50%	Hyperuricaemia, arthritis, nephropathy, stones, tophi

Assay of the erythrocytes reveals some HGPRT activity in most patients. Generally it is less than 5% of the normal level. Thus, these individuals are often referred to as patients with partial deficiency or partial activity of HGPRT. In one patient with gout 60% of normal activity has been found[55].

A variety of other techniques has been used to characterize the abnormal HGPRT proteins[54]. These include kinetic properties and heat stability[50, 51, 54]. Electrophoretic analysis may reveal a mobility slightly faster than that of normal HGPRT[53, 54] or slower than normal[55]. The abnormal enzyme may be unusually sensitive to fluoride or other inhibitors[54]. Assay with antibody prepared against the normal enzyme may indicate the presence[54, 55] or absence[28], of cross-reactive material. In all of these patients, as in patients with the Lesch–Nyhan syndrome, the activity of APTR in erythrocytes is increased.

Most of these patients have no abnormalities of the central nervous system, or behavioural abnormalities. One patient displayed antisocial behaviour and was placed in jail[56], but this may or may not have been related to his defect in HGPRT. It is becoming clear that there is a spectrum of involvement of the nervous system. Patients with cerebral involvement tend to have manifestations reminiscent of those of the Lesch–Nyhan syndrome. Nevertheless, it is our conviction that a patient who appears to have the Lesch–Nyhan syndrome but does not mutilate is likely to have a HGPRT variant. The same may be true of the patient who has normal intelligence. We have recently studied a famous patient who had both of these unusual characteristics and have obtained evidence that he does not have the Lesch–Nyhan syndrome[57]. This 22-year-old male was among the first patients reported with hyperuricaemia and central nervous system symptoms[58, 59]. He has now been found to have a variant of HGPRT distinct from the enzyme present in patients with the Lesch–Nyhan syndrome. He had choreoathetosis, spasticity, dysarthric speech and hyperuricaemia. However, he was of normal intelligence, and there was no evidence of self-mutilation. There was no HGPRT activity in lysates of erythrocytes and cultured fibroblasts when analysed in the usual manner.

We have developed a new method for the study of purine metabolism in intact cultured cells[60]. Cells derived from this patient were found to metabolize some 9% of [8–^{14}C]hypoxanthine, and 90% of the isotope utilized was converted to adenine and guanine nucleotides. In contrast, cells from patients with the Lesch–Nyhan syndrome were unable to convert hypoxanthine to nucleotides. The patient's fibroblasts were even more efficient in the metabolism of [8–^{14}C]guanine, which was utilized to the extent of 27%. Over 80% of the isotope utilized was converted to guanine and adenine nucleotides. The growth of fibroblasts from this patient in culture was intermediate in hypoxanthine–aminopterin–thymidine (HAT) media, whereas the growth of Lesch–Nyhan cells was inhibited, and normal cells grew normally. Similarly, in 8-azaguanine, 6-thioguanine and 8-azahypoxanthine, the growth of the patient's cells was intermediate between that of normal and Lesch–Nyhan cells. These observations provide further evidence for genetic heterogeneity among patients with disorders in purine metabolism involving the HGPRT gene. Thus we can now discuss three phenotypes of deficiency of HGPRT. These studies confirm that this famous patient did not have the Lesch–Nyhan syndrome. He has often been cited as an example of the fact that patients with the Lesch–Nyhan syndrome may have no behavioural abnormalities. The fact that he appears now to be the product of a gene defect different from that of the patient with classic Lesch–Nyhan syndrome illustrates the importance of paying close attention to the clinical phenotype (Table 2.2).

It has seemed intuitively reasonable to assume that the clinical severity of disease among groups of patients with varying defects in a single enzyme might parallel the degree of enzyme deficiency. However, in the only published report, Emmerson and Thompson[61] could find no significant correlation between the level of activity of HGPRT in haemolysates and

TABLE 2.2 **Enlarging spectrum of HPRT deficiency**

Variant	HPRT activity	Clinical features
L–N	Virtually 0 under any conditions	Lesch–Nyhan syndrome
Neurological	May be virtually 0 in erythrocyte assay Unstable or altered kinetics Active in whole cell	Spasticity, choreoathetosis, good mental function, normal behaviour, hyperuricaemia manifestations
Partial	ca. 5 % (1–50 %)	Only the consequences of hyperuricaemia

the clinical features of eight patients. This is not surprising because the conditions of assay under which most determinations, leading to conclusions as to the percentage of normal residual activity, are made under conditions maximizing activity with saturating concentrations of substrate would be expected to minimize difference between variants. Furthermore, other aspects of the conditions in the haemolysate may also be very different from those operating *in vivo*. We have sought methodology for the study of the interrelations of purines under conditions that might be more physiological. It was this methodology that permitted the splitting off of the third category, tentatively designated the neurological phenotype. We have since continued to refine the system and to seek better ways of making sense out of the masses of data generated.

The basic method involves the study of intact cells incubated *in vitro* with a variety of ^{14}C-labelled precursors and then studied using our system of high-pressure liquid chromatography for the analysis of the content of purine products and their isotope content[60, 62]. These studies of phenotype have so far employed fibroblasts cultured in roller bottles in minimal essential medium (MEM) containing 10 % fetal bovine serum. When the cells reach 75 % confluency, they are harvested by brief treatment with trypsin–EDTA solution, washed twice in MEM containing 10 % fetal bovine serum which has been dialysed to deplete it of hypoxanthine, and once in phosphate-buffered saline containing 0.1 % glucose (PBSG). The cells are counted in a Coulter counter and diluted to a concentration of 2×10^6 cells/ml. They are then transferred into plastic culture flasks and incubated for 15 min at 37 C in a shaking water bath. Two microcuries of [8–^{14}C]hypoxanthine (sp. act. 50.4 mCi/mmol) or [8–^{14}C]guanine (sp. act. 44.7 mCi/mmol) are added per millilitre of cell suspension (final concentrations: hypoxanthine 39.7 μmol/l, guanine 44.7 μmol/l). After 2 h of incubation, the suspensions are transferred to centrifuge tubes, quickly chilled to $0°C$ in ice water, and centrifuged at $400 g$ for 5 min. The supernatant medium is removed carefully and the cell pellet extracted with $100 \mu l$ of cold $0.8 mol/l$ $HClO_4$. The precipitated material is removed by centrifugation at $40 000 g$ for 20 min. The supernatant fluid is neutralized to pH 9 with KOH, and $50 \mu l$ of supernatant fluid (equivalent to about 2×10^6 cells) is analysed by high-pressure liquid chromatography (HPLC)[60, 62]. The HPLC system employed separates and quantitates each of the radioactive and non-radioactive purine bases, nucleosides, and nucleotides.

Calculation of the activity of HGPRT has been programmed using an Apple computer to determine the total picomoles of isotope incorporated into all of the purine compounds except for the corresponding nucleoside (i.e. inosine when hypoxanthine is used as a precursor, or guanosine when guanine is used); isotope remaining in the precursor base is also eliminated from the calculations. The nucleosides are not included, because these compounds are produced mainly in reactions catalysed by purine nucleoside phosphorylase (PNP, EC 2.4.2.1). It is recognized that some nucleoside may ensue from the action of nucleotidases on nucleotides, IMP or 6-MP, that are products of HGPRT. The values obtained in this way show considerable variation, even after correcting for cell number and total protein. The total amount of nucleotides per cell varies with cell size[63] and with the phase of growth at harvest[64]. Since the variation in picomoles of isotope incorporated reflects the variation in total purines present in the cell, we compute the final result by dividing these two values, obtaining values in picomoles of isotope incorporated per nanomole of purine compounds present in the cell. Normal cultured fibroblasts incorporate 1.358 ± 0.039 pmol hypoxanthine/nmol and 1.824 ± 0.086 pmol guanine/nmol in 2 h. In order to establish the validity of this method as a measure of the activity of HGPRT, we have measured the K_m for hypoxanthine and guanine in normal fibroblasts. The data obtained were consistent with those reported.

We have now studied a series of 12 unrelated patients[65] with considerable variation in clinical phenotype. The data revealed an apparent inverse correlation between enzyme activity and clinical severity. At this stage of our studies the phenotypes appear to fall into four categories corresponding to four ranges of activity. In this analysis the most severely involved patients, those with the classic Lesch–Nyhan syndrome, have had some activity, as has been the case in most assessments of fibroblasts. The level of activity in our current studies has been less than 1.2 % of normal. In two of the 'partial' variants studied whose symptoms were solely those attributable to hyperuricaemia, the levels of activity were greater than 10% of normal. We have now studied three neurological variants, none of whom had any mutilative or other behavioural abnormalities. Their activities ranged from 1.6 to 10% of normal. Finally, a patient with 1.5% of normal activity represents a 4th group. He has had the neurological syndrome and he does exhibit abnormal behaviour including self-mutilation, but his intelligence is probably normal, and he is able to exert a considerable measure of control over his behaviour. His aggressive activity towards others is quite sophisticated.

In a parallel study of the metabolism of guanine, the correlations were not as good as those obtained using hypoxanthine. It may be that this signifies a closer relationship between the pathogenesis of cerebral abnormality and the disorder of hypoxanthine metabolism. Certainly, concentrations of hypoxanthine are very high in the cerebrospinal fluid of patients with the Lesch–Nyhan syndrome[22, 66]. It is also engaging to consider relevant the fact that the newly discovered diazepam receptors in brain are inhibited by hypoxanthine and inosine[67]. Also relevant to the pathogenesis of the specific neurological manifestations which seem to point to the basal ganglia may be the fact that the specific activity of HGPRT is normally highest in the basal ganglia of the brain[66]. Possibly this area of the brain requires some 10% or more of HGPRT activity for normal neurological function. On the other hand the concentration of uric acid is so close to the limits of its solubility even in normal individuals that one would expect symptoms of hyperuricaemia in the presence of any defect in HGPRT.

ABNORMALITIES IN PHOSPHORIBOSYL PYROPHOSPHATE (PRPP) SYNTHETASE

A small number of families has been reported[68-70] in which clinical gout has been associated with greater than normal activity of phosphoribosyl pyrophosphate (PRPP) synthetase (Figure 2.4). The onset of gouty arthritis has been reported as early as 21 years of age. Renal colic and renal stones have been observed. Patients with this disorder may present in childhood. Some years ago we reported a boy who developed haematuria at 2 months of age and was found to have crystalluria, hyperuricaemia and increased excretion of urate in the urine[7]. He had initially appeared to be retarded and autistic, and was found to be deaf. He also had congenital absence of the lachrymal glands. This patient has more recently been discovered to have an abnormal PRPP synthetase[72].

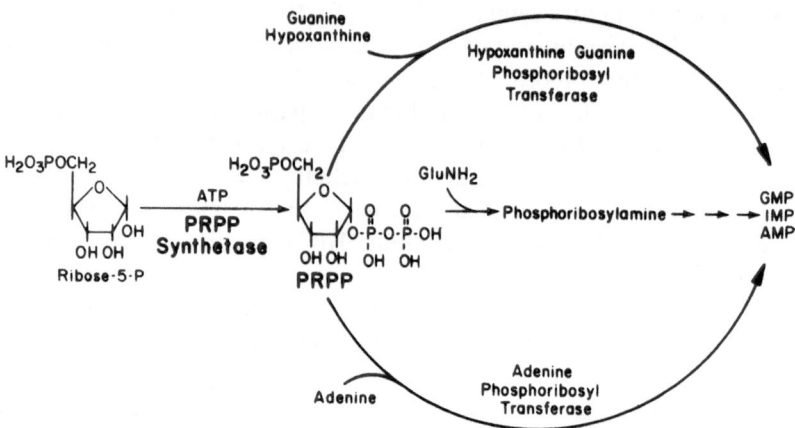

Figure 2.4   Phosphoribosyl pyrophosphate synthetase and the role of its product, phosphoribosyl pyrophosphate, in purine interrelations

Patients with these variant enzymes have increased concentrations of uric acid in the blood and urine. They overproduce purines *de novo*. Intracellular concentrations of PRPP are elevated. Molecular alteration in the PRPP synthetase protein leads to an increase in activity that may be three times that of the normal enzyme[70]. In one family the enzyme displayed increased activity only at low phosphate concentrations[69] and had diminished responsiveness to feedback inhibition by purine nucleotides. In another family the increased activity was demonstrable over a wide range of phosphate concentrations and had normal feedback inhibition[70]. The amounts of immunoreactive enzyme were normal[73]. The problem is a structural alteration in the enzyme that leads to increased specific activity. These observations provide evidence for two sites on the enzyme, a catalytic site altered by one mutation and a regulatory site altered by the other mutation.

Synthesis of PRPP from ATP and ribose-5-P is catalysed by PRPP synthetase. Inherited abnormalities of PRPP synthetase lead either to diminished sensitivity to feedback inhibitors or to excessive reaction velocity. An altered form of PRPP synthetase, which combines feedback resistance and increased catalytic activity, has been found in our patient[71,72]. His fibroblasts showed a four-fold increased PRPP concentration and generation. There was also excessive incorporation of labelled adenine, hypoxanthine, guanine and formate into purine nucleotides. PRPP synthetase activity was twice normal at 32 mol/l inorganic phosphate, but was 10-fold increased at 1 mmol/l inorganic phosphate. Further, the inorganic phosphate activation curve of mutant PRPP synthetase was hyperbolic in contrast to the normal sigmoidal curve. These findings resulted from four- to five-fold diminished responsiveness of the mutant enzyme to inhibition by purine nucleotides. In the absence of inhibitors, partially purified mutant and normal PRPP synthetase showed hyperbolic responses to inorganic phosphate, and mutant PRPP synthetase was twice as active as normal at all inorganic phosphate concentrations. Immune inactivation of the mutant enzyme confirmed the fact that there was increased activity per molecule of enzyme. Thus, in this patient's fibroblasts PRPP synthetase was altered in both regulatory and catalytic properties.

PRPP synthetase is coded for by a gene on the X-chromosome[74]. In some families the abnormality may be fully expressed in the heterozygous female[70]. In others it may be recessive[68], presumably reflecting different degrees of Lyonization. Allopurinol is the treatment of choice for these patients.

SUMMARY

The hyperuricaemic disorders are beginning to yield to biochemical genetic analysis which is defining subpopulations with distinct molecular diseases. The clinical phenotype ranges from the patient with the Lesch–Nyhan syndrome, a classical X-linked defect in which there is a devastating disorder of the central nervous system and abnormal behaviour, to the patient with gout or renal stone disease. Patients with the Lesch–Nyhan syndrome have an abnormality in the HGPRT enzyme which renders it virtually completely inactive. A considerable heterogeneity is being defined at the HGPRT locus and a number of distinct human variants have been described. Molecular alterations in the enzyme PRPP synthetase may increase the activity of this enzyme, generating increased amounts of PRPP which drives the *de novo* synthesis of purines and produces hyperuricaemia. Both enzymes are coded for by genes on the X-chromosome.

Acknowledgements

This work was aided by US Public Health Service Research Grants No. GM-17702, from the National Institute of General Medical Sciences; HDO-4608 from the National Institute of Child Health and Human Development; and No. R-00827, UCSD General Clinical Research Center, NIH/Division of Resources, National Institutes of Health, Bethesda, MD; and Grant NO. MCT-004007 from the Health Services Administration, Department of Health, Education and Welfare, Rockville, MD.

References

1. Lesch, M. and Nyhan, W. L. (1964). A familial disorder of uric acid metabolism and central nervous system function. *Am. J. Med.*, **36**, 561
2. Seegmiller, J. E., Rosenbloom, F. M. and Kelley, W. N. (1967). Enzyme defect associated with a sex-linked human neurological disorder and excessive purine synthesis. *Science*, **155**, 1682
3. Sweetman, L. and Nyhan, W. L. (1972). Further studies of the enzyme composition of mutant cells in X-linked uric aciduria. *Arch. Intern. Med.*, **130**, 214
4. Jeune, M., Hermier, M., Rosenberg, M. M. and Collombel, D. (1967). Encephalopathie familiale avec hyperuricemie. A propos d'une observation. *Pediatrie*, **21**, 663
5. Skyler, J. S., Neelon, F. A., Arnold, W. J., Kelley, W. N. and Lebovitz, H. E. (1974). Growth retardation in the Lesch–Nyhan syndrome. *Acta Endocrinol.*, **75**, 3
6. Nyhan, W. L. (1972). Clinical features of the Lesch–Nyhan syndrome. *Arch. Intern. Med.*, **130**, 186
7. Nyhan, W. L. (1976). Behavior in the Lesch–Nyhan syndrome. *J. Autism Child. Schizophrenia*, **6**, 235
8. Nyhan, W. L., Oliver, W. J. and Lesch, M. (1965). A familial disorder of uric acid metabolism and central nervous system function: II. *J. Pediatr.*, **67**, 257
9. Howard, R. S. and Walzak, M. P. (1968). A new cause for uric acid stones in childhood. *J. Urol.*, **98**, 639
10. Marie, J., Royer, P. and Rappaport, R. (1966). Hyperuricémie congénitale avec troubles neurologiques, rénaux et sanguins. *Arch. Franc. Pediatr.*, **23**, 970
11. Marie, J., Royer, J. M. and Rappaport, R. (1967). Hyperuricémie congénitale avec troubles neurologiques, rénaux et sanguins. *Arch. Franc. Pediatr.*, **24**, 501
12. Manzke, H. (1967). Hyperuricämie mit Cerebralparese. Syndrom eines hereditären Purinstoffwechselleidens. *Helv. Paediatr. Acta*, **22**, 258
13. van der Zee, S. P. M., Lommen, E. J. P., Trijbels, J. M. F. and Schretlen, E. D. A. M. (1970). The influence of adenine on the clinical features and purine metabolism in the Lesch–Nyhan syndrome. *Acta Paediat. Scand.*, **59**, 259
14. Michel, M. (1966) *L'encephalopathie familiale avec hyperuricémie. PhD Thesis*. Lyon, France.
15. Sass, J. K., Itabashi, H. H. and Dexter, R. A. (1965). Juvenile gout with brain involvement. *Arch. Neurol. (Chic.)*, **13**, 639
16. Crussi, F. G. Robertson, D. M. and Hiscox, J. L. (1969). The pathological condition of Lesch–Nyhan syndrome. Report of two cases. *Am. J. Dis. Child.*, **118**, 501
17. Nyhan, W. L., Pesek, J., Sweetman, L., Carpenter, D. G. and Carter, C. H. (1967). Genetics of an X-linked disorder of uric acid metabolism and cerebral function. *Pediatr. Res.*, **1**, 5
18. Sweetman, L., Nyhan, W. L., Klein, P. D. and Szczepanik, P. A. (1973). Glycine 1. 2-^{13}C in the investigation of children with inborn errors of metabolism. In Klein, P. D. and Peterson, S. V. (eds.) *Proceedings of the First*

International Conference on Stable Isotopes in Chemistry, Biology, and Medicine, Argonne Natl. Laboratory, Argonne, IL, pp. 404–409 (Springfield, VA.: US Atomic Energy Commission, Natl. Technical Information Service, US Dept. of Commerce)

19. Nyhan, W. L. (1968). Introduction – clinical and genetic features. In Bland, J. H. (ed.). Seminars on the Lesch–Nyhan Syndrome, pp. 1027–1033 Fed. Proc. 27

20. Sweetman, L. and Nyhan, W. L. (1967). Excretion of hypoxanthine and xanthine in a genetic disease of purine metabolism. Nature (London), 215, 859

21. Balis, M. E., Krakoff, I. H., Berman, P. H., and Dancis, J. (1967). Urinary metabolites in congenital hyperuricosuria. Science, 156, 1122

22. Sweetman, L. (1968). Urinary and CSF oxypurine levels and allopurinol metabolism in the Lesch–Nyhan syndrome. Fed. Proc., 27, 1055

23. Bakay, B., Telfer, M. A. and Nyhan, W. L. (1969). Assay of hypoxanthine-guanine and adenine phosphoribosyl transferases. A simple screening test for the Lesch–Nyhan syndrome and related disorders of purine metabolism. Biochem. Med., 3, 230

24. Berman, P. H., Balis, M. E. and Dancis, J. (1968). Diagnostic test for hyperuricemia with central nervous system dysfunction. J. Lab. Clin. Med., 71, 247

25. Bakay, B. and Nyhan, W. L. (1971). The separation of adenine and hypoxanthine-guanine phosphoribosyltransferase isoenzymes by disc gel electrophoresis. Biochem. Genet., 5, 81

26. Bakay, B. and Nyhan, W. L. (1972). Electrophoretic properties of hypoxanthine-guanine phosphoribosyl transferase in erythrocytes of subjects with Lesch–Nyhan syndrome. Biochem. Genet., 6, 139

27. Bakay, B. and Nyhan, W. L. (1972). Activation of variants of hypoxanthine-guanine phosphoribosyl transferase by the normal enzyme. Proc. Natl. Acad. Sci., USA 69, 2523

28. Bakay, B., Becker, M. A. and Nyhan, W. L. (1976). Reaction of antibody to normal human hypoxanthinephosphoribosyl-transferase with products of mutant genes. Arch. Biochem. Biophys., 177, 415

29. Rubin, C. S., Dancis, J., Yip, L. C., Niwinski, R. C. and Balis, M. E. (1971). Purification of IMP: Pyrophosphate phosphoribosyltransferases, catalytically incompetent enzymes in Lesch–Nyhan disease. Proc. Natl. Acad. Sci. USA, 68, 1461

30. Arnold, W. and Kelley, W. N. (1973). Human hypoxanthine-guanine phosphoribosyltransferase purification and subunit structure. J. Biol. Chem., 246, 7398

31. Nyhan, W. L. (1976). Genetic heterogeneity of human enzymes. N. Engl. J. Med., 294, 781

32. McDonald, J. A. and Kelley, W. N. (1971). Lesch–Nyhan syndrome: Altered kinetic properties of mutant enzyme. Science, 171, 689

33. Upchurch, K. S., Leyva, A., Arnold, W. J., Holmes, E. W. and Kelley, W. N. (1975). Hypoxanthine phosphoribosyltransferase deficiency: association of reduced catalytic activity with reduced levels of immunologically detectable enzyme protein. Proc. Natl. Acad. Sci. USA, 72, 4142

34. Ghangas, G. S. and Milman, G. (1975). Radioimmune determination of

hypoxanthine phosphoribosyltransferase crossreacting material in erythrocytes of Lesch–Nyhan patients. *Proc. Natl. Acad. Sci. USA* **72**, 4147

35. Bakay, B., Francke, U., Nyhan, W. L. and Seegmiller, J. E. (1977). Experience with detection of heterozygous carriers and prenatal diagnosis of Lesch–Nyhan disease. In Müller, M. M., Kaiser, E. and Seegmiller, J. E. (eds.) *Purine Metabolism in Man II: Regulation of Pathways and Enzyme Defects*, pp. 351–358 (New York: Plenum)

36. Migeon, B. R., DerKaloustian, V. M., Nyhan, W. L., Young, W. J. and Childs, B. (1968). X-linked hypoxanthine-guanine phosphoribosyl transferase deficiency: heterozygote has two clonal populations. *Science*, **160**, 425

37. Salzman, J., DeMars, R. and Benke, P. (1968). Single-allele expression at an X-linked hyperuricemia locus in heterozygous human cells. *Proc. Natl. Acad. Sci. USA*, **60**, 545

38. Nyhan, W. L., Bakay, B., Connor, J. D., Marks, J. F. and Keele, D. K. (1970). Hemizygous expression of glucose-6-phosphate dehydrogenase in erythrocytes of heterozygotes for the Lesch–Nyhan syndrome. *Proc. Natl. Acad. Sci. USA* **65**, 214

39. Francke, U., Bakay, B., Connor, J. D., Coldwell, J. G. and Nyhan, W. L. (1974). Linkage relationships of X-linked enzymes glucose-6-phosphate dehydrogenase and hypoxanthine guanine phosphoribosyltransferase: recombination in female offspring of compound heterozygotes. *Am. J. Hum. Genet.*, **26**, 512

40. Felix, J. S. and DeMars, R. (1971). Detection of females heterozygous for the Lesch–Nyhan mutation by 8-azaguanine-resistant growth of cultured fibroblasts. *J. Lab. Clin. Med.*, **77**, 596

41. Migeon, B. R. (1970). X-linked hypoxanthine–guanine phosphoribosyl transferase deficiency: Detection of heterozygotes by selective medium. *Biochem. Genet.*, **4**, 377

42. Gartler, S. M., Scott, R. C., Goldstein, J. L., Campbell, B. and Sparkes, R. (1971). Lesch–Nyhan syndrome: Rapid detection of heterozygotes by use of hair follicles. *Science*, **172**, 572

43. Silvers, D. N., Cox, P., Balis, M. E., and Dancis, J. (1972). Detection of the heterozygote in Lesch–Nyhan disease by hair-root analysis. *N. Engl. J. Med.*, **286**, 390

44. Francke, U., Bakay, B. and Nyhan, W. L. (1973). Detection of heterozygous carriers of the Lesch–Nyhan syndrome by electrophoresis of hair root lysates. *J. Pediatr.*, **82**, 472

45. Greene, M. L., Fujimoto, W. Y. and Seegmiller, J. E. (1969). Urinary xanthine stones – a rare complication of allopurinol therapy. *N. Engl. J. Med.*, **280**, 426

46. Anderson, L. T., Dancis, J., Herrman, L. and Alpert, M. (1977). Punishment learning and self-mutilation in Lesch–Nyhan disease. *Nature (London)*, **265**, 461

47. Mizuno, T.-I. and Yugari, Y. (1974). Self-mutilation in the Lesch–Nyhan syndrome. *Lancet*, **1**, 761

48. Nyhan, W. L., Johnson, H. G., Kaufman, I. A. and Jones, K. L. (1980). Serotonergic approaches to the modification of behavior in the Lesch–Nyhan syndrome. *Appl. Res. Mental Retard.*, **1**, 25

49. Sweetman, L., Borden, M., Kulovich, S., Kaufman, I. and Nyhan, W. L. (1977). Altered excretion of 5-hydroxyindoleacetic acid and glycine in

patients with the Lesch–Nyhan disease. In Müller, M. M., Kaiser, E. and Seegmiller, J. E. (eds.) *Purine Metabolism in Man II: Regulation of Pathways and Enzyme Defects,* pp. 398–404. (New York: Plenum)

50. Kogut, M. D., Donnell, G. N., Nyhan, W. L. and Sweetman, L. (1970). Disorder of purine metabolism due to partial deficiency of hypoxanthine-guanine phosphoribosyltransferase. *Am. J. Med.,* **48,** 148

51. Kelley, W. N., Greene, M. L., Rosenbloom, F. M., Henderson, J. F. and Seegmiller, J. E. (1969). Hypoxanthine–guanine phosphoribosyl transferase deficiency in gout. *Ann. Intern. Med.,* **70,** 155

52. Henderson, J. F., Kelley, W. N., Rosenbloom, F. M. and Seegmiller, J. E. (1969). Inheritance of purine phosphoribosyltransferase in man. *Am. J. Hum. Genet.,* **21,** 61

53. Bakay, B., Nyhan, W. L., Fawcett, N. and Kogut, M. D. (1972). Isozymes of hypoxanthine–guanine phosphoribosyl transferase in a family with partial deficiency of the enzyme. *Biochem. Genet.,* **7,** 73

54. Sweetman, L., Hoch, M. A., Bakay, B., Borden, M., Lesh, P. and Nyhan, W. L. (1978). A distinct human variant of hypoxanthine-guanine phosphoribosyl transferase. *J. Pediatr.,* **92,** 385

55. Sweetman, L., Borden, M., Lesh, P., Bakay, B. and Becker, M. A. (1977). Diminished affinity for purine substrates as a basis for gout with mild deficiency of hypoxanthine quanine phosphoribosyl transferase. In Müller, M. M., Kaiser, E. and Seegmiller, J. E. (eds.) *Purine Metabolism in Man II. Regulation of Pathways and Enzyme Defects,* pp. 319–325. (New York: Plenum)

56. Benke, P. J. and Herrick, N. (1972). Azaguanine-resistance as a manifestation of a new form of metabolic overproduction of uric acid. *Am. J. Med.,* **52,** 547

57. Bakay, B., Nissinen, E., Sweetman, L., Francke, U. and Nyhan, W. L. (1979). Utilization of purines by an HGPRT variant in an intelligent, nonmutilative patient with features of the Lesch–Nyhan syndrome. *Pediatr. Res.,* **13,** 1365

58. Catel, V. W. and Schmidt, J. (1959). Uber familiare gichtische Diathese in Verdendung mit zerebralen und renalen Symptomen bei einem Kleinkind. *Dtsch Med. Wochenschr.,* **84,** 2145

59. Manzke, H., Harms, D. and Dörmer, K. (1971). Zur Problematik der Behandlung der Kongenitalen Hyperurikämie. *Monatssch. Kinderheilk.,* **119,** 424

60. Bakay, B., Nissinen, E., Sweetman, L. and Nyhan, W. L. (1978). Analysis of radioactive and nonradioactive purine bases, purine nucleosides and purine nucleotides by high-speed chromatography on a single column. *Monographs of Human Genetics,* Vol. **10,** pp. 127–134. (Karger: Basel)

61. Emmerson, B. T. and Thompson, L. (1973). The spectrum of hypoxanthine guanine phosphoribosyl transferase deficiency. *Q. J. Med.,* **166,** 423

62. Bakay, B., Nissinen, E. and Sweetman, L. (1978). Analysis of radioactive and nonradioactive purine bases, nucleosides, nucleotides by high-speed chromatography on a single column, *Anal. Biochem.,* **86,** 65

63. Brenton, D. P., Astrin, K. H., Cruikshank, M. K. and Seegmiller, J. E. (1977). Measurement of free nucleotides in cultured human lymphoid cells using high pressure liquid chromatography. *Biochem. Med.,* **17,** 231

64. Snyder, F. F., Henderson, J. F., Kim, S. C., Peterson, A. R. P. and Brox, L. W.

(1973). Purine nucleotide metabolism and nucleotide pool sizes in synchronized lymphoma L5178Y cells. *Cancer Res.*, **33**, 2425

65. Page, T., Bakay, B., Nissinen, R. and Nyhan, W. L. (1981). Hypoxanthine-guanine phosphoribosyl transferase variants: Correlation of clinical phenotype with enzyme activity. *J. Inher. Metab. Dis.*, **4**, 203

66. Rosenbloom, F. M., Kelley, W. N., Miller, J., Henderson, J. F. and Seegmiller, J. E. (1967). Inherited disorder of purine metabolism: Correlation between central nervous system dysfunction and biochemical defects. *J. Am. Med. Assoc.*, **202**, 175

67. Skolnick, P. S., Marangos, P. S. and Goodwin, F. K. (1978). Endogenous inhibitor of diazapam binding. *Life Sci. (Oxford)*, **23**, 1473

68. Sperling, O., Eilam, G., Persky-Broch, S. and DeVries, A. (1972). Accelerated erythrocyte 6-phosphoribosyl-1-pyrophosphate synthesis. A familial abnormality associated with excessive uric acid production and gout. *Biochem. Med.*, **6**, 310

69. Sperling, O., Boer, P., Persky-Broch, S., Kanarek, E. and DeVries, A. (1972). Altered kinetic property of erythrocyte phosphoribosyl pyrophosphate synthetase in excessive purine production. *Eur. J. Clin. Biol. Res.*, **17**, 703

70. Becker, M. A., Meyer, L. J. and Seegmiller, J. E. (1973). Gout with purine overproduction due to increased phosphoribosylpyrophosphate synthetase activity. *Am. J. Med.*, **55**, 232

71. Nyhan, W. L., James, J. A., Teberg, A. J., Sweetman, L. and Nelson, L. G. (1969). A new disorder of purine metabolism with behavioral manifestations. *J. Pediatr.* **74**, 20

72. Becker, M. A., Raivio, K. O., Bakay, B., Adams, W. B. and Nyhan, W. L. (1980). Variant human phosphoribosylpyrophosphate synthetase altered in regulatory and catalytic functions. *J. Clin. Invest.*, **65**, 109

73. Becker, M. A., Kostel, P. J., Meyer, L. J. and Seegmiller, J. E. (1973). Human phosphoribosylpyrophosphate synthetase: Increased enzyme specific activity in a family with gout and excessive purine synthesis. *Proc. Natl. Acad. Sci. USA*, **70**, 2749

74. Becker, M. A., Yen, R. C. K., Goss, S., Seegmiller, J. E., Itkin, P., Lasar, C., and Adams, W. B. (1978). Localization of the structural gene for human phosphoribosyl–pyrophosphate synthetase on the X chromosome. *Clin. Res.*, **26**, 500A

3

Vitamin-responsive inherited metabolic disorders: propionic acidaemia and methylmalonic acidaemia

L. E. Rosenberg

INTRODUCTION

By the end of the 1960's it was clear that most patients with the then-called 'ketotic hyperglycinaemia syndrome' had either of two inherited metabolic disorders – propionic acidaemia due to propionyl CoA carboxylase (PCC) deficiency, or methylmalonic acidaemia due to methylmalonyl CoA mutase (MUT) deficiency[1]. PCC and MUT, each found in the mitochondrial matrix of mammalian cells, act on nearly sequential steps in the 'propionate pathway' by which several essential amino acids, odd-chain fatty acids, the side chain of cholesterol, and certain pyrimidines are catabolized to succinyl CoA and enter the tricarboxylic-acid cycle (Figure 3.1). PCC, a biotin-dependent enzyme, catalyses the conversion of propionyl CoA to D-methylmalonyl CoA; MUT, a cobalamin (vitamin B_{12})-dependent enzyme, catalyses the isomerization of L-methylmalonyl CoA to succinyl CoA. Soon after the delineation of propionic acidaemia and methylmalonic acidaemia as distinct entities, it was shown that some,

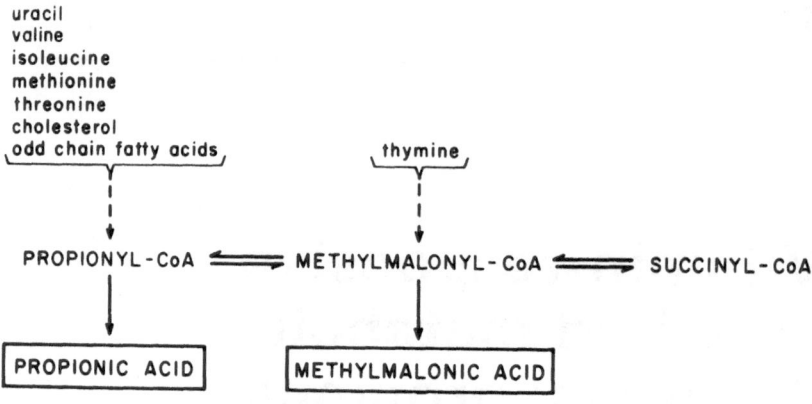

uracil
valine
isoleucine
methionine
threonine
cholesterol
odd chain fatty acids

thymine

PROPIONYL-CoA ⇌ METHYLMALONYL-CoA ⇌ SUCCINYL-CoA

PROPIONIC ACID

METHYLMALONIC ACID

Figure 3.1   The propionate pathway showing the precursors and major catabolic product of propionyl CoA and methylmalonyl CoA. The free acids which accumulate in patients with propionic acidaemia and methylmalonic acidaemia are derived from their CoA esters by hydrolysis. Broken arrows indicate the presence of several reactions

but by no means all, patients with either disorder responded to pharmacological doses of the appropriate vitamin (i.e. biotin in PCC deficiency and cobalamin in MUT deficiency) with a prompt and striking decrease in the concentration of methylmalonate and/or propionate in blood and urine, as well as with a distinctly increased ability to tolerate those amino acids known to precipitate attacks of acute metabolic ketoacidosis in untreated patients[1-4]. The biochemical and genetic bases for such vitamin-responsive variants and their corresponding vitamin-unresponsive counterparts have been pursued vigorously in many laboratories during the past decade. These efforts have taught us much about the significance of the propionate pathway in man, about the enzymes and coenzymes involved, about the ever-increasing complexity of the observed genetic heterogeneity, and about the natural history of these disorders. These efforts, too, have presented us with another example of the value of international co-operation and collaboration in the biomedical sciences.

In this chapter I shall attempt to review, compare, and contrast certain facets of our information about the propionic acidaemias and the methylmalonic acidaemias. In keeping with the theme of this book, I shall concentrate on pathogenetic and pathophysiological mechanisms. Rather than repeating material which has already been reviewed extensively elsewhere[1, 5-8], I shall emphasize work accomplished in our laboratory and elsewhere during the past few years, hoping thereby to focus on the many still unanswered questions in this field. The specific topics to be considered include the structure of human PCC and MUT; the evidence that some forms of propionic acidaemia and some forms of methylmalonic acidaemia result from primary deficiency of the respective PCC and MUT apoproteins, whereas other forms of these disorders are caused by defective metabolism of the biotin or cobalamin vitamers; the biochemical and immunochemical nature of the apocarboxylase and apomutase mutants; and the localization of the defects in vitamin transport or metabolism which underlie the vitamin-responsive forms of these two families of disorders.

ENZYME STRUCTURE

Recently, PCC and MUT from normal postmortem human liver have each been purified to homogeneity in our laboratory[9, 10]. The structural features of these two proteins are shown in Table 3.1. Based on a comparison between the final specific activity of the homogeneous enzymes and their specific activities in crude homogenates, we estimate that mitochondria contain about five to six times as much MUT as PCC.

TABLE 3.1 **Structural features of human hepatic propionyl CoA carboxylase (PCC) and methylmalonyl CoA mutase (MUT)**

Feature	PCC	MUT
Native mol. wt.	540 000	150 000
Quaternary structure	$(\alpha\beta)_4$	α_2
Mol. wt of subunits	$\alpha - 72\,000$	$\alpha - 77\,500$
	$\beta - 56\,000$	
mol coenzyme/mol apoprotein	4	2
mol coenzyme/mol protomer		
or subunit	1	1

Native PCC has a molecular weight of $\sim 540\,000$ and is composed of non-identical subunits, designated α and β, of molecular weights 72 000 and 56 000, respectively. Each mole of native enzyme contains 4 mol of biotin, virtually all of which is bound to the larger (α) subunit. We conclude, therefrom, that the native enzyme consists of four protomers ($\alpha\beta$), each containing one α and one β subunit and each binding 1 mol of biotin per mole of protomer. By analogy with other biotin-dependent carboxylases, a plausible model for the PCC protomer is shown in Figure 3.2. It is not yet known whether the α subunit contains the bicarbonate and ATP binding sites and the β subunit the propionyl CoA site, or vice versa. Since PCC activity is inhibited markedly by phenylglyoxal, an arginine-specific reagent, it is clear that at least one arginine residue is present at or near the enzyme's catalytic site[11].

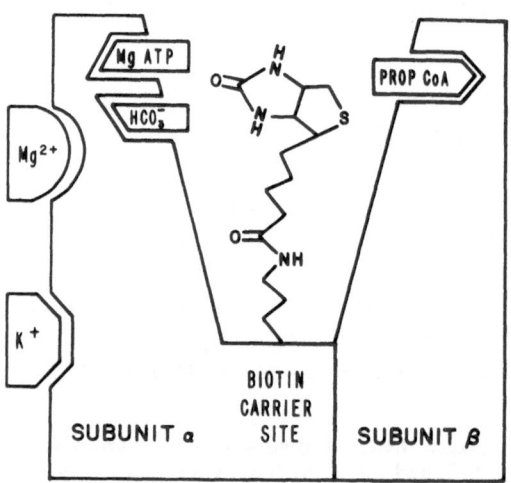

Figure 3.2 A proposed model of the mammalian propionyl CoA carboxylase protomer containing two non-identical subunits (α and β), a biotin carrier site, and multiple substrate and effector sites. See text for details

Native MUT, on the other hand, has a considerably simpler structure (Table 3.1). Its molecular weight is ∼ 150 000 and only one subunit (α) of molecular weight ∼ 77 500 was noted on SDS gel electrophoresis. These results, plus the observation that 2 mol of adenosylcobalamin (AdoCbl) are bound per mole of enzyme, suggest that MUT is composed of two identical subunits (α$_2$), each subunit containing one AdoCbl binding site and presumably one methylmalonyl CoA binding site. Similar findings were obtained by others who purified MUT to homogeneity from human placenta[12]. Despite this apparently simple dimeric structure, MUT appears to be a functionally very complex molecule based on several observations which suggest that, under some conditions, the active sites on the two subunits are not functionally equivalent, that negative co-operativity may exist between the subunits, and that the cobalamin moiety may even be covalently bound to MUT[12, 13].

APOENZYME MUTANTS

In a theoretical sense, reduced or absent activity of an enzyme which requires a coenzyme can result from abnormalities in either the apoprotein or the availability of the required cofactor. It has now been amply demonstrated that both general classes of abnormalities exist among the propionic acidaemias and the methylmalonic acidaemias. In fact, for both disorders, more than one kind of apoenzyme defect and more than one kind of coenzyme defect have been substantiated. Let me discuss the apoenzyme abnormalities first.

MUT mutants

Given the oligomeric structure and the functional complexities of PCC and MUT, it is not surprising that heterogeneity has been defined among apoenzyme mutants for each disorder. In the case of MUT deficiency, all apoenzyme mutants (designated *mut*) thus far identified fall into one complementation group and result from mutations in the structural gene locus for the MUT apoenzyme[8]. One major subclass, denoted *mut*° is characterized by a complete deficiency of MUT activity in fibroblast extracts, regardless of the concentrations of substrate and coenzyme used in the assay system[14]. The *mut*° mutants have been subdivided further by radioimmunoassay techniques as shown in Figure 3.3[15]. Some have no detectable cross-reacting material (CRM⁻) in fibroblast extracts when examined with antibodies prepared against either the human placental or liver enzyme. Others have clearly detectable CRM ranging from 5 to 50% of that noted in control cells.

The other major class of *mut* mutants, denoted *mut*⁻, has residual mutase activity in cell extracts. All *mut*⁻ mutants examined to date have a much reduced affinity for AdoCbl, their K_ms for cofactor being 50–5000-fold greater than that noted in controls. Moreover, this activity exhibits greater thermolability than that found in control cells. As expected for such structural mutants, all *mut*⁻ extracts contain CRM in varying amounts (Figure 3.3). Since these *mut*⁻ mutants differ so much from one another in residual activity, K_m for AdoCbl, and residual CRM, they almost surely differ in more fundamental terms such as the nature of the amino acid substitutions which underlie them.

PCC mutants

The situation with regard to PCC apoenzyme mutants, denoted by the generic abbreviation *pcc*, is more complex and currently less well

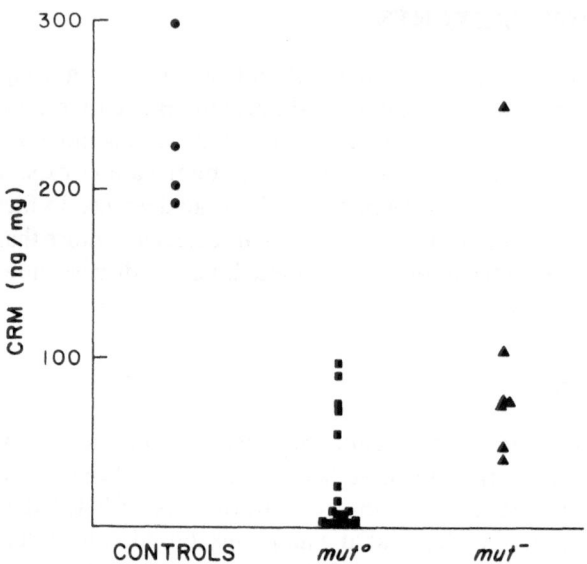

Figure 3.3 Summary of studies aimed at detecting cross-reacting material (CRM) in methylmalonyl CoA mutase apoenzyme mutants (*mut°* and *mut⁻*). CRM was estimated by radioimmunoassay. See text for definition of *mut°* and *mut⁻* designations

understood. All *pcc* mutants retain from 1 to 10% of PCC activity in fibroblast and leukocyte extracts, and fall into two general complementation groups denoted *pcc A* and *pcc BC*[16]. The latter complex class has been further subdivided into *pcc B* and *pcc C* mutants by complementation analysis. Because a detailed analysis of residual PCC activity in *pcc A* and *pcc C* mutants showed that neither class demonstrated increased activity in the presence of added biotin, that neither class had abnormal K_ms for any PCC substrate, and that in both classes, PCC activity showed greater cryolability and thermolability than did control PCC activity, we suggested that such mutants reflected structural abnormalities in one or the other major PCC subunit (α or β)[17, 18]. We proposed, further, that mutants of the *pcc A* class had abnormalities in that subunit which bound potassium, ATP, bicarbonate, and biotin since their K_m of activation by K⁺ and their response to avidin–biotin treatment differed from that of both controls and *pcc C* mutants[17]. By analogy then, it seemed likely that the *pcc C* mutants and, hence, the entire *pcc BC* class had abnormalities in the subunit which bound propionyl CoA. Our recent unpublished immunochemical studies, however, do not fit this formulation. As shown in Figure 3.4, neither the residual PCC activity in several *pcc A* mutants nor

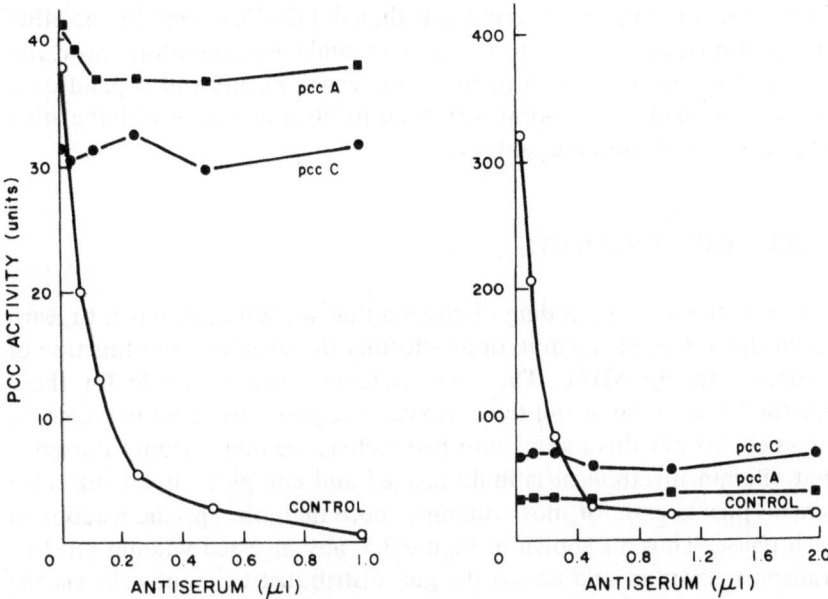

Figure 3.4 Immunotitration studies showing that residual propionyl CoA carboxylase activity in fibroblast extracts of two major classes of apocarboxylase mutants
(*pcc A* and *pcc C*) is not inhibited by anti-carboxylase antiserum. The data on the left
were obtained in experiments aimed at equalizing PCC activity in control and
mutant lines; data on the right were obtained in experiments equalizing amounts of
fibroblast extract protein. See text for details

that in several *pcc C* mutants is inhibited by monospecific, high-titre, anti-
PCC antiserum raised in rabbits either against homogeneous human
hepatic PCC or against PCC purified to homogeneity from pig heart. Since
such antisera strongly inhibit PCC activity from control cells, we are led to
one of two conclusions: either the mutant PCCs in *pcc A* and *pcc C* cells are
so altered as to have lost all of the antigenic determinants displayed by
normal PCC while retaining some catalytic activity; or, as seems more
likely, *pcc* mutant cells lack PCC completely, implying that the residual
propionyl CoA carboxylating activity in mutant cells is produced by other
biotin-dependent carboxylases which can use propionyl CoA as substrate.
However, it should be emphasized that other workers have reported
something very different. They reported that *pcc A* and *pcc C* mutant cells
contain normal amounts of CRM when titrated with rabbit antiserum
prepared against reportedly homogeneous pig-heart PCC[19]. It is conceivable that, in our hands, pure PCC elicited antibodies against a very

different set of antigenic determinants than did the PCC used by the other group of investigators. I find this a most unlikely explanation, however, and suggest that resolution of these discrepant results will depend on a protocol in which each laboratory repeats its titration curves with the other laboratory's cell lines and antisera.

COENZYME MUTANTS

It is clear from the preceding discussion that we still have much to learn about the nature of the mutations affecting the structure and function of apoPCC and apoMUT. The same statement can be made for those inherited defects involving the coenzymes required by these two enzyme moieties. To put this matter into perspective, we must remind ourselves that vitamin metabolism is multi-faceted and complex – involving three general phases and, for most vitamins, more than one specific reaction in each phase. Thus, as shown in Figure 3.5, any ingested vitamin must be transported within and across the gut, distributed to tissue cells via the blood stream, and finally transported and activated in cells before it can function as a cofactor.

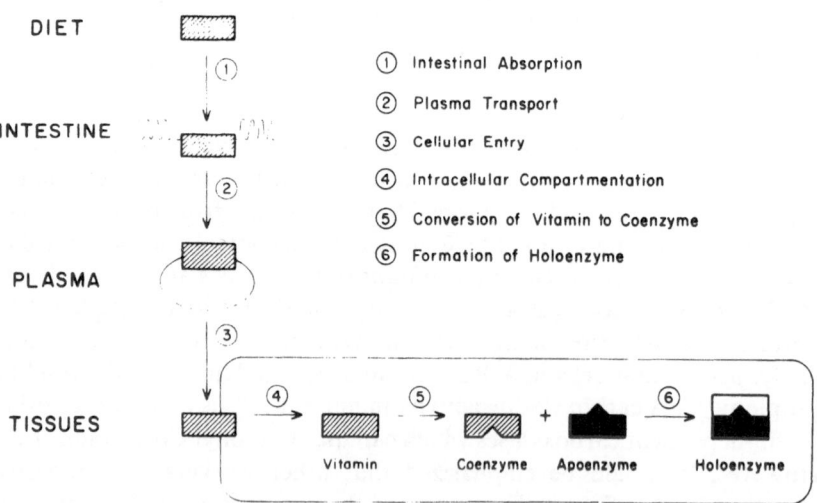

Figure 3.5 Schematic representation of sites at which mutations could interfere with vitamin metabolism and vitamin cofactor-catalysed reactions. (Reproduced from Rosenberg[26] with permission of Plenum Press.)

Transport and metabolism of cobalamin and biotin

We know a great deal more about the details of these several steps for cobalamin (Cbl) than we do for biotin (Bio). Whereas the intra-intestinal transport of Cbl vitamers is facilitated by the well-understood gastric intrinsic factor (IF), and the trans-intestinal transport of Cbl's depends on specific ileal cell membrane receptors[20], there is no detailed information about either the intra- or trans-intestinal transport of Bio. Whereas Cbl vitamers are transported in blood bound to two specific and well-characterized proteins. transcobalamin I (TC I) and transcobalamin II (TC II)[21], it is not yet known whether Bio is transported free or bound in the extracellular compartment. Whereas the uptake of Cbl by some, and probably all, tissue cells has been shown to depend on cell membrane receptor-mediated adsorptive endocytosis of the TC II–Cbl complex[22, 23], the mechanism of Bio uptake by tissue cells is obscure. Whereas the intracellular metabolism of Cbl vitamers has been proposed to proceed via intralysosomal hydrolysis of TC II, efflux of the free vitamer(s) from lysosome to cytosol, and finally diffusion across the mitochondrial membranes into the mitochondrial matrix[24], nothing is known about the mechanisms of subcellular distribution of Bio.

Only at the level of coenzyme synthesis is there considerable data about both these vitamin cofactors, and, here, the mechanisms appear to differ significantly. There are two Cbl coenzymes, methylcobalamin (MeCbl) and adenosylcobalamin (AdoCbl) (Figure 3.6). MeCbl is required by the key cytosolic enzyme, methyltetrahydrofolate:homocysteine methyltransferase (MET) which catalyses the formation of methionine and the conversion of methyltetrahydrofolate to tetrahydrofolate[1, 24]. AdoCbl, as stated previously, is required for methylmalonyl CoA mutase (MUT) holoenzyme activity in the mitochondrial matrix[1, 24]. The formation of these coenzymes depends, in turn, on the activity of other 'activating' systems: at least one cytosolic reductase which acts to reduce the valence of the central cobalt nucleus of the inactive Cbl vitamer, hydroxocobalamin (OH-Cbl) from $3+$ to $2+$ in preparation for methylation; and probably three discrete mitochondrial enzymes (two reductases and an adenosyl-transferase) which convert intramitochondrial OH-Cbl to AdoCbl[1, 24].

Bio, too, is a cofactor for both cytosolic and mitochondrial enzymes (Figure 3.7). In this instance, however, the function of each Bio-dependent enzyme is similar – namely the carboxylation of its preferred substrate[25]. In the cytosol Bio is required for the enzymatic carboxylation of acetyl CoA to malonyl CoA, the critical step in long-chain fatty acid formation. In the mitochondrion Bio is known to be a cofactor for three enzymes:

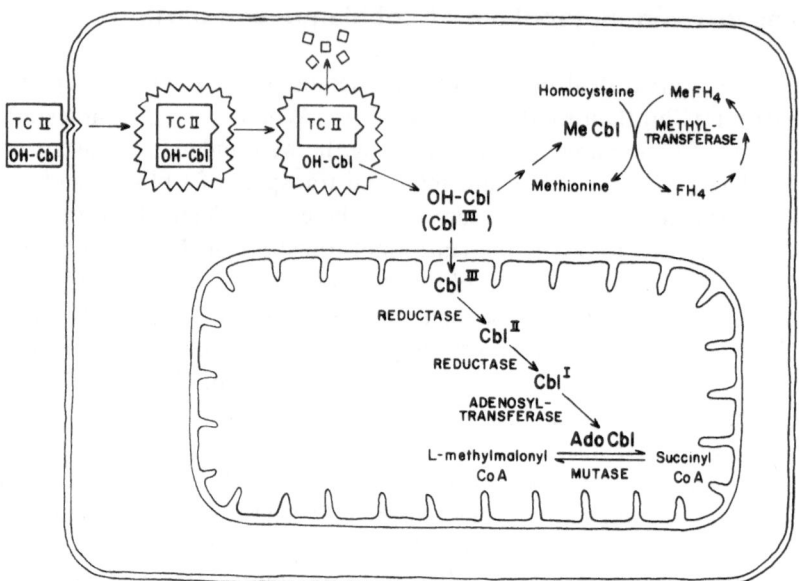

Figure 3.6   Major pathway of cellular uptake and subcellular compartmentation of cobalamins, and of intracellular distribution and enzymatic synthesis of coblamin coenzymes. TC II = transcobalamin II; OH − Cbl = hydroxocobalamin; MeCbl = methylcobalamin; Cbl^{III}, Cbl^{II}, and Cbl^{I} = cobalamins with cobalt valences of 3^+, 2^+, and 1^+, respectively; AdoCbl = adenosylcobalamin

pyruvate carboxylase (PC), a key enzyme in gluconeogenesis; β-methylcrotonyl CoA carboxylase (MCC), required in the catabolic pathway for leucine; and propionyl CoA carboxylase (PCC), whose functional role we considered earlier. It has been established, too, that the structure of the Bio molecule bound to each of these carboxylases is the same, and that this structure does not differ from that of the parent vitamin (as do those of the Cbl coenzymes, MeCbl and AdoCbl). Moreover, only one class of 'activating' enzymes for Bio has been established, an ATP-requiring holocarboxylase synthetase (HS) which first catalyses the formation of a biotinyl adenylate intermediate, and then facilitates the covalent binding of the Bio to an epsilon-amino residue of lysine on the appropriate apoprotein via an amide bond. HS species have been localized to both the cytosol and the mitochondrial matrix, but it has not yet been determined whether these differently distributed synthetases also differ in structure and, therefore, in their genetic control.

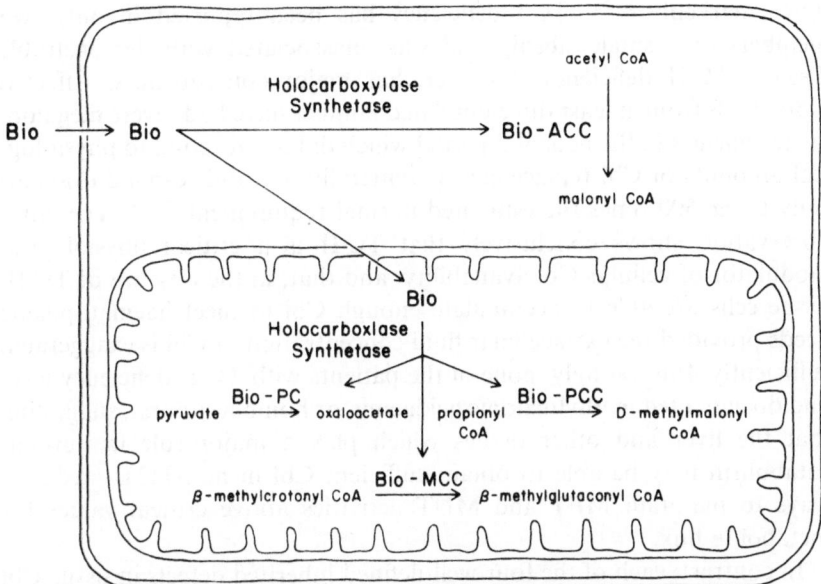

Figure 3.7 General features of cellular uptake and metabolism of biotin. Bio = biotin; ACC = acetyl CoA carboxylase; PC = pyruvate carboxylase; MCC = β-methylcrotonyl CoA carboxylase; PCC = propionyl CoA carboxylase. Neither the mechanism by which biotin is transported across the plasma membrane nor that by which it enters the mitochondrion are understood.

Localization of mutants

Given these pathways of Cbl and Bio transport and metabolism, what can we say about mutants thereof? For Cbl that question has a detailed, albeit still incomplete, answer; for Bio, there are only some interesting clues toward an answer. Inherited disorders of each major phase of Cbl metabolism are well known. At least two different disorders involving gastric IF and one involving ileal Cbl absorption have been delineated[20, 26]. In each case patients present with juvenile megaloblastic anaemia, reduced extracellular and tissue content of Cbl vitamers, and when tested, homocystinuria and methylmalonic aciduria. In each case, too, parenteral administration of physiological amounts of Cbl (approximately 1 µg/day) circumvents the block and leads to sustained chemical and clinical remission. Inherited deficiencies of each Cbl transport protein (TC I and TC II) are known as well; their clinical consequences differ markedly[21, 26]. TC I deficiency has been reported in only two members of a single sibship and was unassociated with demonstrable disease. TC II deficiency, however, has major consequences. Affected individuals from at least three unrelated families have had severe megaloblastic anaemia in the neonatal period which did not respond to physiological amounts of Cbl replacement parenterally, but did respond dramatically to *ca.* 500 times the estimated normal requirement[27, 28]. The latter observation shows conclusively that TC II is a critical physiological modulator of cellular Cbl availability, and that, in the absence of TC II, tissue cells are able to accumulate enough Cbl to meet haematopoietic needs provided the extracellular fluid concentration of Cbl is exaggerated sufficiently. Interestingly, none of the patients with TC II deficiency have had documented methylmalonic acidaemia or homocystinuria, suggesting that the liver and other tissues which play a major role in nutrient catabolism may be able to obtain sufficient Cbl in non-TC II-mediated ways to maintain MET and MUT activities above critical values for metabolite flux.

In contrast, each of the four well-defined inherited defects in tissue Cbl metabolism lead to abnormalities in either sulphur amino acid metabolism and/or methylmalonate isomerization. These defects, denoted *cbl A*, *cbl B*, *cbl C* and *cbl D*, result from four biochemically and genetically distinct lesions[24]. The *cbl A* and *cbl B* mutants are defective in different steps in the intramitochondrial pathway of AdoCbl formation and, secondarily, of MUT holoenzyme activity: the *cbl A* defect most likely being at the level of a mitochondrial reductase; the *cbl B* lesion being due to a defective adenosyltransferase. In these two classes MeCbl formation and MeCbl-requiring MET activity are normal. In the *cbl C* and *cbl D* classes, however, synthesis of both MeCbl and AdoCbl is deficient, leading to impaired activities of cytosolic MET and mitochondrial MUT. In neither *cbl C* nor *cbl D* mutants is the precise metabolic defect known, but abnormalities in one or more cytosolic Cbl reductases appear likely[29]. With the exception of some *cbl B* mutants, none of these cellular mutants are 'tight', as evidenced by their response *in vivo* and in culture to far greater than physiological amounts of Cbl vitamers. Whether such vitamin responsiveness reflects mass action 'drive' of a partially deficient enzyme or, alternatively, circumvention of a completely blocked reaction by 'recruitment' of a usually minor pathway remains to be determined.

More than 50 patients with one of the Cbl-responsive defects are now known. In contrast, fewer than ten patients with Bio-responsive metabolic lesions have been described, but progress in their understanding is accelerating. Summarizing this group of patients is difficult because neither their clinical nor their chemical phenotypes have been reported to be consistent. Some, for instance, were reported as cases of Bio-responsive propionic acidaemia[4,30]; others, as cases of Bio-responsive methyl-crotonylglycinuria[31-33]. When one of the latter patients (J. R.)[31] was shown subsequently to excrete metabolites consistent with both propionic and β-methylcrotonic acidaemia[34] and to have reduced activities of both PCC and MCC in fibroblast extracts[35, 36], it was recognized that at least some of these Bio-responsive patients might have abnormalities in Bio metabolism leading to deficiencies of several carboxylases. During the past three to four years more patients with now-called 'multiple carboxylase deficiency' have been described[37-40]. Each of these patients excretes urinary metabolites consistent with deficiency of PC, MCC and PCC. Each, too, has responded to oral administration of 10 mg Bio daily (about 1000 times the estimated normal requirement) with a prompt and dramatic fall in excretion of abnormal metabolites.

Studies with cultured fibroblasts from these patients are providing most interesting biochemical and genetic data. First, those cells tested fall into a unique complementation group (called *bio*), distinct from that for any of the PCC apocarboxylase defects[41, 42]. Second, two patterns of Bio-dependent carboxylase activities have been reported in cell extracts. When cells from two of these patients are grown in Bio-depleted medium, PC, MCC and PCC activities are only a tiny fraction of those in control cells; when the same cells are grown in Bio-supplemented medium, however, activities of these Bio-dependent enzymes are in the normal or near-normal range[35, 36, 41]. A defect in cellular Bio transport or in the mitochondrial form of HS has been suggested to explain this pattern of results, but no direct test of these theses has yet been reported. In contrast, cell extracts from two other affected patients have reportedly had normal activities of all Bio-dependent enzymes in Bio-depleted as well as Bio-supplemented media[39, 40]. Since serum and urine Bio content has been reported recently to be much reduced in one such patient[43], it has been proposed that this entity may be due to an abnormality in intestinal absorption of Bio, which is not expressed in cultured cells. The hypotheses put forth for these proposed variants of multiple carboxylase deficiency are eminently testable, and answers should soon be forthcoming. It will not be surprising to find, as has already been shown for inherited defects of Cbl metabolism, that patients with Bio-responsive disorders will have distinct abnormalities in each of the compartments (gut, blood plasma, cell) in which this vitamin is utilized.

References

1. Rosenberg, L. E. (1978). Disorders of propionate, methylmalonate and cobalamin metabolism. In Stanbury, J. B. , Wyngaarden, J. B. and Fredrickson D. S. (eds.) *The Metabolic Basis of Inherited Disease*, 4th Edn., pp. 411–429. (New York: McGraw-Hill)

2. Rosenberg, L. E., Lilljeqvist, A.-C. and Hsia, Y. E. (1968). Methylmalonicaciduria: Metabolic block localization and vitamin B_{12} dependency. *Science*, **162**, 805

3. Lindblad, B., Lindstrand, K., Svanberg, B. and Zetterstrom, R. (1969). The effect of cobamide coenzyme in methylmalonic acidemia. *Acta Paediatr. Scand.*, **58**, 178

4. Barnes, N. D., Hull, D., Balgobin, L. and Gompertz, D. (1970). Biotin-responsiveness propionicacidaemia. *Lancet*, **2**, 244

5. Rosenberg, L. E. and Scriver, C. R. (1980). Disorders of amino acid metabolism. In Bondy, P. K. and Rosenberg, L. E. (eds.). *Metabolic Control and Disease*, 8th Edn., pp. 583–776. (Philadelphia: Saunders)

6. Ando, T. and Nyhan, W. L. (1974). Propionic acidemia and the ketotic hyperglycinemia syndrome. In Nyhan, W. L. (ed.). *Heritable Disorders of Amino Acid Metabolism*, pp. 37–60. (New York: John Wiley)

7. Galjaard, H. (1980). *Genetic Metabolic Diseases*, p. 743. (Amsterdam: Elsevier/North-Holland Biomedical)

8. Willard, H. F. and Rosenberg, L. E. (1979). Inherited deficiencies of methylmalonyl CoA mutase activity: Biochemical and genetic studies in cultured skin fibroblasts. In Hommes, F. (ed.). *Models for the Study of Inborn Errors of Metabolism*, pp. 297–310. (Amsterdam: Elsevier/North-Holland Biomedical)

9. Kalousek, F., Darigo, M. D. and Rosenberg, L. E. (1980). Isolation and characterization of propionyl CoA carboxylase from normal human liver: Evidence for a protomeric tetramer of non-identical subunits. *J. Biol. Chem.*, **255**, 60

10. Fenton, W. A., Hack, A., Willard, H. F., Gertler, A. and Rosenberg, L. E. (1982). Purification and properties of methylmalonyl CoA mutase from human liver. *Arch. Biochim. Biophys.* (In press)

11. Wolf, B., Kalousek, F. and Rosenberg, L. E. (1979). Essential arginine residues in the active sites of propionyl CoA carboxylase and β-methylcrotonyl CoA carboxylase. *Enzyme*, **24**, 302

12. Kolhouse, J. F., Utley, C. and Allen, R. H. (1980). Isolation and characterization of methylmalonyl-CoA mutase from human placenta. *J. Biol. Chem.*, **255**, 2708

13. Willard, H. F. and Rosenberg, L. E. (1980). Interactions of methylmalonyl CoA mutase from normal human fibroblasts with adenosylcobalamin and methylmalonyl CoA: Evidence for non-equivalent active sites. *Arch. Biochem. Biophys.*, **200**, 130

14. Willard, H. F. and Rosenberg, L. E. (1980). Inherited methylmalonyl CoA mutase apoenzyme deficiency in human fibroblasts: Evidence for allelic heterogeneity, genetic compounds, and codominant expression. *J. Clin. Invest.*, **65**, 690

15. Kolhouse, J. F., Utley, C., Fenton, W. A. and Rosenberg, L. E. (1981). Immunochemical studies on cultured fibroblasts from patients with inherited methylmalonic acidemia. *Proc. Natl. Acad. Sci. USA*, **78**, 7737

16. Gravel, R. A., Lam, K.-F., Scully, K. J. and Hsia, Y. E. (1977). Genetic complementation of propionyl-CoA carboxylase deficiency in cultured human fibroblasts. *Am. J. Human Genet.*, **29**, 378

17. Wolf, B., Hsia, Y. E. and Rosenberg, L. E. (1978). Biochemical differences between mutant propionyl CoA carboxylases from two complementation groups. *Am. J. Human Genet.*, **30**, 455

18. Hsia, Y. E., Scully, K. J. and Rosenberg, L. E. (1979). Human propionyl CoA carboxylase: Some properties of the partially purified enzyme in fibroblasts from controls and patients with propionic acidemia. *Pediatr. Res.*, **13**, 746

19. McKeon, C., Eanes, R. Z., Fall, R. R., Tasset, D. M. and Wolf, B. (1980). Immunological studies of propionyl CoA carboxylase in livers and fibroblasts of patients with propionic acidemia. *Clin. Chim. Acta*, **101**, 217

20. Donaldson, Jr., R. H. (1975). Mechanisms of malabsorption of cobalmin. In Babior, B. (ed.). *Cobalamin: Biochemistry and Pathophysiology*, pp. 335–368. (New York: John Wiley)

21. Allen, R. H. (1975). Human vitamin B_{12} transport proteins. *Prog. Hematol.*, **IX**, 57

22. Youngdahl-Turner, P., Rosenberg, L. E. and Allen, R. H. (1978). Binding and uptake of transcobalamin II by human fibroblasts. *J. Clin. Invest.*, **61**, 133

23. Youngdahl-Turner, P., Mellman, I. S., Allen, R. H. and Rosenberg, L. E. (1979). Protein mediated vitamin uptake: Adsorptive endocytosis of the transcobalamin II–cobalamin complex by cultured human fibroblasts. *Exp. Cell Res.*, **118**, 127

24. Fenton, W. A. and Rosenberg, L. E. (1978). Genetic and biochemical analysis of human cobalamin mutants in cell culture. *Annu. Rev. Genet.*, **12**, 233

25. Moss, J. and Lane, M. D. (1971). The biotin-dependent enzymes. *Adv. Enzymol.*, **35**, 321

26. Rosenberg, L. E. (1976). Vitamin responsive inherited metabolic disorders. In Hirschhorn, H. and Harris, H. (eds.). *Advances in Human Genetics*, Vol. 6, pp. 1–74. (London: Plenum)

27. Hakami, N., Neiman, P. E., Canellos, G. P. and Lazerson, J. (1971). Neonatal megaloblastic anemia due to inherited transcobalamin II deficiency in two siblings. *N. Engl. J. Med.*, **285**, 1163

28. Gimpert, E., Jakob, M. and Hitzig, W. H. (1975). Vitamin B_{12} transport in blood. I. Congenital deficiency of transcobalamin II. *Blood*, **45**, 71

29. Mellman, I. S., Willard, H. F., Youngdahl-Turner, P. and Rosenberg, L. E. (1979). Cobalamin coenzyme synthesis in normal and mutant human fibroblasts: Evidence for a processing enzyme activity deficient in *cbl C* cells. *J. Biol. Chem.*, **254**, 11847

30. Hillman, R. E., Keating, J. P. and Williams, J. C. (1978). Biotin-responsive propionic acidemia presenting as the rumination syndrome. *J. Pediatr.*, **92**, 439

31. Gompertz, D., Draffan, G. H., Watts, J. L. and Hull, D. (1971). Biotin-responsive-methylcrotonyl-glycinuria. *Lancet*, **2**, 22

32. Gompertz, D., Bartlett, K., Blair, D. and Stern, M. M. (1973). Child with a

defect in leucine metabolism associated with β-hydroxyisovaleric aciduria and
β-methylcrotonylglycinuria. *Arch. Dis. Child.*, **48,** 975

33. Lehnert, W., Niederhoff, H., Junker, A., Saule, H. and Frasch, W. (1979). A
case of biotin-responsive 3-methylcrotonylglycin- and 3-hydroxyisovaleric
aciduria. *Eur. J. Pediatr.*, **132,** 107

34. Sweetman, L., Bates, S. P., Hull, D. and Nyhan, W. L. (1977). Propionyl-CoA
carboxylase   deficiency   in   a   patient   with   biotin-responsive   3-
methylcrotonylglycinuria. *Pediatr. Res.*, **11,** 1144

35. Bartlett, K. and Gompertz, D. (1976). Combined carboxylase defect: Biotin-
responsiveness in cultured fibroblasts. *Lancet,* **2,** 804

36. Weyler, W., Sweetman, L., Maggio, D. C. and Nyhan, W. L. (1977).
Deficiency of propionyl-CoA carboxylase and methylcrotonyl-CoA carboxylase in a patient with methylcrotonylglycinuria. *Clin. Chim. Acta,* **76,** 321

37. Roth, K., Cohn, R., Yandrasitz, J., Preti, G., Dodd, P. and Segal, S. (1976).
Beta-methylcrotonic aciduria associated with lactic acidosis. *J. Pediatr.*, **88,**
229

38. Cowan, M. J., Wara, D. W., Packman, S., Ammann, A. J., Yoshino, M.,
Sweetman, L. and Nyhan, W. (1979). Multiple biotin-dependent carboxylase
deficiencies associated with defects in T-cell and B-cell immunity. *Lancet,* **2,**
115

39. Charles, B. M., Hosking, G., Green, A., Pollitt, R., Bartlett, K. and Taitz, L.
E. (1979). Biotin-responsive alopecia and developmental regression. *Lancet,*
2, 118

40. Thoene, J., Yoshino, M. and Sweetman, L. (1979). Biotin-responsive multiple
carboxylase deficiency. *Am. J. Human Genet.*, **31,** 64A (abstr)

41. Saunders, M., Sweetman, L., Robinson, B., Roth, K., Cohn, R. and Gravel,
R. A. (1979). Biotin-response organicaciduria. Multiple carboxylase defects
and complementation studies with propionicacidemia in cultured fibroblasts.
J. Clin. Invest., **64,** 1695

42. Wolf, B., Willard, H. F. and Rosenberg, L. E. (1980). Kinetic analysis of
genetic complementation in heterokaryons of propionyl CoA carboxylase-
deficient human fibroblasts. *Am. J. Human Genet.*, **32,** 16

43. Thoene, J., Baker, H., Yoshino, M. and Sweetman, L. (1981). Biotin-
responsive carboxylase. Deficiency apparently due to a defect in biotin
absorption. *N. Engl. J. Med.*, **304,** 817

4

Homocystinuria: clinical and biochemical heterogeneity
N. A. J. Carson

INTRODUCTION

Some years ago it appeared to those of us interested in inherited metabolic disorders that a characteristic clinical and biochemical syndrome corresponded to the inactivity of a specific enzyme in the intermediary metabolism of a substance. As our knowledge of these hereditary disorders continued to expand, it became obvious that we must modify these earlier views. It is now common experience among the inborn errors of metabolism that similar phenotypes, both clinical and biochemical in nature, are often caused by a variety of different genotypes; in other words, heterogeneity abounds. One such disorder demonstrating heterogeneity is the condition first described as homocystinuria.

CLASSICAL HOMOCYSTINURIA

When a new disease is discovered, one of the problems one faces is finding an appropriate name for it. This decision is made more difficult by the fact that experience of the new disorder is initially limited to the study of only a few patients. When, in 1962, in Northern Ireland we discovered two mentally retarded sisters to be excreting a large quantity of homocystine in their urine, it seemed appropriate to call the disorder homocystinuria, as this condition had never previously been described[1]. With the discovery of more patients in Northern Ireland and in different parts of the world, a clinical and biochemical pattern emerged. The major clinical features are found in the central nervous system, the eye, the skeletal and the vascular systems. Of 31 patients discovered in Northern Ireland, all are mentally retarded, with the exception of those treated from an early age, and have IQs varying from < 30 to 70. This is contrary to the experience of other workers. For example, in the series of patients described by McKusick and his co-workers[2], 41 of 84 patients had at least average intelligence. Similarly, Wilcken and Turner[3] report 13 of 27 patients to have normal IQ. One reason for this difference may be the manner in which these patients were discovered. In Northern Ireland many of our patients were detected whilst screening the mentally retarded population for amino-acid disorders, whereas McKusick and his co-workers[2] found most of their cases by screening patients with ectopia lentis and/or presumed Marfan syndrome.

Developmental delay is rarely manifest before the first to second year of life. Walking tends to be delayed and patients have a wide based gait. Two of our young patients found great difficulty rising from a sitting position and climbed up their legs or the legs of furniture, like a child with muscular dystrophy. Convulsions, both major and minor; occur but seldom present a problem in the clinical management of the patient. About 50% of our patients had a history of convulsions. It is difficult to know how much of the brain damage is due to the abnormal chemical milieu surrounding the developing brain and how much is secondary to intra-cranial thrombosis. Some patients have been described with schizophrenia-like illnesses and extreme nervousness.

Ectopia lentis is the hallmark of classical homocystinuria and many cases have been diagnosed because of it. It is not present at birth and in our own series of patients it was diagnosed as early as 18 months and as late as seven years, the last being a patient who had been under the care of an ophthalmologist for three years before it was diagnosed. Other workers report it as not being recognized in mild cases until over 20 years of age. Eye complications occur in the older children and adults with glaucoma secondary to complete anterior dislocation of the lens. Myopia is common and retinal detachment, buphthalmos, staphyloma and cataract formation may occur.

The skeletal features are not evident in infants and very young children. The first signs are usually the appearance of genu valgum and pes cavus. As they near puberty, dolichostenomelia becomes evident and their limbs appear to grow out of proportion to the trunk, anterior chest deformities may occur taking the form of pectus excavatum or carinatum and kyphosis or scoliosis may be present. These skeletal manifestations give older patients an appearance similar to that of Marfan's syndrome. One of the distinguishing features of homocystinuria is the presence of osteoporosis, which may occur at an early age and involves the vertebrae and the long bones; arachnodactyly is a classical feature of Marfan's syndrome and in our experience is only sometimes noted in homocystinuria. Radiology of the vertebral column shows further distinguishing features with the homocystinuric patients displaying biconcavity and flattening of the intervertebral discs. There is marked widening of the metaphyses and epiphyses, most easily noted at the knees, the metaphyses showing the most pronounced changes.

The cardinal vascular sign in cystathionine synthase-deficient homocystinuria is thrombosis, occurring in both arterial and venous systems and affecting most major arteries and veins of the body; this is not a feature of Marfan's syndrome. Cerebrovascular thrombosis has occurred as early as six months of age in our series of patients. It is because of this tendency that most of us treating patients with this form of homocystinuria are very wary about stopping treatment as we would do in older patients with phenylketonuria. The pathological findings in the arterial walls show marked fibrous thickening in the intima, with splitting of the muscle fibres in the media and fragmentation of elastic fibres in both media and the internal elastic laminae.

As the eye defects, the skeletal manifestations and the microscopic appearance of the arterial walls were suggestive of Marfan's syndrome, we examined the urine of patients with this syndrome in Northern Ireland for the presence of homocystine. We did not find any, but we did discover that two of our homocystinuric patients had been written up in the literature as suffering from Marfan's syndrome. We have, therefore, the first indication of heterogeneity with this clinical association with Marfan's syndrome. Genetically, as well as biochemically, they can be distinguished as the latter is of autosomal dominant inheritance and homocystinuria is an autosomal recessive disorder. There is a marked variation in the severity of the clinical manifestations in classical homocystinuria, some patients being severely affected with brain damage, eye defects, severe skeletal abnormalities with osteoporosis and life threatening thrombotic episodes. At the other end of the scale there are those described with normal intelligence, late diagnosed eye defects and minimal skeletal changes. All our untreated patients were severely affected.

The amino acid profile shows an increased plasma concentration of methionine, homocyst(e)ine and the mixed disulphide of homocysteine and cysteine, with a lack of cystathionine and greatly reduced plasma cyst(e)ine. There is a marked overexcretion of homocystine in the urine, the presence of the mixed disulphide and varying quantities of methionine and cystine. The urine of patients with homocystinuria gives a positive cyanide/nitro-prusside colour reaction which is a useful screening test, but as this is also positive with other disulphides such as cysteine further tests using high voltage electrophoresis, thin layer or paper chromatography must be undertaken for positive identification of homocystine.

Two years after the discovery of homocystinuria, Mudd and his co-workers[4] demonstrated a deficiency of hepatic crystathionine β-synthase, a pyridoxine-dependent enzyme on the trans-sulphuration pathway (Figure 4.1) which converts methionine to cysteine and inorganic sulphate. In this pathway methionine adenosyltransferase catalyses the formation of S-adenosylmethionine, which is the primary methyl group donor in man, and this is then transmethylated to form S-adenosylhomocysteine which is enzymatically cleaved to adenosine and homocysteine. Homocysteine may then be condensed with serine to form

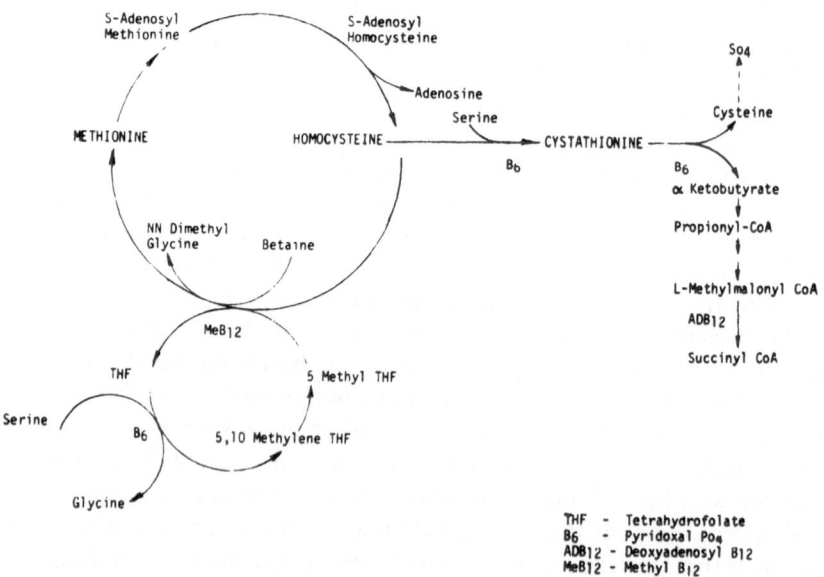

Figure 4.1   The methionine trans-sulphuration and remethylation pathway in man

cystathionine through the activity of cystathionine β-synthase (CS) or be re-methylated to form methionine. In the normal individual the metabolic flow is through cystathionine, which is then cleaved to cysteine and α-ketobutyrate by α-cystathionase, thus completing the trans-sulphuration pathway. In homocystinuria, due to CS deficiency, there is overproduction of homocysteine; the re-methylation pathway back to methionine then becomes active causing a rise in plasma methionine. At least two enzymes take part in this re-methylation step:

(1) Homocysteine reacts with betaine catalysed by the enzyme betaine-homocysteine methyltransferase; this is an irreversible reaction.
(2) 5-Methyltetrahydrofolate (5-Me THF) acts as the methyl donor reacting with homocysteine through N5-methyltetrahydrofolate-homocysteine methyltransferase, a cobalamin containing enzyme. The co-substrate, 5-Me THF, is formed by a further enzyme, i.e. N5,10-methylenetetrahydrofolate reductase (5,10-Methylene THF).

Deficiency of either of these enzymes results in an inability to reform methionine, also causing homocysteinaemia and homocystinuria.

CS deficiency resulting in the classical clinical and biochemical picture has been confirmed by other investigators[5-7]. The defect is not confined to the liver, but has also been demonstrated in the brain[8], in fibroblasts cultured from skin biopsies[9] and phytohaemagglutinin-stimulated lymphocytes[10]. Other enzymes of the trans-sulphuration and the re-methylation pathways have been reported in normal concentrations in these patients[11]. Available evidence indicates that CS-deficient homocystinuria is inherited as an autosomal recessive disorder as established by analysis of published pedigrees[2] and from the study of enzyme activity in liver biopsy and in cultured skin fibroblasts from parents of affected individuals[11].

CYSTATHIONINE SYNTHASE AND PYRIDOXINE

The first indication of the presence of genetic heterogeneity in the CS enzyme protein was the report by Barber and Spaeth in 1967[12] of three patients with CS-deficient homocystinuria who responded to pharmacological doses of pyridoxine by showing a reduction in plasma methionine and almost complete disappearance of homocystine from plasma and urine. Following this observation, other workers reported their experiences with pyridoxine therapy[13-17]. It soon became obvious that not all patients responded to pyridoxine. Moreover, responsiveness or non-responsiveness was constant within sibships, suggesting that there were at least two different genetic mutations in the enzyme protein. Mudd and Levy[11] in a survey of the literature, found 24 sibships with a total of 54 patients in which B_6 responsiveness was constant within sibships. Less than 50 % of CS deficient patients respond to pyridoxine. In our own series of 31 patients, 21 were given a challenge of pyridoxine; 14 patients were resistant and seven responded. Further heterogeneity was suggested by Brenton and Cusworth[18] when they described the response of 18 patients to pyridoxine and divided them into three groups, those that were biochemically completely responsive to B_6, those that were partially responsive and those that were resistant.

It is still not known with certainty in what manner the activity of the mutant CS apoenzyme is enhanced by the availability of excess co-enzyme. Uhlendorf et al.[19] using fibroblast extracts reported that those grown from pyridoxine-responsive patients had detectable levels of activity which were stimulated 3–4 % by the addition in vitro of pyridoxine. In pyridoxine-unresponsive patients they found no detectable activity and no in vitro response to pyridoxine in the cell cultures. These workers claim that the small percentage increase in the activity of CS would be sufficient to reactivate the methionine–cysteine pathway. Kim and Rosenberg[20], studying CS kinetics and thermostability in cultured fibroblasts from pyridoxine-responsive patients, suggested from their studies that in CS pyridoxine-responsive cell lines the mutation had altered the apoenzyme in such a way that its affinity for co-enzyme was markedly reduced. This leads to reduced holoenzyme activity and to reduced apoenzyme content as the mutant apoenzyme turns over more rapidly than normal. In this situation, pyridoxine stimulation in vivo will lead to only a small increase in enzyme activity because there is only a very small amount of apoenzyme which can be converted to active holoenzyme. This investigation was extended by the same group[21]. They studied CS activity in cultured fibroblasts from seven pyridoxine-responsive and seven non-responsive patients and came to the conclusion that there are three general classes of CS mutants; those with no residual activity, those with reduced activity and normal affinity for pyridoxine, and those with reduced activity and a reduced affinity for the co-factor. More research is required in this field as precise knowledge of the molecular defects in this disorder may help us to understand the other vitamin-dependent metabolic disorders.

The presence or absence of pyridoxine responsiveness is of great importance to the patient, and makes the difference between taking tablets and enjoying a normal diet with a moderate protein intake or a low methionine diet which is very monotonous and difficult to cope with. The long-term use of large doses of pyridoxine does not seem to cause any ill effects in the patients; seven of our patients have received 100–450 mg pyridoxine daily from 11.5–13.5 years without any untoward effects.

In keeping with other inborn errors of metabolism, the earlier the diagnosis the more successful the treatment. We have had 31 patients with homocystinuria from 19 families, of whom 19 were male and 12 female. Their ages at diagnosis varied from four days to 28 years. Seven were treated with pyridoxine and eight of the younger pyridoxine non-responsive patients were placed on a low methionine diet.

Results of therapy with either pyridoxine or diet show that those patients first treated up to the age of nine months have had a good clinical response, but those treated from one year eight months already showed signs of the disorder which were not reversed by treatment. Twelve of our patients have been under treatment for 8–13 years, the oldest patients now being 31 and 35 years old, without suffering any thrombotic episodes and without any obvious signs of progression of the disorder. In contrast to the treated patients, all 15 untreated patients are now dead, the oldest patients being 29 and 30 years of age at death and the youngest being six months. Six patients died as the result of a thrombotic episode, five of which were proven by post mortem; two died after a major fit; two died in congestive heart failure; one in status asthmaticus and one from uraemia as a sequel to hypertension.

HOMOCYSTEINE METHYLTRANSFERASE DEFECTS

Homocyst(e)ine, as indicated earlier, could become increased in plasma and urine due to the inactivity of enzymes in the re-methylating pathway from homocysteine back to methionine. Three genetically determined defects are now known which act by interfering with the cobalamin-dependent enzyme N5-Me THF-homocysteine methyltransferase. In two instances this is due to lack of available methylcobalamin, the co-factor necessary for this reaction and in the third case due to lack of formation of the co-substrate, N5-Me THF, through the inactivity of the enzyme N5,10-Methylene THF reductase.

Congenital homocystinuria due to decreased activity of N5-Me THF-homocysteine methyltransferase was first described in 1969 by Mudd et al.[22]. They were investigating an infant with homocystinuria who deteriorated clinically from birth, dying at seven and a half weeks of age. The fact that the infant had decreased concentration of plasma methionine and increased plasma homocysteine and cystathionine suggested the possibility that he was unable to methylate homocysteine to methionine at a normal rate. The enzyme N5-Me THF-homocysteine methyltransferase was found to have very low activity in the patient's liver. In 1970 the same group of workers[23] reported decreased activity of this enzyme in cultured fibroblasts which was restored to normal by *in vitro* addition of methylcobalamin, suggesting that the enzyme defect was due to lack of formation of its co-factor methylcobalamin, rather than a defect in the apoenzyme itself. The only other cobalamin derivative known to act as a co-factor is adenosylcobalamin, required for the activity of the enzyme methylmalonyl CoA mutase which catalyses methylmalonyl CoA to succinyl CoA. Decreased activity of this enzyme leads to the excretion of excessive amounts of methylmalonic acid in the urine. Urine collected before death in this infant was found in retrospect to cóntain methylmalonic acid. His cultured fibroblasts showed a reduction in the mutase which could be overcome by the addition of high concentrations of hydroxocobalamin. This inability to accumulate normal tissue concentrations of the methyl and adenosylcobalamin in these patients explains the homocystinuria and methylmalonic aciduria.

HOMOCYSTEINE TRANSFERASE AND COBALAMIN

Fenton and Rosenberg[24] have made a detailed study of the genetic and biochemical features of these human cobalamin mutants in cell culture (see p. 45). Genetic complementation studies indicate that within the group of patients with N5-Me THF-homocysteine methyltransferase deficiency there are at least two different genetic entities, termed cobalamin C and D. These appear to result from an inability to synthesize both methyl and adenosylcobalamin at different steps in intracellular cobalamin metabolism. The C mutation represents a more severe biochemical and clinical defect than the D form.

Including the original case described by Mudd *et al.*[22], seven patients in six families have been reported to date[25-28]. Typical findings in all seven patients were homocystinuria, methylmalonic aciduria, low plasma methionine with normal serum B_{12} and transcobalamin II levels, but low tissue levels of total B_{12} and normal folate concentration. Carmel *et al.*[29] compare the clinical picture of all seven cases. Two of the patients had milder clinical and biochemical abnormalities with no megaloblastosis, and were thought to belong to the cobalamin D mutation. The other five patients showed some similarity in their clinical picture. They presented between the ages of birth to three years with failure to thrive, poor feeding, lethargy, vomiting and poor growth. Neurological sequelae were present with microcephaly, mental retardation, atypical fits and hypotonia. Death occurred in three patients at the ages of seven and a half weeks, four months and seven years. Postmortem findings in these three patients showed similar vascular lesions, but in different areas of the body. These take the form of disruption and splitting of the elastic lamina and patchy fibrous thickening of the intima, similar to features seen in CS homocystinuric patients[28]. In patients with methylmalonic aciduria unassociated with homocystinuria due to decreased activity of methylmalonyl CoA mutase, vascular pathology has not been present. This leads to the speculation that it is the raised serum and tissue levels of homocysteine which causes the thrombotic episodes in CS-deficient homocystinuria and in the cobalamin-dependent homocystinuria. Cobalamin C mutation may have haematological abnormalities characteristic of Vitamin B_{12} deficiency; these abnormalities seem to vary with age, the younger patients showing only myeloid hyperplasia and segmentation of neutrophils and normocytic anaemia. It would appear from the patient reports that massive doses of parenteral B_{12} in the hydroxo form are required for biochemical improvement, which was not always accompanied by clinical improvement. The methionine intake in these patients is critical, and lowering the daily intake as one would do in CS deficiency could lead to negative nitrogen balance.

In 1960 two independent observers described patients with acquired juvenile-type megaloblastic anaemia secondary to a specific malabsorption of vitamin B_{12}. They had low serum B_{12}, normal intrinsic factor and normal B_{12} binding capacity. The anaemia responded to physiological doses of parenteral B_{12} [30, 31]. Homocystine and methylmalonic acid were reported in the urine of one such patient which disappeared within two weeks after a total of 3 mg parenteral B_{12}[32]. The reason for the homocystinuria and methylmalonic aciduria was presumably lack of formation of cellular methyl and adenosylcobalamin due to deficient B_{12}. These patients all had megaloblastic anaemia and this was invariably the reason for their discovery. This is unlike the patients with N5-Me THF-homocysteine methyltransferase deficiency who only rarely presented with macrocytic anaemia and megaloblastic marrow. Insufficient data is at hand to establish whether homocystinuria and methylmalonic aciduria is a rare or common association in untreated patients with this type of B_{12} malabsorption.

5,10-METHYLENE THF REDUCTASE

A further congenital defect associated with the excretion of homocystine was described in three teenage patients by Mudd et al. in 1972[33]. They had no increase in plasma methionine distinguishing them from CS-deficient patients, and unlike patients with the methyltransferase deficiency did not excrete methylmalonic acid. Studies on cultured fibroblasts showed that N5-Me THF-homocysteine methyltransferase and CS enzymes were not markedly decreased and that the patients' fibroblasts were unable to grow as rapidly as control fibroblasts when methionine in the culture media was replaced by homocystine. The enzyme N5,10-methylene THF-reductase which converts N5, 10-methylene THF to N5-Me THF was significantly reduced.

We now have knowledge of eleven patients with this disorder[34−38]. All had an amino-acid profile similar to that described above. All had low folate and normal or greater than normal serum B_{12} concentrations and did not excrete methylmalonic acid. Of five patients given folate medication, three responded and two were resistant, suggesting further heterogeneity within this group. Two infants were severely affected clinically and died aged 38 days and nine months with apnoeic attacks and coma indicating the presence of a severe neonatal form of the disease. Seven patients were not diagnosed until the ages of eight to 17 years and all were mentally retarded with neurological sequelae. Five patients have died and postmortems were performed on three. In two of them extensive vascular thromboses were present[35,39].

Rosenblatt and Erbe[38] studied 5,10-methylene THF reductase in cultured cells in four patients from three families. All showed decreased activity of the reductase. In heat-inactivation studies at 55°C two of the unrelated patients also showed reduced thermal stability, whereas the results in the two related siblings resembled those in normal control subjects. This implies that the reduced deficiency of the reductase in these families is due to different alleles; the altered thermal stability suggesting a structural defect in the apoenzyme. Table 4.1 gives a list of the distinguishing features of the three different genetic disorders resulting in homocystinuria.

DRUG-INDUCED HOMOCYSTINURIA

Homocystinuria has also been noted in patients with psoriasis treated with the drug Azaribine (Triazine)[40]. The use of this drug has recently been prohibited because of the possibility of an association with thromboembolism. Five of 13 patients receiving Azaribine developed homocystinuria and homocysteinaemia and one of the five developed a thrombotic episode. When the drug was discontinued, homocyst(e)ine disappeared from blood and urine.

TABLE 4.1 Summary of biochemical findings in genetic forms of homocystinuria

	Cystathionine synthase	5-Me THF-homocysteine transferase	5,10-Methylene THF reductase
Plasma and urinary homocyst(e)ine	Increase	Increase	Increase
Plasma methionine	Increase	Low normal or decreased	Low normal or decreased
Methylmalonic aciduria	Absent	Increased	Absent
Serum B_{12}	Normal	Normal or increased	Normal or increased
Serum folate	Low normal	Normal	Decreased
Anaemia	None	None (3) Normocytic (3) Macrocytic (1)	None
Vitamin responsiveness	B_6	B_{12}	Folate
No. of patients	> 300	7	9

Homocystinuria has also been described as an artefact in the urine of a patient who was excreting cystathionine in her urine. Contamination of the urine specimen and bacterial conversion of urinary cystathionine to homocyst(e)ine[41] was shown to be the reason.

CONSEQUENCES OF GENETIC HETEROGENEITY

Appreciating the extent of genetic heterogeneity in any inherited metabolic disorder can have far reaching implications for the treatment of the patient and in genetic counselling.

Genetic mutations in three different enzymes on the methionine trans-sulphuration and remethylation pathways have been shown to result in the excretion of homocystine, an amino acid not normally present in man. Because of this heterogeneity it is therefore no longer appropriate to use the term homocystinuria without qualification as to which enzyme-defect it relates to. Precise definition of the genotype is of considerable therapeutic importance, as each enzyme defect is known to exist in co-enzyme responsive and non-responsive forms.

CS deficiency, the first disorder to be described and so far the commonest cause of homocystinuria is present as B_6 responsive and B_6 non-responsive forms.

Patients with 5-Me THF-homocysteine methyltransferase deficiency require large doses of parenteral B_{12} which appears to be most effective in the hydroxocobalamin form. Some patients described failed to respond to parenteral B_{12} but they were severely affected clinically and the dosage may not have been adequate. Therefore it is not clear if they should be classified as B_{12} non-responsive.

Deficiency of 5,10-methylene THF reductase has been reported in 11 patients, but only documented in detail in nine. Three of five patients responded to folate medication.

As stated above, a low methionine intake could be dangerous in patients with the 5-Me THF-homocysteine methyltransferase deficiency or 5,10-methylene THF reductase deficiency, whereas it is the treatment of choice in CS deficient patients who are B_6 non-responsive.

The following investigations are helpful in distinguishing the various forms of homocystinuria: amino acid studies; the presence or absence of methylmalonic acid; B_{12} and folate studies. After a methionine-load test, normal subjects and patients with 5-Me THF methyltransferase and 5,10-methylene THF reductase deficiency will excrete $> 65\%$ of the load as inorganic sulphate in 24 h, whereas CS deficient patients will excrete $< 10\%$ of the load.

CS deficiency has characteristic clinical manifestations in older children and adults but so far, apart from neurological involvement, the two remethylating enzyme deficiencies show a complexity of clinical findings. The final diagnosis can, for all three defects, where necessary be made by appropriate enzyme assays on cultured skin fibroblasts or lymphocytes.

References

1. Carson, N. A. J. and Neill, D. W. (1962). Metabolic abnormalities detected in a survey of mentally backward individuals in Northern Ireland. *Arch. Dis. Child.*, **37**, 505
2. McKusick, V. A., Hall, J. G. and Char, F. (1971). The clinical and genetic characteristics of homocystinuria. In Carson, N. A. J. and Raine, D. N. (eds.) *Inherited Disorders of Sulphur Metabolism*, pp. 179–203. (London: Churchill Livingston)

3. Wilcken, B. and Turner, G. (1978). Homocystinuria in New South Wales. *Arch. Dis. Child.,* **53,** 242
4. Mudd, S. H., Finkelstein, J. D., Irreverre, F. and Laster, L. (1964). Homocystinuria: an enzymatic defect. *Science,* **143,** 1443
5. Holowell, J. G. Jr., Coryell, M. E., Hall, W. K., Findley, J. K. and Thevos, T. G. (1968). Homocystinuria as affected by pyridoxine, folic acid and vitamin B_{12}. *Proc. Soc. Exp. Biol. Med.,* **129,** 327
6. Yoshida, T., Tada, K., Yokoyama, Y. and Arakawa, T. (1968). Homocystinuria of vitamin B_6 dependent type. *Tohoku J. Exp. Med.,* **96,** 235
7. Gaull, G. E., Rassin, D. K. and Sturman, J. A. (1969). Enzymatic and metabolic studies of homocystinuria: effects of pyridoxine. *Neuropadiatrie,* **1,** 199
8. Mudd, S. H., Finkelstein, J. D., Irreverre, F. and Laster, L. (1965). Transsulfuration in mammals: Microassays and tissue distribution of three enzymes of the pathway. *J. Biol. Chem.,* **240,** 4382
9. Uhlendorf, B. W. and Mudd, S. H. (1968). Cystathionine synthase in tissue culture derived from human skin: Enzyme defect in homocystinuria. *Science,* **160,** 1007
10. Goldstein, J. L., Campbell, B. K. and Gartler, S. M. (1972). Cystathionine synthase activity in human lymphocytes, induction by phytohemagglutinin. *J. Clin. Invest.,* **51,** 1034
11. Mudd, S. H. and Levy, H. L. (1978). Disorders of transsulfuration. In Stanbury, Wyngaarden and Fredrickson (eds.) *The Metabolic Basis of Inherited Disease.* 4th Edn., pp. 458–527. (New York: McGraw Hill)
12. Barber, G. W. and Spaeth, G. L. (1967). Pyridoxine therapy in homocystinuria. *Lancet,* **1,** 337
13. Hooft, C., Carton, D. and Samyn, W. (1967). Pyridoxine treatment in homocystinuria. *Lancet,* **1,** 1384
14. Turner, B. (1967). Pyridoxine treatment in homocystinuria. *Lancet,* **2,** 1151
15. Hagberg, B. and Hambraeus, L. (1968). Some aspects of the diagnosis and treatment of homocystinuria. *Devel. Med. Child. Neurol.,* **10,** 479
16. Carson, N. A. J. and Carre, I. J. (1969). Treatment of homocystinuria with pyridoxine. A preliminary study. *Arch. Dis. Child.,* **44,** 387
17. Cusworth, D. C., and Dent, C. E. (1969). Homocystinuria. *Br. Med. Bull.,* **25,** 42
18. Brenton, D. P. and Cusworth, D. C. (1971). The response of patients with cystathionine synthase deficiency to pyridoxine. In Carson, N. A. J. and Raine, D. N. (eds.) *Inherited Disorders of Sulphur Metabolism,* pp. 264–274. (London: Churchill Livingston)
19. Uhlendorf, B. W., Conerly, E. B. and Mudd, S. H. (1973). Homocystinuria: Studies in tissue culture. *Pediatr. Res.,* **7,** 645
20. Kim, Y. J. and Rosenberg, L. E. (1974). On the mechanism of pyridoxine responsive homocystinuria, II properties of normal and mutant cystathionine-β-synthase from cultured fibroblasts. *Proc. Natl. Acad. Sci. USA,* **71,** 4821
21. Fowler, B., Kraus, J., Packman, S. and Rosenberg, L. E. (1978). Evidence for three distinct classes of cystathionine-β-synthase mutants in cultured fibroblasts. *J. Clin. Invest.,* **61,** 645
22. Mudd, S. H., Levy, H. L. and Abeles, R. H. (1969). A derangement in B_{12}

metabolism leading to homocysteinemia, cystathioninemia and methyl-malonic aciduria. *Biochem. Biophys. Res. Commun.*, **35**, 121

23. Mudd, S. H., Uhlendorf, B. W., Hinds, K. R. and Levy, H. L. (1970). Deranged B_{12} metabolism: studies of fibroblasts grown in tissue culture. *Biochem. Med.*, **4**, 215

24. Fenton, W. A. and Rosenberg, L. E. (1978). Genetic and biochemical analysis of human cobalamin mutants in cell culture. *Annu. Rev. Genet.*, **12**, 223

25. Goodman, S. I., Moe, P. G., Hammond, K. B., Mudd, S. H. and Uhlendorf, B. W. (1970). Homocystinuria with methylmalonic aciduria: two cases in a sibship. *Biochem. Med.*, **4**, 500

26. Dillon, M. J., England, J. M., Gompertz, D., Goodey, P. A., Grant, D. B., Hussein, H. A. A., Linnell, J. C., Matthews, D. M., Mudd, S. H., Newns, G. H., Seakins, J. W. T., Uhlendorf, B. W. and Wise, I. J. (1974). Mental retardation, megaloblastic anaemia, methylmalonic aciduria and abnormal homocysteine metabolism due to an error in vitamin B_{12} metabolism. *Clin. Sci. Mol. Med.*, **47**, 43

27. Anthony, M. and McLeay, A. C. (1976). A unique case of derangement of vitamin B_{12} metabolism. *Proc. Aust. Assoc. Neurol.*, **13**, 61

28. Baumgartner, E. R., Wick, H., Maurer, R., Egli, N. and Steinmann, B. (1979). Congenital defect in intracellular cobalamin metabolism resulting in homo-cystinuria and methylmalonic aciduria. I. case report and histopathology. *Helv. Paediatr. Acta*, **34**, 465

29. Carmel, R. Bedros, A. A., Mace, J. W. and Goodman, S. I. (1980). Congenital methylmalonic aciduria – homocystinuria with megaloblastic anaemia. Observations on response to hydroxocobalamin and on the effect of homocysteine and methionine on the deoxyuridine suppression test. *Blood*, **55**, 570

30. Imerslund, O. (1960). Idiopathic chronic megaloblastic anaemia in children. *Acta Paediatr. Scand.*, **119** (Suppl.), 1

31. Grasbeck, R., Gordin, R., Kantero, I. and Kuhlback, B. (1960). Selective vitamin B_{12} malabsorption and proteinuria in young people. *Acta Medi. Scand.*, **167**, 289

32. Hollowell, J. G. Jr., Hall, W. K., Coryell, M. E., McPherson, J. Jr. and Hahn, D. A. (1969). Homocystinuria and organic aciduria in a patient with vitamin B_{12} deficiency. *Lancet*, **2**, 1428

33. Mudd, S. H., Uhlendorf, B. W., Freeman, J. M., Finkelstein, J. D. and Shih, V. E. (1972). Homocystinuria associated with decreased methylenetetrahyd-rofolate reductase activity. *Biochem. Biophys. Res. Commun.*, **46**, 905

34. Freeman, J. M., Finkelstein, J. D. and Mudd, S. H. (1975). A defect in methylation due to deficient 5,10-methylenetetrahydrofolate reductase ac-tivity. *N Engl. J. Med.*, **292**, 491

35. Wong, P. W. K., Justice, P., Hruby, M., Weiss, E. B. and Diamond, E. (1977). Folic acid non-responsive homocystinuria due to methylenetetrahydrofolate reductase deficiency. *Pediatrics*, **59**, 749

36. Wong, P. W. K., Justice, P. and Berlow, S. (1977). Detection of homozygotes and heterozygotes with methylenetetrahydrofolate reductase deficiency. *J. Lab. Clin. Med.*, **90**, 283

37. Narisawa, K., Wada, Y., Saito, T., Suzuki, H., Kudo, M., Arakawa, T., Atsushima, K. and Tsuboi, R. (1977). Infantile type of homocystinuria with

N5,10-methylenetetrahydrofolate reductase defect. *Tohuku J. Exp. Med.,* **121,** 185

38. Rosenblatt, D. S. and Erbe, R. W. (1977). Methylenetetrahydrofolate reductase in cultured human cells. II. Genetic and biochemical studies of methylenetetrahydrofolate reductase deficiency. *Pediatr. Res.,* **11,** 1141
39. Kanwar, Y. S., Manaligod, J. and Wong, W. K. (1976). Morphologic studies in a patient with homocystinuria due to 5,10-methylenetetrahydrofolate reductase deficiency. *Pediatr. Res.,* **10,** 598
40. Shupack, J. L., Grieco, A. J., Epstein, A. M., Sansaric, Q. C. and Snyderman, S. (1977). Azaribine, homocysteinaemia and thrombosis. *Arch. Dermatol.,* **113,** 1301
41. Levy, H. L., Mudd, S. H., Uhlendorf, B. W. and Madigan, P. M. (1975). Cystathioninuria and homocystinuria. *Clin. Chim. Acta,* **58,** 51

5

Hereditary defects of steroid biosynthesis

A. Prader and M. Zachmann

INTRODUCTION

The adrenocortical and gonadal hormones are synthesized through a common initial pathway from acetyl coenzyme A and cholesterol. Certain steps of their subsequent synthesis also occur in the placenta, in the liver and in other tissues. Several hereditary enzyme defects are known. Many more are theoretically possible, but have not yet been described. Best known are those of the adrenal steroids which cause adrenal insufficiency and the adrenogenital syndrome, and those of testosterone which cause male pseudohermaphroditism, i.e. incomplete prenatal differentiation of the male genitalia. Certain defects have also been described in other tissues. Interestingly, hardly anything is known about hereditary defects of the ovarian steroids.

This is a short review of the localization of the enzyme blocks in the biosynthetic pathway, the clinical manifestations and the genetics, with emphasis on some new aspects. Space does not allow us to discuss the technical details of the diagnostic steroid analyses. Table 5.1 lists the presently known enzyme defects in order of the year in which clinical and laboratory evidence of the defect was first reported.

TABLE 5.1   Discovery of hereditary steroid defects

Date of first report	Defect	Reference
1953	21-Hydroxylase	Jailer[1]
1955	11-Hydroxylase	Eberlein and Bongiovanni[2]
1957	22, 22-Desmolase	Prader and Siebenmann[3]
1961	3 β-Dehydrogenase	Bongiovanni[4]
1964	18-Hydroxylation	Visser and Cost[5]
1964	18-Dehydrogenase	Ulick et al[6]
1966	17-Hydroxylase	Biglieri et al.[7]
1966	17-Reductase	Neher and Kahnt[8]
1969	Steroid-sulphatase	France and Liggins[9]
1972	17, 20-Desmolase	Zachmann et al.[10]
1974	5 α-Reductase	Imperato-McGinley et al.[11]

BIOCHEMISTRY

In order to understand the biosynthesis of the steroid hormones, it is essential to know the precursor cholesterol (Figure 5.1). Cholesterol has four rings and a side chain at C-17 which is cleaved first at C-20 to form the C-21 steroids and then at C-17 to form the C-19- and C-18-steroids. Two methyl groups are in positions 18 and 19. There is a hydroxy group at C-3 of ring A and a double bond $\Delta 5$ in ring B which will be shifted to $\Delta 4$ in ring A.

The glucocorticoid cortisol and the mineralocorticoid aldosterone (Figure 5.1), which are produced by the adrenals, are steroids with a keto group at C-3 and a $\Delta 4$ double bond in ring A. The sex hormones testosterone and oestradiol are produced in the gonads, but also in the adrenals. Testosterone and the other androgenic steroids are C-19-steroids. Through aromatization in ring A they are converted into the C-18-steroid oestradiol and the other oestrogenic steroids.

BIOSYNTHESIS OF THE ADRENAL STEROIDS

Figure 5.2 gives the simplified biosynthetic pathway of the gluco- and mineralocorticoids in the adrenals. Cholesterol is transformed along a vertically indicated pathway to pregnenolone through a cleavage enzyme system designated 20,22-desmolase, to progesterone through a 3β-dehydrogenase and $\Delta 5$–$\Delta 4$ isomerase system, to deoxy-corticosterone

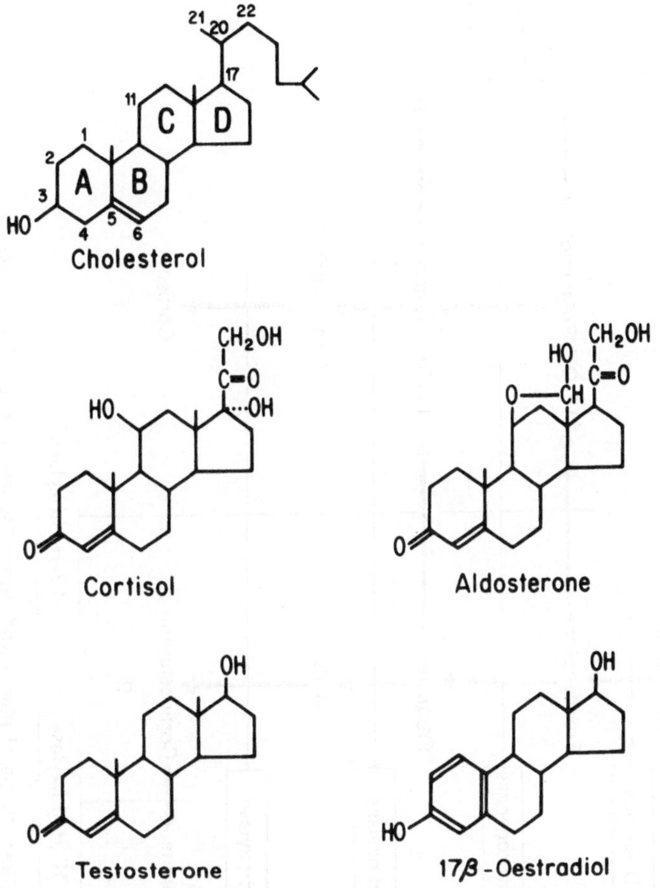

Figure 5.1 Structure of cholesterol, indicating conventional alphabetical order of cyclopentanophenanthren rings and numbering of carbon atoms. Structures of cortisol, aldosterone, testosterone, and oestradiol

(DOC) through a 21-hydroxylase system, and finally to corticosterone through an 11β-hydroxylase system. This is the *17-deoxy pathway*. At the level of pregnenolone and progesterone, a 17-hydroxylase system leads to the parallel 17-hydroxy pathway with 17-hydroxy-pregnenolone, 17-hydroxy-progesterone, cortexolone or compound S, and finally cortisol. 17-Hydroxy-pregnenolone and 17-hydroxy-progesterone are the precursors of the androgens and oestrogens, as will be discussed later. The 17-deoxy compounds DOC and corticosterone can be hydroxylated at C-18 which yields 18-hydroxy DOC and 18-hydroxy-corticosterone and from

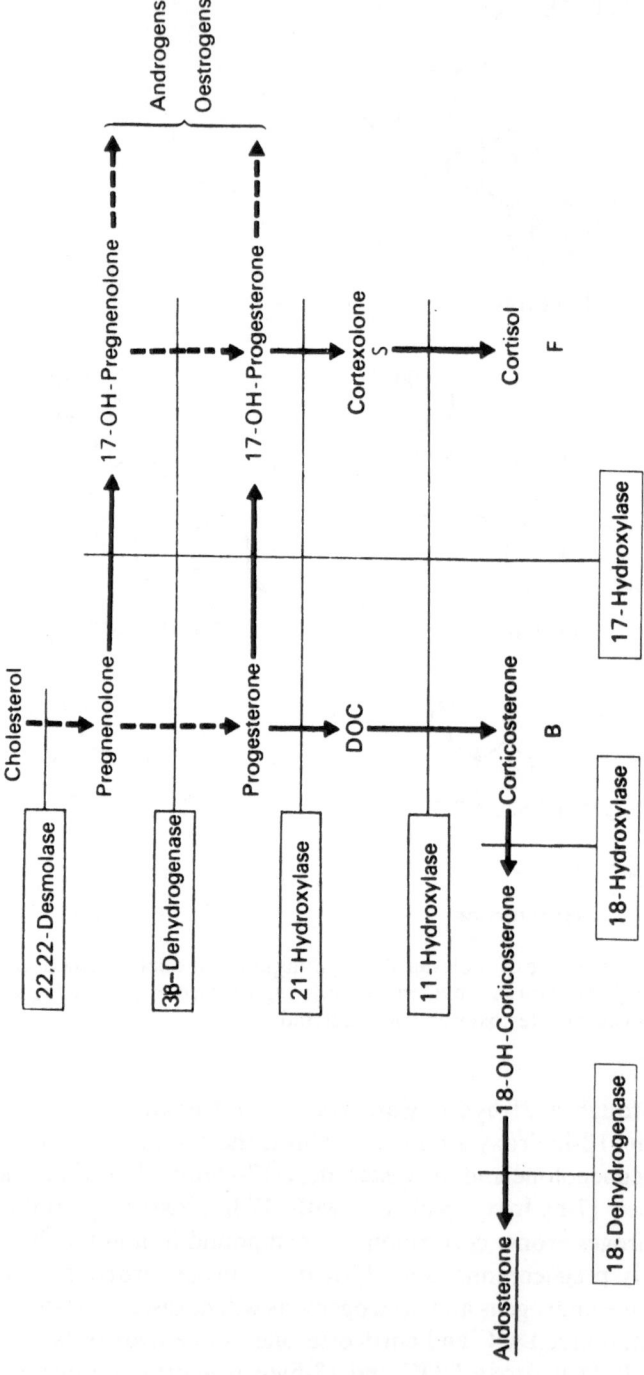

Figure 5.2 Biosynthesis of gluco- and mineralocorticoids (C-21 steroids)

the latter, finally aldosterone. Cortisol and corticosterone are produced mainly in the zona fasciculata and aldosterone mainly in the zona glomerulosa. Stimulation- and suppression-studies have shown that these two zones are, to a large extent functionally independent, aldosterone being stimulated mainly by the renin–angiotensin system, and cortisol by adrenocorticotrophic hormone (ACTH).

GENERAL ASPECTS OF ADRENAL STEROID DEFECTS

Heredity defects of all enzymatic steps indicated in Figure 5.2 are known. They affect both sexes, and their hereditary pattern is uniformly autosomal recessive. For all of them there is suggestive evidence of considerable genetic heterogeneity, a field which so far has been little explored.

The clinical manifestations can be easily predicted from the localization of the defect. Their presence will lead the informed clinician to suspect the site of the defect, and an appropriate analysis of plasma and urinary steroids will confirm or rule out the clinical suspicion.

The defects which compromise the production of cortisol are those of the 20, 22-desmolase, the 3β-dehydrogenase, the 21-hydroxylase and the 11β-hydroxylase systems. With the exception of the 11β-hydroxylase defect, they cause *adrenal insufficiency* with salt loss and failure to thrive in the neonatal period, and death in early infancy if the defect is severe. The characteristic symptoms are Addisonian pigmentation, anorexia, weight loss and vomiting. The biochemical findings are decreased values of plasma cortisol and aldosterone, urinary salt loss with hyponatraemia, hyperkalaemia, hypovolaemia and increased plasma renin activity. Untreated survivors frequently show craving for salt and instinctively correct their salt loss by an increased intake. *Salt loss* may be a passive process if aldosterone is lacking, as in the defects of the 18-hydroxylase and 18-dehydrogenase systems, or it may be an active process caused by an excess of mineralocorticoid antagonists or saluretic steroids, a hypothesis which is discussed later. Too little cortisol stimulates ACTH secretion which leads to adrenal hyperplasia with partial compensation of cortisol production and overproduction of androgens, provided that the pathway from cholesterol to the androgens is open. This is the background of the *adrenogenital syndrome* or congenital virilizing adrenal hyperplasia (CAH).

The three defects causing the *adrenogenital syndrome* are those of the 3β-dehydrogenase, 21-hydroxylase and the 11β-hydroxylase systems. The overproduction of androgens masculinizes the female external genitalia prenatally in affected girls, accelerates growth and bone maturation postnatally, causes premature development of male secondary sex characteristics in both sexes, and inhibits gonadal maturation and fertility (in girls more commonly than in boys) by suppression of the gonadotropins. Prenatal virilization of the female external genitalia presents at birth as ambiguity of the external genitalia with normal female internal genitalia, called female pseudohermaphroditism. The acceleration of growth and bone maturation causes tall stature in childhood and premature closure of the epiphyses, resulting in premature cessation of growth before normal adult height has been reached. The aspect of the external female genitalia varies from simple enlargement of the clitoris to full masculinization. We have proposed subdivision of this spectrum into five arbitrary stages[12] which probably correspond to different degrees of the enzyme defect (Figure 5.3).

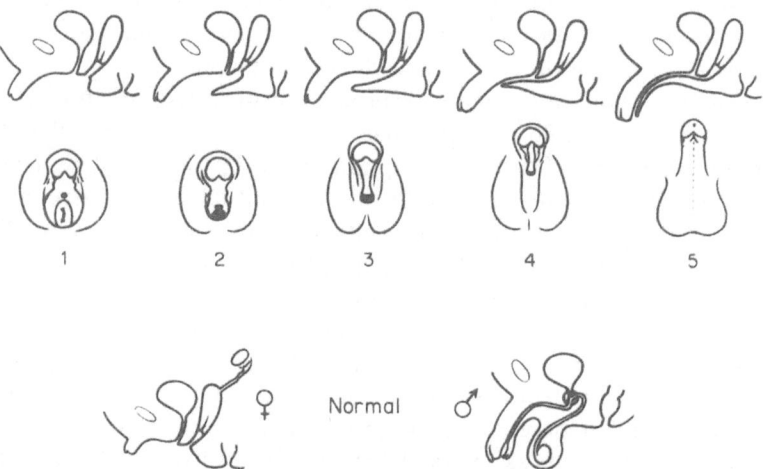

Figure 5.3 Stages of development of the external genitalia. 1 = clitoral enlargement; 5 = full masculinization; 2, 3 and 4 = varying degrees of intersexuality

Therapy is possible in an almost ideal way. The female external genitalia can be corrected by plastic surgery in infancy. Adrenal insufficiency and the overproduction of androgens with all their consequences can be prevented by lifelong replacement therapy with cortisol, beginning in early infancy. In general, fludrocortisone is added to prevent salt loss and to reduce the amount of cortisol required.

Another manifestation of certain enzyme defects is *hypertension*. This is seen in the 17-hydroxylase[7] and the 11β-hydroxylase[2] defects. Hypertension is probably caused by the accumulation of the mineralocorticoid DOC, which also explains the absence of salt loss.

17-Hydroxylase deficiency also prevents the production of sex steroids. The same is true for the 20,22-desmolase defect[3], and in part also for the 3β-dehydrogenase defect[4]. These defects will be discussed later together with other defects in the biosynthesis of the sex steroids.

21-HYDROXYLASE DEFECT

The 21-hydroxylase defect is by far the most frequent cause of the adrenogenital syndrome. Its prevalence is estimated to be about 1 in 12000 births[13]. In addition to the general aspects of the adrenogenital syndrome which have been mentioned, there are several interesting specific aspects. One is the fact that in some families, affected children do not manifest salt loss in infancy and that girls with salt loss tend to be more severely masculinized than girls without salt loss. There is controversy as to whether the two forms result from different enzyme defects or whether they are part of a spectrum varying from manifest to compensated salt loss. In this respect it is of interest that salt losers tend to have low levels of aldosterone whereas non-salt losers have increased levels in spite of the absence of other signs of hyperaldosteronism[14-18]. This may be explained by the accumulation of a mineralocorticoid antagonist causing salt loss, which is compensated in the non-salt losers by an increase of aldosterone through stimulation of the renin angiotensin system. The accumulated 17-hydroxyprogesterone and some other steroids have, in fact, a mild salt losing effect. An increase of aldosterone appears possible only if the 21-hydroxylase defect is limited to the zona fasciculata and is absent from the zona glomerulosa[19]. This suggests different 21-hydroxylase systems in the two adrenal zones.

The problem of genetic heterogeneity and the genetic aspects in general have become even more interesting since the recent finding of a close *linkage between the 21-hydroxylase gene and the B locus of the histocompatibility gene HLA* on the short arm of chromosome No. 6[20-22]. The determination of the HLA genotype of an affected child and its parents allows recognition of the HLA haplotype which is linked with the mutant 21-hydroxylase gene. This permits identification of the heterozygote siblings of that patient. This is more reliable than the diagnosis of heterozygosity by sophisticated steroid analysis, which does not completely separate heterozygotes from normal homozygotes[23]. It is rather remarkable that, in this situation, the identification of heterozygotes is achieved by studying not the product of the mutant gene, but the product of the neighbouring gene. The HLA linkage also offers the possibility of prenatal diagnosis, although this may raise serious ethical dilemmas[24].

We have studied two *unusual families* in which the index patients had the classical complete manifestation of the 21-hydroxylase defect and some other family members a mild expression of the same defect[25]. HLA studies have confirmed our assumption that in these unusual families the classical defect corresponded to homozygosity and the mild defect to hetero-zygosity[26]. On the other hand, HLA studies of salt losers and non-salt losers have not given additional information. Both forms show the same HLA linkage, which suggests that the two mutant genes are on the same locus. It seems likely that they represent different alleles with the unexplored possibility of compound heterozygosity. Little is known about the so called *'acquired' adrenogenital syndrome*. It is a very mild manifes-tation of the 21-hydroxylase deficiency in girls and may represent a separate genotype[27]. Further studies, especially on HLA linkage, are necessary to establish the genetic basis of this variant.

11β-HYDROXYLASE DEFECT

About 10–20% of all patients with the adrenogenital syndrome (and probably more than 50% in Israel and Turkey) have an 11β-hydroxylase deficiency. In addition to the general symptoms of the adrenogenital syndrome they classically present with hypertension and absence of salt loss, which is probably caused by an excess of the mineralocorticoid DOC. However, hypertension is not obligatory and if present it appears only in late childhood or adolescence. Treatment with cortisol may precipitate salt loss because DOC no longer accumulates and aldosterone production is low.

From our own experience with 25 patients we find that they can be divided into *severe* and *mild* defect groups. DOC and compound S are increased in both groups, though to a different degree, indicating that both the 17-deoxy and the 17-hydroxy pathways are involved. In patients with the severe defect, hypertension may be present and the masculinization of the female external genitalia is severe. In patients with the mild defect, hypertension is always absent, and the masculinization of the female external genitalia is minor. In addition, we have found patients, in whom the defect was only present in the 17-hydroxy pathway and not in the 17-deoxy pathway. This confirms earlier reports from ourselves and others about patients in whom the 11β-hydroxylase defect was limited to the 17-deoxy[28] or to the 17-hydroxy pathway[29]. and supports *in vitro* evidence for different 11β-hydroxylase systems in these two pathways[30]. Further genetic heterogeneity is suggested by the recent demonstration that in some patients the 11β-hydroxylase defect is limited to the zona fasciculata and does not involve the zona glomerulosa[19]. In contrast to the 21-hydroxylase gene, there is no linkage of the 11β-hydroxylase gene with the HLA system[31].

UNKNOWN DEFECTS OF ADRENAL STEROIDS

Before considering the gonadal steroids, the probable existence of as yet unknown hereditary defects of adrenal steroids should be mentioned. Intriguing examples are adrenal hirsutism without any of the known defects, low renin-hypertension in young children, and adrenoleukodystrophy, a sex linked disorder, in which affected boys develop primary adrenal insufficiency and progressive demyelinization of the brain.

During the last 10 years, we[32] and others[33-35] have tried unsuccessfully to solve the mystery of low renin hypertension in childhood. Clinical findings correspond to those found with hyperaldosteronism, yet plasma aldosterone and renin concentrations are reduced. Nevertheless, the hypertension can be corrected with the aldosterone antagonist spironolactone, as well as with cortisone. We still assume that these patients produce an excess of an unidentified mineralocorticoid. *Adrenoleukodystrophy* is a sex linked recessive disorder in which the affected boys develop severe adrenal insufficiency with adrenal atrophy and progressive diffuse demyelinization of the brain[36, 37]. A common defect in cerebral myelin and in adrenal steroid biosynthesis must be postulated.

BIOSYNTHESIS OF THE SEX STEROIDS

In Figure 5.4, a simplified pathway of the biosynthesis of the sex steroids is presented. To the left are shown, in abbreviated form, the biosynthesis of the gluco- and mineralocorticoids from cholesterol through the 17-deoxy and the 17-hydroxy pathways already discussed. The upper horizontal line is the Δ5-pathway. 17-Hydroxy-pregnenolone is transformed to dehydroepiandrosterone (DHA) through the 17,20-desmolase system and to androstenediol through the 17-reductase system. All compounds on that pathway are 3-hydroxy-Δ5-compounds. Through the combined 3β-

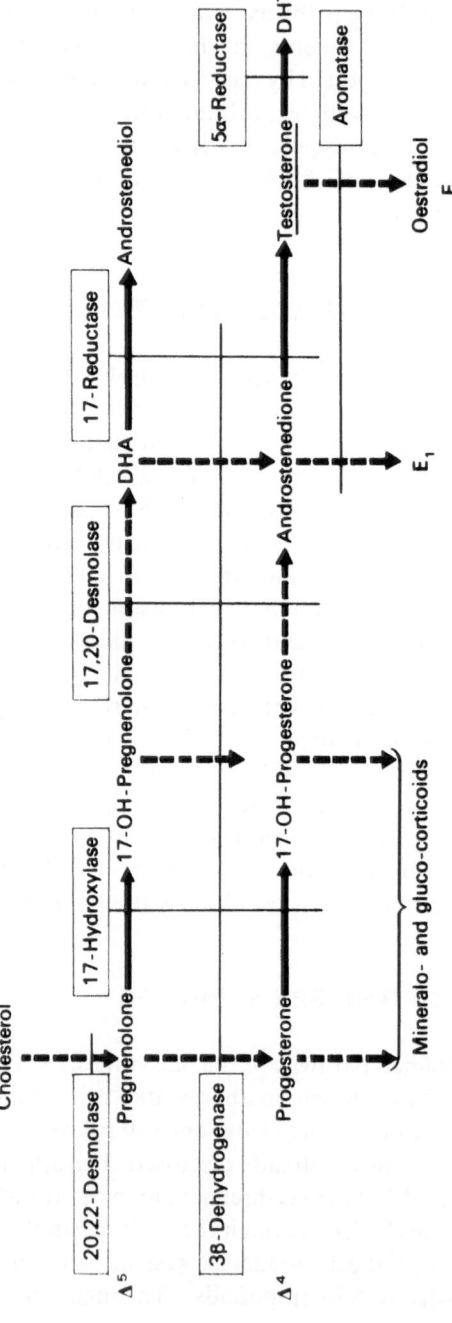

Figure 5.4 Biosynthesis of sex steroids (C-18 and C-19 steroids)

dehydrogenase and Δ5−Δ4 isomerase systems, they are transformed to the 3-keto-Δ4-compounds, 17-hydroxy-progesterone, androstenedione and testosterone on the Δ4-pathway. DHA and androstenedione are the main androgens of the adrenals. Through aromatization, androstenedione and testosterone are converted to the oestrogens oestrone (E_1) and oestradiol (E_2). These pathways are present in the gonads as well as in the adrenals. In the target cells of the periphery, testosterone is reduced in ring A to dihydrotestosterone (DHT) through the 5α-reductase system. Testosterone and DHT are necessary for the male sex differentiation in the fetus, which is a *hormone dependent* process[38], and, of course, also for the development of male puberty. The differentiation of the external male genitalia in the fetus depends mainly on DHT[39]. Oestradiol is mainly produced in the ovaries. It is not necessary for female sex differentiation, which is a *hormone-independent* process, but it is, of course, required for the development of female puberty.

GENERAL ASPECTS OF SEX STEROID DEFECTS

Table 5.1 lists the inherited enzyme defects. They affect the adrenals and the testes, sometimes also the ovaries and, in the case of the 5α-reductase the target cells. The pattern of inheritance in most of them is autosomal-recessive. In the case of the 17,20-desmolase and the 17-reductase blocks, where only male patients have been reported, it may be X-chromosomal-recessive.

The clinical manifestations can again be predicted from knowledge of the physiological effects of the accumulated and the deficient steroids. The enzyme blocks which affect the biosynthesis of all sex steroids cause *primary hypogonadism* with absent or incomplete puberty and sterility. These are the defects of the 20,22-desmolase, the 17-hydroxylase, and the 17,20-desmolase systems, and in part also that of the 3β-dehydrogenase system. Furthermore, the deficiency of testosterone in males prevents the normal differentiation of the male external genitalia leading to *male pseudohermaphroditism*. Male patients have testes which usually are undescended and female or ambiguous external genitalia, depending on the degree of the defect. They may be regarded as girls. Affected females have normal genitalia. The diagnostic test to demonstrate a defect in testosterone biosynthesis is to stimulate testosterone production with human chorionic gonadotropin (HCG)[40]. This test is useful at any age. An inadequate testosterone production with a marked increase of certain precursors allows confirmation and identification of the defect. If the defect affects also the biosynthesis of the mineralo- and glucocorticoids, the clinical manifestations include those of adrenal insufficiency. Thus these patients may present with hypogonadism, male pseudohermaphroditism, and adrenal insufficiency. Hormone substitution, and under certain circumstances, surgical corrections will allow a normal physical development. The delicate problem which cannot be discussed here, is reaching a decision about the male or female gender role in affected males.

20,22-DESMOLASE DEFECT

The 20,22-desmolase defect[3] is the cause of the very rare lipoid adrenal hyperplasia. The adrenals are hyperplastic, because the same feed-back mechanism is operative as in the adrenogenital syndrome. The adrenal cells are large and packed with lipids and cholesterol, which explains the bright orange colour of the adrenals. Most reported patients with this defect have died in infancy from adrenal insufficiency. The affected males have male pseudohermaphroditism with female or ambiguous genitalia. There are no reports of adolescent or adult patients, but one can safely predict that there would be no spontaneous puberty. There is probably marked genetic heterogeneity because the 20,22-desmolase system appears to be very complex, involving also a 20- and a 22-hydroxylase.

3β-DEHYDROGENASE DEFECT

As mentioned, the 3β-dehydrogenase defect is a rare cause of the adrenogenital syndrome with salt loss[4]. In both sexes, an abnormal development of the external genitalia is seen. In girls, the accumulation of the androgen DHA frequently leads to some degree of masculinization. In boys, the deficiency of testosterone does not allow full masculinization. Early appearance of male secondary sex characteristics caused by the excess of DHA is seen in both sexes. Spontaneous puberty in boys in spite of a relative deficiency of testosterone has been reported[41]. In girls one would expect the absence of female pubertal development. We have recently re-examined one of our patients, a girl aged 15, who has had cortisol replacement therapy since infancy[42, 43]. In spite of pubertal bone age, she had no breast development and had not menstruated. Hormone stimulation studies showed her, as expected, to be unable to produce normal amounts of oestradiol and progesterone.

17-HYDROXYLASE DEFECT

In the 17-hydroxylase defect[7], accumulation of DOC and corticosterone compensates for the cortisol deficiency and causes hypertension with hypokalaemic alkalosis as in classical hyperaldosteronism, although plasma aldosterone is low. Affected males present with female or intersexual[44] external genitalia. If the genitalia are female, they are considered normal girls and diagnosis is missed until late childhood, when hypertension and lack of puberty become conspicuous.

17,20-DESMOLASE DEFECT

The 17,20-desmolase defect[10] blocks the production of all sex steroids. Affected males show male pseudohermaphroditism and hypogonadism with lack of puberty. Affected females have not been reported. If the defect does exist in girls, one would expect hypogonadism with lack of puberty as in the boys. Different patterns in the accumulation of 17-hydroxy-progesterone and its urinary metabolites suggest genetic heterogeneity[48]. In fact, the 17,20-desmolase system is complex and also involves a 20-hydroxylase.

17-REDUCTASE DEFECT

The 17-reductase defect[8] causes a deficiency of the main sex hormones testosterone and oestradiol and an accumulation of the androgens DHA and androstenedione as well as of oestrone (E_1) Affected boys present with male pseudohermaphroditism caused by the lack of testosterone. Their secondary sex characteristics are male due to the high plasma levels of adrenal androgens, but gynaecomastia may also be present and is mainly caused by the accumulated E_1[45,46]. Affected females have not been reported.

5α-REDUCTASE DEFECT

The 5α-reductase[11] defect blocks the conversion of testosterone to DHT in peripheral cells. Affected boys have male pseudohermaphroditism because the differentiation of the male external genitalia depends mainly on DHT.

In contrast puberty, which depends mainly on testosterone, is of a male pattern, and fertility is possible[47]. Affected females are clinically normal.

AROMATASE DEFECT

So far, we have discussed mainly defects of the adrenal and testicular steroids. If the defect concerns precursors of the oestrogens, the block is also present in the ovaries. It is, however, peculiar that defects concerning specifically the biosynthesis of the oestrogens, such as those of the 17-reductase, and the aromatase systems are not known. As mentioned, the 17-reductase defect has been observed in boys only. An aromatase defect has been discussed in the Stein–Leventhal syndrome with polycystic ovaries. but the fact that this defect develops only during adolescence and is not present in ovarian cells studied *in vitro* raises doubts about a primary aromatase defect in this disorder.

We have recently studied an adolescent girl affected with the hereditary syndrome of virilization, acanthosis nigricans and insulin resistance[49]. In spite of pubertal bone age she had no spontaneous breast development. E_2 was low. Testosterone was increased and was not of adrenal origin. Under prolonged stimulation with human menopausal gonadotropin (HMG), which increases ovarian oestrogen production, E_2 did not increase but, surprisingly, testosterone increased markedly. We regard this as suggestive evidence of an aromatase defect in the ovaries and as the cause of the high testosterone levels as well as the clinical virilization found in this syndrome.

STEROID DEFECTS IN THE FETO-PLACENTAL UNIT

Figure 5.5 is a simplified illustration of oestrogen biosynthesis in the feto-placental unit. The placenta has a sulphatase and an aromatase system, which is necessary for the biosynthesis of oestrogens from fetal DHA, DHA sulphate and their 16-hydroxylated compounds. Pregnancy urine contains large amounts of oestriol (E_3). Decreased oestriol excretion is found mainly in placental insufficiency and fetal distress, but also if the fetal adrenals are unable to produce DHA, and theoretically if any of the enzyme steps indicated in Figure 5.5 are blocked. So far, only the sulphatase defect[9], which is X-chromosomal recessive, has been described. This steroid sulphatase defect is combined with a defect of the aryl sulphatase C. It has no influence on the wellbeing of the fetus, but is associated with and possibly the cause of the X-linked type of ichthyosis[50].

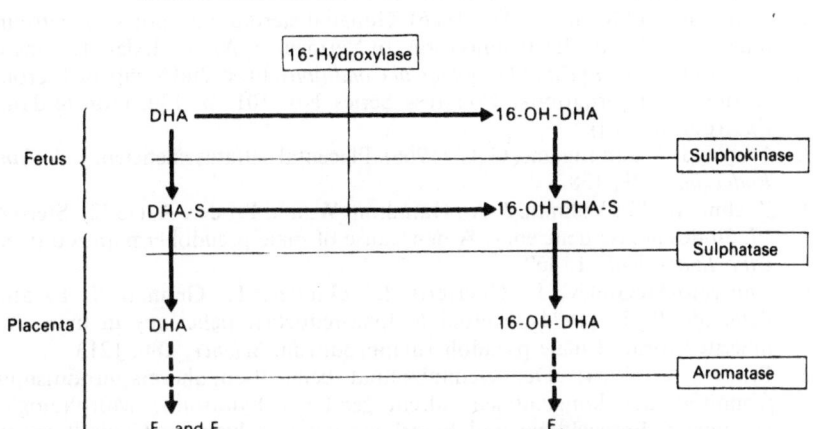

BIOSYNTHESIS OF ESTROGENS IN THE FETOPLACENTAL UNIT

Figure 5.5   Biosynthesis of oestrogens in the feto-placental unit

As expected in such a skin condition, the defect is not limited to the placenta, but is also present in fibroblasts. Steinmann *et al.* in our department have recently found that this defect is also present in multiple sulphatase deficiency, a metabolic disorder, clinically characterized by a combination of metachromatic leukodystrophy and mucopolysaccharidosis[51].

References

1. Jailer, J. W. (1953). Virilism. *Bull. N. Y. Acad. Med.*, **29,** 377
2. Eberlein, W. R. and Bongiovanni, A. M. (1955). Congenital adrenal hyperplasia with hypertension: unusual steroid pattern in blood and urine. *J. Clin. Endocrinol.,* **15,** 1531
3. Prader, A. and Siebenmann, R. E. (1957). Nebenniereninsuffizienz bei kongenitaler Lipoidhyperplasie der Nebennieren. *Helv. Paediatr. Acta,* **12,** 569
4. Bongiovanni, A. M. (1961). Unusual steroid pattern in congenital adrenal hyperplasia: deficiency of 3-beta-hydroxy dehydrogenase. *J. Clin. Endocrinol.,* **21,** 860
5. Visser, H. K. A. and Cost, W. S. (1964). A new hereditary defect in the biosynthesis of aldosterone: urinary C21-corticosteroid pattern in three related patients with a salt-losing syndrome, suggesting an 18-oxidation defect. *Acta Endocrinol.,* **47,** 589
6. Ulick, S., Gautier, E., Vetter, K. K., Markello, J. R., Yaffe, S. and Lowe, C. U. (1964). An aldosterone biosynthetic defect in a salt-losing disorder. *J. Clin. Endocrinol.,* **24,** 669

7. Biglieri, E. G., Herron, M. A. and Brust, N. (1966). 17-Hydroxylation deficiency in man. *J. Clin. Invest.*, **45**, 1946
8. Neher, R. and Kahnt, F. W. (1966). Gonadal steroid biosynthesis *in vitro* in four cases of testicular feminisation. In Vermeulen, A. and Exley, D. (eds.). *Androgens in Normal and Pathological Conditions*. Proc. 2nd Symp. on Steroid Hormones. International Congress Series No. 101, p. 130, (Amsterdam: Excerpta Medica)
9. France, J. T. and Liggins, G. C. (1966). Placental sulfatase deficiency. *J. Clin. Endocrinol.*, **29**, 138
10. Zachmann, M., Völlmin, J. A., Hamilton, W. and Prader, A. (1972). Steroid 17, 20-desmolase deficiency. A new cause of male pseudohermaphroditism. *Clin. Endocrinol.*, **1**, 369
11. Imperato-McGinley, J., Guerrero, L., Gautier, T., German, J. L. and Peterson, R. E. (1974). Steroid 5-alpha-reductase deficiency in man. An inherited form of male pseudohermaphroditism. *Science*, **186**, 1213
12. Prader, A. (1954). Der Genitalbefund beim Pseudohermaphroditismus femininus des kongenitalen adreno-genitalen Syndroms. Morphologie, Häufigkeit, Entwicklung und Vererbung der verschiedenen Genitalformen. *Helv. Paediatr. Acta*, **9**, 231
13. Werder, E. A., Siebenmann, R. E., Knorr-Mürset, G., Zimmermann, A., Sizonenko, P. C., Theintz, P., Girard, J., Zachmann, M. and Prader, A. (1980). The incidence of congenital adrenal hyperplasia in Switzerland – a survey of patients born in 1960 to 1974. *Helv. Paediatr. Acta*, **35**, 5
14. Bryan, G. T., Kliman, B. and Bartter, F. C. (1965). Impaired aldosterone production in 'salt-losing' congenital adrenal hyperplasia. *J. Clin. Invest.*, **44**, 957
15. Degenhart, H. J., Visser, H. K. A., Wilmink, R. and Croughs, W. (1965). Aldosterone and cortisol secretion rates in infants and children with congenital adrenal hyperplasia suggesting different 21-hydroxylation defects in 'salt-losers' and 'non-salt-losers'. *Acta Endocrinol. (Kbh.)*, **48**, 587
16. New, M. I., Miller, B. and Peterson, R. E. (1966). Aldosterone excretion in normal children and in children with adrenal hyperplasia. *J. Clin. Invest.*, **45**, 412
17. Bartter, C., Henkin, R. I. and Bryan, G. T. (1968). Aldosterone hypersecretion in 'non-salt-losing' congenital adrenal hyperplasia. *J. Clin. Invest.*, **47**, 1742.
18. Simopoulos, A. P., Marshall, J. R., Delea, C. S. and Bartter, F. C (1971). Studies on the deficiency of 21-hydroxylation in patients with congenital adrenal hyperplasia. *J. Clin. Endocrinol.*, **32**, 438
19. New, M. I., Dupont, B., Pang, S., Pollack, M. and Levine, L. S. (1981). An update of congenital adrenal hyperplasia. *Rec. Prog. Horm. Res.*, **37**, 105
20. Dupont, B., Oberfield, S. E., Smithwick, E. M., Lee, T. D. and Levine, L. S. (1977). Close genetic linkage between HLA and congenital adrenal hyperplasia (21-hydroxylase deficiency). *Lancet*, **2**, 1309
21. Levine, L. S., Zachmann, M., New, M. I., Prader, A., Pollack, M. S., O'Neill, G. J., Yang, S. Y., Oberfield, S. E. and Dupont B. (1978). Genetic mapping of the 21-hydroxylase-deficiency gene within the HLA linkage group. *N. Engl. J. Med.*, **299**, 911

22. Lorenzen, F., Pang, S., New, M., Pollack, M., Oberfield, S., Dupont, B., Chow, D., Schneider, B. and Levine, L. (1980). Studies of the C-21 and C-19 steroids and HLA genotyping in siblings and parents of patients with congenital adrenal hyperplasia due to 21-hydroxylase deficiency. *J. Clin. Endocrinol.*, **50,** 572

23. Knorr, D., Bidlingmaier, F., Butenandt, O., von Schnakenburg, K. and Wagner, W. (1977). Test for heterozygosity of congenital adrenal hyperplasia. In Lee, P. A., Plotnick, L. P., Kowarski, A. A. and Migeon, C. J. (eds.). *Congenital Adrenal Hyperplasia*, p. 495. (Baltimore, London, Tokyo: University Park Press)

24. Levine, L. S., New, M. I., Pollack, M. and Dupont, B. (1979). Prenatal diagnosis of congenital adrenal hyperplasia. *Lancet*, **2,** 637

25. Zachmann, M. and Prader, A. (1978). Unusual heterozygotes of congenital adrenal hyperplasia due to 21-hydroxylase deficiency. *Acta Endocrinol. (Kbh)*, **87,** 557

26. Zachmann, M. and Prader, A. (1979). Unusual heterozygotes of congenital adrenal hyperplasia due to 21-hydroxylase deficiency confirmed by HLA tissue typing. *Acta Endocrinol. (Kbh.)*, **92,** 542

27. New, M. I., Lorenzen, F., Pang, S., Gunczler, P., Dupont, B. and Levine, L. S. (1979). 'Acquired' adrenal hyperplasia with 21-hydroxylase deficiency is not the same genetic disorder as congenital adrenal hyperplasia. *J. Clin. Endocrinol. Metab.*, **48,** 356

28. Gregory, T., and Gardner, L. I. (1976). Hypertensive virilizing adrenal hyperplasia with minimal impairment of synthetic route to cortisol. *J. Clin. Endocrinol.*, **43,** 769

29. Zachmann, M., Völlmin, J. A., New, M. I., Curtius, H. C. and Prader, A. (1971) Congenital adrenal hyperplasia due to deficiency of 11-beta-hydroxylation of 17-alpha-hydroxylated steroids. *J. Clin. Endocrinol.*, **33,** 501

30. Klein, A., Curtius, H. C. and Zachmann, M. (1974). Difference in 11-beta-hydroxylation of deoxycortisol and deoxy-corticosterone by human adrenals. *J. Steroid Biochem.*, **5,** 557

31. Brautbar, C., Rösler, A., Landau, H., Cohen, I., Nelken, D., Cohen, T., Levine, L. S. and New, M. I. (1979). No linkage between HLA and congenital adrenal hyperplasia due to 11-beta-hydroxylase deficiency. *N. Engl. J. Med.*, **300,** 205

32. Werder, E. A., Zachmann, M., Völlmin, J. A., Veyrat, R. and Prader, A. (1975). Unusual steroid excretion in a child with low renin hypertension. *Res. steroids*, **6,** 385

33. Ulick, S., Ramirez, L. C. and New, M. I. (1977). An abnormality in steroid reductive metabolism in a hypertensive syndrome. *J. Clin. Endocrinol.*, **44,** 799

34. New, M. I., Bradlow, L., Fishman, J., Gunczler, P., Zanconato, G., Rauh, W., Levine, L. S. and Ulick, S. (1978). Deficiency of cortisol 11-beta-ketoreductase – a new metabolic defect. *Pediatc. Res.*, **12,** 416

35. Shackleton, C. H. L., Honour, J. W., Dillon, M. J., Chantler, C. and Jones, R. W. (1980). Hypertension in a four year old child: gas chromatographic and mass spectrometric evidence for deficient hepatic metabolism of steroids. *J. Clin. Endocrinol.*, **50,** 786

36. Davis, L. E., Snyder, R. D., Orth, D. N., Nicholson, W. E., Kornfeld, M. and Seelinger, D. F. (1979). Adrenoleukodystrophy and adrenomyeloneuropathy associated with partial adrenal insufficiency in three generations of a kindred. *Am. J. Med.*, **66**, 342

37. Ramsey, R. B., Banik, N. L. and Davison, A. N. (1979). Adrenoleukodystrophy brain cholesteryl esters and other neutral lipids. *J. Neurol. Sci.*, **40**, 189

38. Jost, A. (1953). Problems of fetal endocrinology. The gonadal and hypophyseal hormones. *Recent Prog. Hormone Res.*, **8**, 379

39. Siiteri, P. and Wilson, J. D. (1974). Testosterone formation and metabolism during male sexual differentiation in the human embryo. *J. Clin. Endocrinol.*, **38**, 113

40. Zachmann, M. (1972). The evaluation of testicular endocrine function before and in puberty. Effect of a single dose of human chorionic gonadotropin on urinary steroid excretion under normal and pathological conditions. *Acta Endocrinol. (Kbh.)*, **70** (Suppl.), 164

41. Parks, G. A., Bermudez, J. A., Anast, C. S., Bongiovanni, A. M. and New, M. I. (1971). Pubertal boy with the 3-beta-hydroxysteroid dehydrogenase defect. *J. Clin. Endocrinol.*, **33**, 269

42. Zachmann, M., Völlmin, J. A., Mürset, G., Curtius, H. C. and Prader, A. (1970). Unusual type of congenital adrenal hyperplasia probably due to deficiency of 3-beta-hydroxysteroid dehydrogenase. Case report of a surviving girl and steroid studies. *J. Clin. Endocrinol.*, **30**, 719

43. Zachmann, M., Forest, M. G. and De Peretti, E. (1979). 3-beta-hydroxysteroid dehydrogenase deficiency. Follow-up study in a girl with pubertal bone age. *Hormone Res.*, **11**, 292

44. New, M. I. (1970). Male pseudohermaphroditism due to 17-alpha-hydroxylase deficiency. *J. clin. Invest.*, **49**, 1930

45. Saez, J. M., De Peretti, E. and Morera, A. M. (1971). Familial male pseudohermaphroditism with gynecomastia due to a testicular 17-ketosteroid reductase defect. I. Studies *in vivo*. *J. Clin. Endocrinol.*, **32**, 604

46. Saez, J. M., Morera, A. M., De Peretti, E. and Bertrand, J. (1972). Further *in vivo* studies in male pseudohermaphroditism with gynecomastia due to a testicular 17-steroid reductase defect (compared to a case of testicular feminization). *J. Clin. Endocrinol.*, **34**, 598

47. Imperato-McGinley, J., Guerrero, L., Gautier, T., German, J. L. and Peterson, R. E. (1975). Steroid 5-alpha-reductase deficiency in man. An inherited form of male pseudohermaphroditism. In Bergsma, D. (ed.) *Genetic Forms of Hypogonadism*, p. 91. (New York: Stratton)

48. Goebelsmann, U., Zachmann, M., Davajan, V., Israel, R., Mestman, I. H. and Mishell, D. R. (1976). Male pseudohermaphroditism consistent with 17, 20-desmolase deficiency. *Gynecol. Invest.*, **7**, 138

49. Zachmann, M., Manella, B., Santamaria, L., Andler, W. and Prader, A. (1981). Plasma steroid response of pubertal girls to human menopausal gonadotropin. *Res. Steroids*, **9**, 266

50. Shapiro, L. J., Weiss, R., Webster, D. and France, J. T. (1978). X-linked ichthyosis due to steroid-sulphatase deficiency. *Lancet*, **1**, 70

51. Steinmann, B., Mieth, D. and Gitzelmann, R. (1980). A newly recognized cause of low urinary estriol in pregnancy: multiple sulfatase deficiency of the fetus. *Gynecol. Obstet. Invest.* (In press)

6

Blood–brain barrier amino-acid transport: clinical implications

W. M. Pardridge

INTRODUCTION

The carrier systems mediating neutral and basic amino-acid transport through the brain capillary wall, i.e. the blood–brain barrier (BBB), have an influence on, nerve cell function and on a variety of clinical disorders. The physiological principles underlying this influence are two-fold. Firstly, as shown principally by the work of Wurtman and his colleagues, a large number of cerebral pathways of amino-acid metabolism, e.g. monoamine synthesis, branched chain amino-acid axidation, and S-adenosyl methionine synthesis[1–5], are influenced by precursor availability in brain. Secondly, as originally shown by Guroff and Udenfriend[6] and later by Fernstrom and Wurtman[7] and by Oldendorf[8], amino-acid supply in brain is a function of amino-acid competition at the BBB. Therefore, amino-acid availability in brain is not influenced simply by plasma supply of the amino acid, but is also acutely regulated by the plasma concentrations of other amino acids, which compete for a common BBB transport site. Competition for neutral amino-acid transport sites under physiological conditions appears to be unique for the central nervous system (CNS) and forms the basis for the close connection between BBB transport and a variety of clinical situations affecting the CNS[9]. The purpose of this chapter is to discuss the physiological basis for the unique sensitivity of the CNS to amino-acid competition and to point out relevant clinical implications.

OVERVIEW OF BLOOD–BRAIN
BARRIER NUTRIENT TRANSPORT

Nine specific transport systems have been identified in the BBB using the tissue sampling–carotid injection technique of Oldendorf[10]. As shown in Table 6.1, the affinity constants (K_m) of the transport systems generally parallel the plasma substrate concentration. Moreover, as the affinity of the system increases (K_m decreases), the transport capacity (V_{max}) decreases, so that the V_{max}/K_m ratio is about the same for all nine transport systems. Each BBB transport system mediates the trans capillary flux of a group of substrates. The hexose carrier[14] transports 2-deoxy-glucose (K_m = 6 mmol/l), glucose (K_m = 9 mmol/l), 3-O-methyl glucose (K_m = 10 mmol/l), mannose (K_m = 22 mmol/l), and galactose (K_m = 40 mmol/l). The monocarboxylic-acid carrier transports lactate (K_m = 1.9 mmol/l), pyruvate (K_m = 0.4 mmol/l), butyrate and the ketone bodies, acetoacetate and β-hydroxybutyrate[16, 17]. The α-keto acids of amino acids, e.g. phenylpyruvate or the branched chain keto acids, probably also have an affinity for the monocarboxylic-acid carrier, but these compounds have not yet been tested. Since the α-keto acids reach plasma concentrations greater than 1 mmol/l in such diseases as phenylketonuria (PKU) and maple syrup urine disease (MSUD), it may be that these α-keto acids inhibit the BBB transport of ketone bodies, compounds which act as a

TABLE 6.1   Blood–brain barrier transport systems

Transport system	Representative substrate	K_m (mmol/l)	V_{max} (nmol min^{-1} g^{-1})
Hexose	glucose	9	1600
Monocarboxylic acid	lactate	1.9	120
Neutral amino acid	phenylalanine	1.12	30
Amine	choline	0.44	10
Basic amino acid	lysine	0.10	6
Purine	adenine	0.027	1
Nucleoside	adenosine	0.018	0.7
Acidic amino acid	glutamate	0.04	0.4
Thyroid hormone	T$_3$	0.0011	0.1

Sources: References 11–15

major source of carbon to the brain during states of physiological ketosis[18]. The choline carrier transports Deanol, a drug precursor of choline[19]; therefore, if plasma levels of Deanol exceed 100 μmol/l, it is likely the drug will competitively inhibit choline transport into brain. The thyroid hormone carrier transports triiodothyronine (T_3), thyroxine (T_4; $K_i = 2.5$ μ mol/l), and reverse T_3 ($K_i = 5.4$ μ mol/l), but not tyrosine or leucine[13]. Owing to large magnitude of the K_m relative to plasma thyronine values, it is unlikely physiological changes in T_4 levels influence brain T_3 uptake[13].

Much quantitative information has been obtained over the past 10 years on the BBB transport systems. However, relatively little is known about modulation of the carriers. Developmental or pathological inductions or repressions of carrier activity can be expected to have a pronounced influence on those pathways of brain metabolism that are limited by precursor availability. (For review of substrate-limited pathways of brain metabolism, see ref. 20.) Known examples of modulations of BBB transport systems are listed in Table 6.2. The most striking inductions of carrier activity are those seen for the basic amino acid, the purine base, and the choline carriers in the newborn period[29]. While basic amino acids are generally regarded as essential nutrients, choline and adenine bases are often viewed as non-essential compounds. The dramatic increases in BBB transport activity of choline and purine bases in the newborn period is compelling evidence that these compounds are essential nutrients for the developing brain. If so, then consideration by clinical neonatologists should be given to including choline and purine bases as essential nutrients for infants receiving parenteral nutrients.

TABLE 6.2   Modulations of blood–brain barrier transport systems

Transport system	Activation	Inhibition
Hexose	? seizures	neonatal period hypo-thyroidism anoxia
Monocarboxylic acid	ketosis? thiamine deficiency	liver disease
Neutral amino acid	liver disease	hypo-thyroidism mercury intoxication
Basic amino acid	neonatal period	—
Choline	neonatal period	—
Purine base	neonatal period	—

Sources: References 17, 21- 29

AMINO-ACID TRANSPORT: ROLE OF COMPETITION

The K_m values for neutral and basic amino-acid transport through the BBB are shown in Table 6.3. The close approximation of the K_m and plasma amino-acid level provides the physiological basis for the important role played by competition in regulating amino-acid transport into brain. Much insight into the nature of transport competition is provided by studying the following equation.

$$K_m(\text{app}) = K_m\left(1 + \sum \frac{[AA]}{K_m^{AA}}\right) \qquad (1)$$

TABLE 6.3   **Blood–brain barrier amino acid transport**

Amino acid	Plasma levels (mmol l)	K_m (mmol l)	app K_m (mmol l)	V_{max} (nmol min^{-1} g^{-1})	Influx (nmol min^{-1} g^{-1})
Neutral amino acids					
Phenylalanine	0.05	0.12	0.45	30	3.0
Leucine	0.10	0.15	0.53	33	5.2
Tyrosine	0.09	0.16	0.58	46	6.2
Tryptophan	0.10	0.19	0.71	33	4.1
Methionine	0.04	0.19	0.77	33	1.6
Histidine	0.05	0.28	1.1	38	1.6
Isoleucine	0.07	0.33	1.3	57	2.9
DOPA	0.004	0.44	1.9	64	0.1
Valine	0.14	0.63	2.5	49	2.5
Threonine	0.19	0.73	3.0	37	2.2
Basic amino acids					
Arginine	0.10	0.09	0.40	9	1.8
Lysine	0.30	0.10	0.25	6	3.3
Ornithine	0.09	0.23	1.2	11	0.8

Sources: References 30, 31. The plasma level of DOPA is a representative therapeutic concentration

The apparent (app) K_m of a given amino acid (i.e. in the presence of competing amino acids) deviates from the absolute K_m of the amino acid (i.e. in the absence of competing amino acids) in proportion to the sum of the ratio of amino-acid concentration [AA] to absolute K_m for each competing amino acid. Inspection of equation 1 indicates if the plasma amino-acid concentration$<<K_m$, then $K_m(\text{app}) \simeq K_m$, i.e. competition

does not effectively occur *in vivo*. This point deserves emphasis since the K_m of neutral amino-acid transport in virtually all organs other than brain is about 5–10 mmol/l or greater (Table 6.4), which is 10–100 times the physiological concentration of plasma amino acids (Table 6.3). These considerations suggest competition effects do not occur under physiological conditions *in vivo* in tissues other than brain, although competition can be readily demonstrated in peripheral tissues *in vitro* using 5–50 mmol/l concentrations of amino acids.

TABLE 6.4 Neutral amino-acid transport K_m in peripheral tissues (mmol/l)

Amino acid	Renal tubule	Exocrine pancreas	Intestinal epithelia	Red blood cell	Liver
Phenylalanine			1	4	4
Leucine			2	2	6
Tryptophan	4				
Methionine		3	5	5	
Histidine	5		6		
Valine		7	3	7	43

Sources: References 32–38

Substitution of amino-acid plasma levels, apparent K_m, and transport V_{max} into the Michaelis–Menten equation results in predicted rates of amino-acid influx into brain (Table 6.3). These estimates correlate well ($r = 0.8$–0.9) with experimentally observed values[31], and Fernstrom and associates[39] have shown that influx rates predicted on the basis of the K_m values in Table 6.3 correlate with brain amino-acid pool sizes. In addition, James *et al.* and Mans *et al.* have utilized the K_m values in Table 6.3 to estimate competition effects and to predict rates of amino-acid influx into brain of normal and cirrhotic rats[40, 41]. Therefore, the kinetic parameters listed in Table 6.3 provide the necessary data for quantitative predictions of amino-acid influx into brain under a variety of conditions.

COMPETITION BETWEEN THE BLOOD–BRAIN BARRIER NEUTRAL AMINO-ACID TRANSPORT SYSTEM AND ALBUMIN FOR TRYPTOPHAN

In the previous section the view was emphasized that by virtue of the close approximation of transport K_m and plasma amino-acid level, different ligands (amino acids) compete for a common binding site on the brain endothelial wall. The converse is also true. Given an appropriate kinetic situation, two binding sites existing within the capillary lumen, e.g. the neutral amino-acid carrier and albumin may compete for binding of a common ligand. The extent to which two binding sites compete for a common ligand is determined by the binding index, i.e. the ratio of binding capacity/binding affinity, of each site. The albumin-binding index for tryptophan is equal to A_T/K_D, where A_T = the total albumin concentration and K_D = the affinity (dissociation) constant. The binding index of the BBB carrier = app C/app K_m, where app K_m is defined according to equation (1) and app C = the apparent binding capacity of the BBB tryptophan carrier[42]. An important insight into the role of a capillary transport system as a binding system which competes with albumin is the recognition that the apparent binding capacity of the carrier system greatly exceeds the local capillary concentration (C_T) of the carrier. Previously reported derivations[42] indicate

$$\text{app } C = C_T(1 + k_5 t) \qquad (2)$$

where k_5 = the rate constant of the movement of the carrier–ligand complex through the BBB membrane and t = the brain capillary transit time (~ 1 s). In order for a transport system to function effectively, k_5 must greatly exceed the capillary transit time. Otherwise, no effective transmembrane movement of solute would occur. Therefore, the apparent binding capacity greatly exceeds C_T and the carrier system is able to effectively compete with albumin for tryptophan binding, despite the large molar excess of albumin. Stated differently, the binding of tryptophan by albumin at the brain capillary is inhibited by the carrier and this inhibition results in a decrease in the apparent affinity of albumin binding of tryptophan. These considerations may be quantitatively expressed as follows

$$\text{app } K_D = K_D\{1 + (\text{app}C/\text{app } K_m)\} \qquad (3)$$

where app K_D refers to the apparent K_D of albumin binding of tryptophan in the presence of the competing BBB tryptophan carrier, and app C and app K_m are defined as in equations 2 and 1, respectively. Previous studies in the adult rat brain indicate app $K_D = 1.4$ mmol/l, $K_D = 0.13$ mmol/l, and app $C = 1.9$ mmol/l[42].

A different way of expressing the ability of the BBB tryptophan carrier to compete with albumin and thereby inhibit the binding of tryptophan by albumin is by defining the apparent free (non-protein bound) tryptophan in brain capillaries *in vivo*[42]

$$\text{app free } (in \ vivo) = \frac{1 + (\text{app } C/\text{app } K_m)}{1 + (A_T/K_D) + (\text{app } C/\text{app } K_m)} \tag{4}$$

Given app $C/$app $K_m = 0$, i.e. the *in vitro* situation where no BBB carrier exists, then equation 4 reduces to,

$$\text{free } (in \ vitro) = \frac{1}{1 + A_T/K_D} \tag{5}$$

Substitution into equations 4 and 5 of hypothetical but likely values for K_D, which is directly related to the plasma-free fatty-acid level, and K_m, which is directly related to the plasma level of large neutral amino acids, and given $A_T = 500 \ \mu\text{mol/l}$ and app $C = 1900 \ \mu\text{mol/l}$, then estimates of app free (*in vivo*) and free (*in vitro*) tryptophan may be predicted (Table 6.5). The data indicate that the app free tryptophan (*in vivo*) greatly exceeds the *in vitro* estimate except in the presence of gross hyperaminoacidaemia. Therefore, as suggested by Wurtman[43] and Fernstrom[44] and their associates, in many situations the total plasma tryptophan concentration provides a better index of available amino acid than does the *in vitro* free tryptophan measurement.

TABLE 6.5 Comparison of free, non-albumin bound tryptophan *in vivo* in brain capillaries with *in vitro* values

Condition or diet	app K_m ($\mu\text{mol/l}$)	K_D ($\mu\text{mol/l}$)	% free in vitro	% free in vivo
Carbohydrate/fat	400	300	38	77
Basal	700	300	38	69
Carbohydrate	400	100	17	53
Protein	900	100	17	38
Phenylketonuria	5000	100	17	21

Source: Reference 42

AMINO-ACID TRANSPORT THROUGH THE BLOOD–BRAIN BARRIER OF THE NEWBORN

The preceding discussion pertained to amino-acid transport through the adult rat BBB. Amino-acid transport through the BBB of the newborn rabbit (< 24 h old) is currently being investigated. The BBB of the newborn is fully developed and amino acids and other nutrients effectively enter brain from blood only by carrier-mediation[29]. The neutral amino-acid transport system of the newborn rabbit is a somewhat lower affinity, higher capacity, system than that of the adult rat. For example, tryptophan transport through the newborn rabbit BBB is characterized by a $K_m = 0.5$ mmol/l, $V_{max} = 55$ nmol min^{-1} g^{-1} (W. M. Pardridge, unpublished observations). Therefore, the V_{max}/K_m ratio (0.11) of the newborn BBB is about the same as the V_{max}/K_m ratio of tryptophan transport through the adult rat BBB (Table 6.3). The V_{max}/K_m ratio of the basic amino-acid carrier is several times greater in the newborn rabbit than in the adult[29].

CLINICAL IMPLICATIONS

A number of neutral amino-acids are either being used presently or may be used in the future as centrally acting pharmacological agents. Since these compounds enter the brain via the BBB neutral amino-acid carrier, brain clearance is subject to the effects of competition. For example, patients on a high protein diet would be expected to have a relative hyperaminoacidaemia and to have a reduced transport of neutral amino acid (drug) into brain. Indeed, it is well known that the therapeutic efficacy of L-DOPA in the treatment of Parkinson's disease is decreased in patients on a high protein diet[45]. Moreover, α-methyldopa has been shown to be less effective in reducing blood pressure in the spontaneously hypertensive rat when animals are placed on a high protein meal[46]. Similarly, the use of tryptophan for depression[47], tyrosine for reducing blood pressure[48], on 5-hydroxytryptophan for the treatment of myoclonus[49], would be expected to be influenced by dietary induced changes in plasma amino acids. The use of α-methyltyrosine, an inhibitor of tyrosine hydroxylase, for the treatment of pheochromocytoma is occasionally associated with Parkinson-like side effects due to the central dopaminergic antagonism of the drug[50]. Since it is probable that the K_m of neutral amino-acid transport into adrenal medullary cells is high relative to plasma amino-acid levels, it may be that competition effects have no influence on drug action in peripheral tissues, but do regulate drug side effects in the CNS.

The unique sensitivity of the CNS to the hyperaminoacidaemias associated with inborn errors of amino-acid metabolism may also be related to the unusual susceptibility of the brain to transport competition effects. Phenylketonuria (PKU) has a marked effect on brain neutral amino-acid uptake[8], because phenylalanine has the greatest affinity for the BBB transport system (Table 6.3). Conversely, histidinaemia often presents as a benign disease[51]. However, this disease should not be regarded as evidence that plasma hyperaminoacidaemias, *per se*, are benign. Due to the nearly 2.5-fold greater affinity of the BBB carrier for phenylalanine relative to histidine (Table 6.3), the plasma level of histidine would have to reach 2.5 times the concentrations of phenylalanine found in PKU for the two diseases to have equivalent effects on amino-acid uptake by the CNS. However, plasma histidine concentrations in histidinaemia are generally less than half that of the plasma phenylalanine in PKU[51].

If competition effects at the BBB do play a major role in the pathogenesis of brain disease associated with inborn errors, then it is likely that the most effective therapy would be achieved by (i) dietary restriction of the amino acid in excess, and (ii) dietary supplementation of those amino acids that enter brain via the same transport system as the amino acid in excess[52]. For example, the treatment of PKU or homocystinuria might include dietary supplementation of large neutral amino acids in addition to the restriction of dietary phenylalanine and methionine, respectively. Similarly, the treatment of hyperargininaemia might best be achieved by dietary restriction of arginine and supplementation with lysine.

Competition effects at the BBB may also be involved in the pathogenesis of several metabolic encephalopathies. For example, plasma lysine is markedly elevated in Reye's syndrome to levels of 1.7 mmol/l or greater[53], which would fully saturate the BBB basic amino-acid carriers (Table 6.3), and deprive the brain of arginine needed for protein synthesis. The encephalopathy of chronic liver disease and the associated increase in brain tryptophan is probably not related to competition effects. The decreased concentrations of plasma branched chain amino-acids observed in patients with cirrhosis is offset by an increase in aromatic amino acids[40]. Moreover, the V_{max} of the BBB neutral amino-acid carrier is enhanced in cirrhosis and this appears to be the major factor leading to the elevated brain tryptophan in hepatic encephalopathy[26, 40].

The extension of concepts regarding amino-acid competition effects at the BBB of the rat to similar situations in man is based on the assumption that BBB amino-acid transport in man, like that of the rat, is characterized by absolute K_m values in the 0.1–0.5 mmol/l range. With the introduction of positron emission tomography, the kinetics of brain uptake of positron-labelled amino acids can now be estimated in man. Based on studies reported by Oldendorf 10 years ago, in which the brain uptake of labelled seleno-methionine was reduced in untreated PKU[54], it is likely that the K_m of BBB amino-acid transport in man is of the order of 0.1–0.5 mmol/l.

Finally, in future considerations of the role of competition effects at the BBB in clinical conditions, it will probably be unnecessary to calculate apparent K_m values as in Table 6.3. Fernstrom and associates[39] have shown that, in most situations, amino-acid ratios (e.g. tryptophan/Σ large neutral amino acids) provide excellent indices of amino-acid availability in brain.

Acknowledgements

The author is indebted to Larry Mietus for superior technical assistance and to Charlotte Limberg for preparing the manuscript. These studies are supported by a Basil O'Connor grant from the National Foundation-March of Dimes, Research Career Development Award AM-00783 and grant AM-25744 from the National Institute of Health.

References

1. Wurtman, R. J. and Fernstrom, J. D. (1976). Control of brain neurotransmitter synthesis by precursor availability and nutritional state. *Biochem. Pharmacol.*, **25**, 1691
2. Chaplin, E. R., Goldberg, A. L. and Diamond, I. (1976). Leucine oxidation in brain slices and nerve endings. *J. Neurochem.*, **26**, 701
3. Rubin, R. A., Ordonez, L. A. and Wurtman, R. J. (1974). Physiological dependence of brain methionine and S-adenosylmethionine concentrations on serum amino acid pattern. *J. Neurochem.*, **23**, 227
4. Schwartz, J. C., Lampart, C. and Rose, C. (1972). Histamine formation in rat brain *in vivo*: Effects of histidine loads. *J. Neurochem.*, **19**, 801
5. Chung-Hawang, E., Khurana, H. and Fisher, H. (1976). The effect of dietary histidine level on the carnosine concentration of rat olfactory bulbs. *J. Neurochem.*, **26**, 1087
6. Guroff, G. and Udenfriend, S. (1962). Studies on aromatic amino acid uptake by rat brain *in vivo*. *J. Biol. Chem.*, **237**, 803
7. Fernstrom, J. D. and Wurtman, R. J. (1972). Brain serotonin content: Physiological regulation by plasma neutral amino acids. *Science*, **178**, 414
8. Oldendorf, W. H. (1973). Saturation of blood–brain barrier transport of amino acids in phenylketonuria. *Arch. Neurol.*, **28**, 45
9. Pardridge, W. M. (1977). Regulation of amino acid availability to the brain. In Wurtman, R. J. and Wurtman, J. J., (eds.) *Nutrition and the Brain*, Vol. 1, pp. 141–204. (New York: Raven Press)
10. Oldendorf, W. H. (1970). Measurement of brain uptake of radiolabeled substances using a tritiated water internal standard. *Brain Res.*, **24**, 372
11. Pardridge, W. M. and Oldendorf, W. H. (1977). Transport of metabolic substrates through the blood–brain barrier. *J. Neurochem.*, **28**, 5
12. Pardridge, W. M. (1979). Regulation of amino acid availability to brain: selective control mechanisms for glutamate. In Filer L. J., Jr. *et al* (eds.) *Glutamic Acid: Advances in Biochemistry and Physiology*, pp. 125–137. (New York: Raven Press)

13. Pardridge, W. M. (1979). Carrier-mediated transport of thyroid hormones through the rat blood–brain barrier: Primary role of albumin-bound hormone. *Endocrinology,* **105,** 605
14. Cornford, E. M., Braun, L. D. and Oldendorf, W. H. (1978). Carrier mediated blood–brain barrier transport of choline and certain choline analogs. *J. Neurochem.,* **30,** 299
15. Pardridge, W. M. and Oldendorf, W. H. (1975). Kinetics of blood–brain barrier transport of hexoses. *Biochim. Biophys. Acta,* **382,** 377
16. Oldendorf, W. H. (1973). Carrier-mediated blood–brain barrier transport of short-chain monocarboxylic organic acids. *Am. J. Physiol.,* **224,** 1450
17. Cremer, J. E., Braun, L. D. and Oldendorf, W. H. (1976). Changes during development in transport processes of the blood–brain barrier. *Biochim. Biophys. Acta,* **448,** 633
18. Hawkins, R. A. and Biebuyck, J. F. (1979). Ketone bodies are selectively used by individual brain regions. *Science,* **205,** 325
19. Millington, W. R., McCall, A. L. and Wurtman, R. J. (1978). Deanol acetamidobenzoate inhibits the blood–brain barrier transport of choline. *Ann. Neurol.,* **4,** 302
20. Pardridge, W. M. (1981). Transport of nutrients and hormones through the blood–brain barrier. *Diabetologia,* **20,** 246
21. Chapman, A. G., Meldrum, B. S. and Siesjo, B. K. (1977). Cerebral metabolic changes during prolonged epileptic seizures in rats. *J. Neurochem.,* **28,** 1025
22. Moore, T. J., Lione, A. P. and Regen, D. M. (1973). Effect of thyroid hormone on cerebral glucose metabolism in the infant rat. *Am. J. Physiol.,* **225,** 925
23. Betz, A. L., Gilboe, D. D. and Drewes, L. R. (1975). Accelerative exchange diffusion kinetics of glucose between blood and brain and its relation to transport during anoxia. *Biochim. Biophys. Acta,* **401,** 416
24. Warnock, L. G. and Burkhalter, V. J. (1968). Evidence of malfunctioning blood–brain barrier in experimental thiamine deficiency in rats. *J. Nutr.,* **94,** 256
25. Sarna, G. S., Bradbury, M. W. B., Cremer, J. E., Lai, J. C. K. and Teal, H. M. (1979). Brain metabolism and specific transport at the blood–brain barrier after portocaval anastomosis in the rat. *Brain Res.,* **160,** 69
26. James, J. H., Escourrou, J. and Fischer, J. E. (1978). Blood brain neutral amino acid transport activity is increased after portacaval anastomosis. *Science,* **200,** 1395
27. Daniel, P. M., Love, E. R. and Pratt, O. E. (1975) Hypothyroidism and amino acid entry into brain and muscle. *Lancet,* **2,** 872
28. Pardridge, W. M. (1976). Inorganic mercury: selective effects on blood–brain barrier transport systems. *J. Neurochem.,* **27,** 333
29. Braun, L. D., Cornford, E. M. and Oldendorf, W. H. (1980). Newborn rabbit blood–brain barrier is selectively permeable and differs substantially from the adult. *J. Neurochem.,* **34,** 147
30. Pardridge, W. M. and Oldendorf, W. H. (1975). Kinetic analysis of blood–brain barrier transport of amino acids. *Biochim. Biophys. Acta,* **401,** 128
31. Pardridge, W. M. (1977). Kinetics of competitive inhibition of neutral amino acid transport across the blood–brain barrier. *J. Neurochem,* **28,** 103
32. Larsen, P. R., Ross, J. E. and Tapley, D. F. (1964). Transport of neutral, dibasic and *N*-methyl substituted amino acids by rat intestine. *Biochim. Biophys. Acta,* **88,** 570

33. Lingard, J., Rumrich, G. and Young, J. A. (1973) Kinetics of L-histidine transport in the proximal convolution of rat nephron studied using the stationary microperfusion technique. *Pfluegers Arch.*, **342**, 13

34. Chang, Y. Z. and Huang, K. C. (1971). Microperfusion studies on renal tubular transport of tryptophan derivatives in rats. *Am. J. Physiol.*, **221**, 575

35. Begin, N. and Scholefield, P. G. (1965). The uptake of amino acids by mouse pancreas *in vitro*. II. The specificity of the carrier systems. *J. Biol. Chem.* **240**, 332

36. Winter, C. G. and Christensen, H. N. (1964). Migration of amino acids across the membrane of the human erythrocyte. *J. Biol. Chem.*, **239**, 872

37. LeCam, A. and Freychet, P. (1977). Neutral amino acid transport. Characterization of the A and L system in isolated rat hepatocytes. *J. Biol. Chem.*, **252**, 148

38. Seglen, P. O. and Solheim, A. E. (1978). Valine uptake and incorporation into protein in isolated rat hepatocytes. *Eur. J. Biochem.*, **85**, 15

39. Fernstrom, J. D. and Faller, D. V. (1978). Neutral amino acids in the brain: changes in response to food ingestion. *J. Neurochem.*, **30**, 1531

40. James, J. H., Ziparo, V., Jeppsson, B. and Fischer, J. E. (1979). Hyperammonaemia, plasma amino acid imbalance and blood–brain amino acid transport: A unified theory of portal-systemic encephalopathy. *Lancet*, **2**, 772

41. Mans, A. M., Biebuyck, J. F., Saunders, S. J., Kirsch, R. E. and Hawkins, R. A. (1979). Tryptophan transport across the blood–brain barrier during acute hepatic failure. *J. Neurochem.*, **33**, 409

42. Pardridge, W. M. (1979). Tryptophan transport through the blood–brain barrier: *in vivo* measurement of free and albumin-bound amino acid. *Life Sci.*, **25**, 1519

43. Madras, B. K., Cohen, E. L. Messing, R., Munro, H. N. and Wurtman, R. J. (1974). Relevance of free tryptophan in serum to tissue tryptophan concentrations. *Metabolism*, **23**, 1107

44. Fernstrom, J. D., Hirsch, M. J. and Faller, D. V. (1976). Tryptophan concentrations in rat brain. Failure to correlate with free serum tryptophan or its ratio to the sum of other serum neutral amino acids. *Biochem. J.*, **160**, 589

45. Mena, I. and Cotzias, G. C. (1975). Protein intake and treatment of Parkinson's disease with levodopa. *N. Engl. J. Med.*, **292**, 181

46. Sved, A. F., Goldberg, I. M. and Fernstrom, J. D. (1980). Dietary protein intake influences the antihypertensive potency of methyldopa in spontaneously hypertensive rats. *J. Pharmacol. Exp. Ther.*, **214**, 147

47. Shaw, D. M., Blazek, R., Tidmarsh, S. F., Riley, G. J., Johnson, A. L. and Michalakeas, A. (1979). Distribution of tryptophan and tyrosine in unipolar affective disorders as defined by multicompartmental analysis. In Baumann, P. (ed.) *J. Neural Transmission*, pp. 197–207. (New York: Springer)

48. Sved, A. F., Fernstrom, J. D. and Wurtman, R. J. (1979). Tyrosine administration reduces blood pressure and enhances brain norepinephrine release in spontaneously hypertensive rats. *Proc. Natl. Acad. Sci. USA*, **76**, 3511

49. Chadwick, D., Harris, R., Jenner, P., Reynolds, E. H. and Marsden, C. D. (1975). Manipulation of brain serotonin in the treatment of myoclonus. *Lancet*, **2**, 434

50. Gillow, S. E., Pertsemlidis, D. and Bertani, L. M. (1971). Management of patients with pheochromocytoma. *Am. Heart J.*, **82**, 557

51. Levy, H. L., Shih. V. E. and Madigan, P. M. (1974). Routine newborn screening for histidinemia. Clinical and biochemical results. *N. Engl. J. Med.*, **291**, 1214

52. Andersen, A. E. and Avins, L. (1976). Lowering brain phenylalanine levels by giving other large neutral amino acids. A new experimental therapeutic approach to phenylketonuria. *Arch. Neurol.*, **33**, 684

53. Hilty, M. D., Romshe, C. A. and Delamater, P. V. (1974). Reye's syndrome and hyperaminoacidemia. *J. Pediatr.* **84**, 362

54. Oldendorf, W. H., Sisson, W. B. and Silverstein, A. (1971). Brain uptake of selenomethionine Se75. II. Reduced brain uptake of selenomethionine Se75 in phenylketonuria. *Arch Neurol.*, **24**, 524

SECTION TWO

Treatment: New Aspects and Limits, Transplantation, Replacement Therapy, Genetic Engineering

7

Recent studies on the maturation of lysosomal enzymes

E. F. Neufeld

The class of enzymes called 'lysosomal' refers in general to hydrolases with an acid pH optimum, which reside in lysosomes but which may also be found in body fluids and sometimes in microsomes. Recent work has shown that the fine structure of these hydrolases determines their location, and conversely, that the location and history of the hydrolases affects their structure. Because acid hydrolases are glycoproteins, the structural variations may be in the polypeptide or the carbohydrate portions of the molecule.

Our studies of the synthesis and maturation of hydrolases have made use of the following technology. Human diploid fibroblasts in culture were administered an isotopic precursor of hydrolases such as an amino acid, a sugar or a phosphate. The enzyme of interest was isolated by immunoprecipitation and subjected to polyacrylamide gel electrophoresis under denaturing and reducing conditions. The radioactive polypeptides were visualized by fluorography or autoradiography.

When this technique was applied to the enzyme β-hexosaminidase[1], the radioactive polypeptides seen after an extended period of labelling with [^{3}H]leucine included not only the two chains seen in placental enzyme (α-chain, $M_r = 54K$; β-chain, $M_r = 29K$), but also chains of higher molecular weight. Pulse–chase experiments showed that these larger chains

($M_r = 67K$ and 63K) appeared in early labelling, and were gradually replaced during a 20 h period by chains with molecular weights similar to the placental type. Smaller chains, of M_r 24K, 22K and 19K were also formed during the chase. By the use of cells from appropriate mutants (patients with Tay–Sachs and Sandhoff disease) and of antibodies against the isolated 54K and 29K polypeptides, the 67K chain was shown to be the precursor of the 54K α-chain, and the 63K to be a precursor of the 29K β-chain as well as of smaller pieces. A transient band of 52K was seen occasionally, and was interpreted to be an intermediate in the maturation of β-chains; this intermediate would be nicked to give rise to the 29K polypeptide from one side, and 24K, which would be degraded further from the other. In electrophoresis under denaturing but non-reducing conditions, the pieces of the nicked β-chain remained associated, presumably by disulphide linkages[1,2]. β-Hexosaminidase from Chinese hamster ovary (CHO) cells showed the same kind of processing of α and β chains, except that the β-chain remained in the 52K (un-nicked) form[3].

Several other hydrolases have been shown, in our laboratory and elsewhere, to undergo a reduction in size (Table 7.1)[4–6]. Enzyme secreted into the medium was in all cases of approximately the same size as the precursor. Of particular interest is the very slow maturation of α-L-iduronidase[4]; complete conversion of the 75K precursor to the 60K form took 5 days, in contrast to the few hours required for the processing of cathepsin D or the one day for the full processing of β-hexosaminidase in human fibroblasts.

The slowness of the maturation process indicated that size reduction was a late event, occurring after the enzyme had been inserted into lysosomes. In agreement with this postulate, a partial degradation of β-hexosaminidase was shown to be catalysed by an acid protease, activated by thiols and inhibited by leupeptin and antipain, which was in the 3000–12000 g fraction of fibroblasts[7]. The protease converted the β-hexosaminidase precursor chains to products of 56K and 52K. The larger product was similar, but not identical to the mature α-chain of intact fibroblasts, whereas the smaller one corresponded to the intermediate in β-chain maturation. The lysosomal protease appeared to be similar to lysosomal thiol proteases such as cathepsin B, L and H. Purified cathepsin B itself did not catalyse the reaction. On the other hand, trypsin and chymotrypsin generated similar 56K and 52K products as did the acid protease[8]. These results show that β-hexosaminidase has a protease-resistant core and portions that are easily cleaved by proteolytic enzymes. To date, we have failed to produce cleavage of the β-chain to the 29K size of the mature β-hexosaminidase. It may be that this second cleavage requires prior steps, such as changes in the carbohydrate content or in the conformation of the protein.

Other important changes concern the glycosylation of acid hydrolases and the attachment of the 'recognition marker' which is necessary to ensure the localization of enzymes with lysosomes[9,10]. It had been shown, first by indirect, kinetic experiments[11][14] and later by sensitive enzymatic and chemical analysis[15][19] that the marker includes mannose 6-phosphate residues. Labelling experiments with [^{3}H]-mannose and $^{32}PO_4$ confirmed the presence of mannose 6-phosphate residues on oligosaccharides of the high mannose type in β-hexosaminidase and cathepsin D[19]. This year, workers at two laboratories independently found that the mannose 6-phosphate was at times covered by N-acetylglucosamine in phosphodiester linkage[20,21]. Whether such groups represent biosynthetic precursors of the recognition marker or have some independent function is not known as yet.

The relationship of the recognition marker, localization of the enzyme and proteolytic processing has been clarified by studies of I-cell disease. In this mutation, acid hydrolases are deficient from fibroblasts (and probably from other connective tissue cells) but present in excess in extracellular fluids[22]. Early experiments demonstrated that the acid hydrolases elaborated by I-cell fibroblasts were defective in that they failed to be recognized and taken up by other fibroblasts[23]. As the molecular basis of recognition was understood to be mannose 6-phosphate, it was established that I-cell enzymes were not phosphorylated, in contrast to their normal counterparts[19,24].

Other differences have been noted between the I-cell and normal enzymes. I-cell enzymes were synthesized as precursors of the correct size in a 3 h pulse, but were secreted almost in their entirety into the medium[19]. If enzyme remained inside the cell, it appeared to be processed, albeit incompletely. The acid protease that catalyses the cleavage of β-hexosaminidase precursor to the 56K and 52K pieces has been found in homogenates of I-cell fibroblasts[8]. Thus the failure of I-cell enzymes to be processed proteolytically is probably the result of their failure to reach lysosomes, which in turn is a consequence of the phosphorylation defect. This concept is in keeping with the temporal sequence of events observed in normal cells (i.e. phosphorylation precedes proteolytic processing).

It has also been noted that enzymes secreted by I-cell fibroblasts have more sialic acid than their normal counterparts[25,26]. This is readily understood in terms of current concepts of the synthesis of complex (i.e. sialylated) oligosaccharides from high mannose oligosaccharide precursors[27,28]. The latter presumably also serve as precursors to the phosphorylated oligosaccharides. Thus the absence of phosphorylation of

TABLE 7.1 Apparent molecular weight ($\times 10^3$) of isolated chains of acid hydrolases

Enzyme	Reference	Cell	Precursor form	Processed form	Intermediate form	Secreted form
β-Hexosaminidase	1	Human fibroblasts				
α-chain			67	54	—	67
β-chain			63	29, 22, 19	52	63
β-Hexosaminidase	3	CHO* cells				
α-chain			68	55	—	68
β-chain			63	52	—	63
α-L-Iduronidase	4	Human fibroblasts	75	66	72	76
α-Glucosidase	1	Human fibroblasts	95	79, 76	several	95
Cathepsin D	1	Human fibroblasts	53	31	47	53
Cathepsin D	5	Porcine kidney	46	44, 30	—	?
β-Galactosidase	6	Mouse macrophages	82	63	?	?
β-Glucuronidase	6	Mouse macrophages	75	75	?	?

* Chinese hamster ovary

I-cell enzymes could allow their carbohydrate branches to be processed to the complex form.

Mucolipidosis III (pseudo-Hurler polydystrophy) has been considered a clinically and biochemically attenuated form of I-cell disease[22,23]. In keeping with this view we have found some phosphate in β-hexosaminidase, some retention of the enzyme within fibroblasts and proteolytic processing of the intracellular fraction in fibroblasts from patients with this disorder[29].

If it is clear that the mannose phosphate residues are needed to target hydrolases to lysosomes, the role of the extra polypeptide is not yet known. It is not the unique site of attachment of mannose 6-phosphate, since mature enzyme has been found to remain phosphorylated[4,19,29]. Nor does the extra peptide determine catalytic activity; β-hexosaminidase and α-L-iduronidase secreted in precursor form are as active as the enzymes processed by intact cells or by cell-free systems[4,8].

Could the extra peptide be a co-recognition marker, acting in conjunction with mannose 6-phosphate to guide enzymes to lysosomes? This had been suggested[30] because of discrepancies between expected and observed kinetic constants of uptake of a mannose 6-phosphate–albumin conjugate[31] and because of evidence that arginine residues may participate in the binding of enzyme to its receptor[32]. However, both precursor and processed forms of β-hexosaminidase were taken up equally well by fibroblasts[8]. An alternative function for the extra peptide might be as a signal for the enzymes transferring the mannose 6-phosphate recognition marker to the newly formed enzyme. A priori, it seems plausible that there might be a specific signal to distinguish would-be lysosomal hydrolases (to which a recognition marker must be attached) from other glycoproteins destined for secretion, incorporation into plasma membrane or retention in microsomes. Such a signal should be common to a number of hydrolases and should be recognized either by the enzymes attaching the recognition marker or by some area of the endoplasmic reticulum or Golgi membranes where such attachment would occur.

The extra polypeptide which is cleaved in the maturation of lysosomal hydrolases should not be confused with the signal or leader sequence which introduces proteins into the cisternae of the endoplasmic reticulum, and which is usually cleaved co-translationally[33]. As glycoproteins, lysosomal enzymes must enter the endoplasmic reticulum, where glycosylation occurs[27], and have therefore been expected to be synthesized with such a signal sequence. This has been shown to be true by in vitro translation of cathepsin D[5].

Phosphorylation is a relatively early step in the life of a hydrolytic enzyme; limited proteolysis occurs later. But the half-life of hydrolytic enzymes in lysosomes may be long, and still other changes may take place – dephosphorylation, removal of some carbohydrate residues, further proteolysis – before the enzymes finally lose all catalytic activity. Thus the heterogeneity of hydrolases extracted from tissues, the variability of 'subunit' molecular weights sometimes found in apparently homogeneous enzymes and the differences between hydrolases in tissues and body fluids are readily understood as a consequence of the history of the enzymes between the time of their synthesis and that of their isolation by the experimenter.

References

1. Hasilik, A. and Neufeld, E. F. (1980). Biosynthesis of lysosomal enzymes in fibroblasts; synthesis as precursors of higher molecular weight. *J. Biol. Chem.*, **255**, 4937
2. Puchalski. C. and Neufeld, E. F. (1981). Polypeptides of processed β-hexosaminidase remain associated under non-reducing conditions. *Fed. Proc.*, **40**, 1551
3. Robbins. A. R. and Myerowitz, R. (1981). The mannose 6-phosphate receptor of Chinese hamster ovary cells. *J. Biol. Chem.*, **256**, 10623
4. Myerowitz. R. and Neufeld, E. F. (1981). Maturation of α-L-iduronidase in cultured human fibroblasts. *J. Biol. Chem.*, **256**, 3044
5. Erickson. A. H. and Blobel, G. (1979). Early events in the biosynthesis of the lysosomal enzyme cathepsin D. *J. Biol. Chem.*, **254**, 11771
6. Skudlarek. M. D. and Swank, B. T. (1979). Biosynthesis of two lysosomal enzymes in macrophages. *J. Biol. Chem.*, **254**, 9939
7. Frisch, A. and Neufeld, E. F. (1980). Limited proleolysis of β-hexosaminidase in a cell-free system. *Fed. Proc.*, **39**, 1866
8. Frisch, A. and Neufeld, E. F. (1981). Limited proteolysis of the β-hexosaminidase precursor in a cell-free system. *J. Biol. Chem.*, **256**, 8242
9. Hickman. S., Shapiro, L. J. and Neufeld, E. F. (1974). A recognition marker required for uptake of a lysosomal enzyme by cultured fibroblasts. *Biochem. Biophys. Res. Commun.*, **57**, 55
10. Neufeld, E. F., Sando, G. N., Garvin, A. J. and Rome, L. H. (1977). The transport of lysosomal enzymes. *J. Supramol. Struct.*, **6**, 95
11. Kaplan, A., Achord, D. T. and Sly, W. S. (1977). Phosphohexosyl components of a lysosomal enzyme are recognized by pinocytosis receptors on human fibroblasts. *Proc. Natl. Acad. Sci. USA*, **74**, 2026
12. Sando, G. N. and Neufeld, E. F. (1977). Recognition and receptor-mediated uptake of a lysosomal enzyme. α-L-iduronidase, by cultured human fibroblasts. *Cell* **12**, 619
13. Kaplan, A., Fischer, D., Achord, D. and Sly, W. (1977). Phosphohexosyl recognition is a general characteristic of pinocytosis of lysosomal glycosidases by human fibroblasts. *J. Clin. Invest.*, **60**, 1088 .
14. Ullrich, K., Mersmann, G., Weber, E. and von Figura, K. (1978). Evidence

for lysosomal enzyme recognition by human fibroblasts via a phosphorylated carbohydrate moiety. *Biochem. J.,* **170,** 643

15. Natowicz, M. R., Chi, M. M-Y., Lowry, O. H. and Sly, W. S. (1979). Enzymatic identification of mannose 6-phosphate on the recognition marker for receptor-mediated pinocytosis of β-glucuronidase by human fibroblasts. *Proc. Natl. Acad. Sci. USA,* **76,** 4322

16. Distler, J., Hieber, V., Sahagian, G., Schmickel, R. and Jourdian, G. W. (1979). Identification of mannose 6-phosphate in glycoproteins that inhibit the assimilation of β-galactosidase by fibroblasts. *Proc. Natl. Acad. Sci. USA,* **76,** 4235

17. von Figura, K. and Klein, U. (1979). Isolation and characterization of phosphorylated oligosaccharides from α-N-acetyl-glucosaminidase that are recognized by cell surface receptors. *Eur. J. Biochem.,* **94,** 347

18. Sahagian, G., Distler, J., Hieber, V., Schmickel, R., and Jourdian, G. W. (1979). Role of mannose-6-phosphate in β-galactosidase assimilation. *Fed. Proc.,* **38,** 467

19. Hasilik, A. and Neufeld, E. F. (1980). Biosynthesis of lysosomal enzymes in fibroblasts; phosphorylation of mannose residues. *J. Biol. Chem.,* **255,** 4946

20. Tabas, I. and Kornfeld, S. (1980). Biosynthetic intermediates of β-glucuronidase contain high mannose oligosaccharides with blocked phosphate residues. *J. Biol. Chem.,* **255,** 6633

21. Hasilik, A., Klein, U., Waheed, A., Strecker, G. and von Figura, K. (1980). Phosphorylated oligosaccharides in lysosomal enzymes: identification of α-N-acetylglucosamine(1)phospho(6)mannose diester groups. *Proc. Natl. Acad. Sci. USA,* **77,** 7074

22. McKusick, V. A., Neufeld, E. F. and Kelly, T. E. (1978). The mucopolysaccharide storage diseases. In Stanbury, J. B., Wyngaarden, J. B. and Fredrickson, D. S. (eds.) *The Metabolic Basis of Inherited Disease,* pp. 1282–1307. (New York: McGraw-Hill).

23. Hickman, S. and Neufeld, E. F. (1972). A hypothesis for I-Cell disease: defective hydrolases that do not enter lysosomes. *Biochem. Biophys. Res. Commun.,* **49,** 992

24. Bach, G., Bargal, R. and Cantz, M. (1979). I-Cell disease: deficiency of extracellular hydrolase phosphorylation. *Biochem. Biophys. Res. Commun.,* **91,** 976

25. Vladutiu, G. D. and Rattazzi, M. C. (1975). Abnormal lysosomal hydrolases excreted by cultured fibroblasts in I-Cell disease (mucolipidosis II). *Biochem. Biophys. Res. Commun.,* **67,** 956

26. Miller, A. L., Freeze, H. S. and Kress, B. C. (1981). I-Cell disease. In Callahan, J. W. and Lowden, J. A. (eds.) *Lysosomes and Lysosomal Storage Diseases,* p. 271. (New York: Raven Press)

27. Struck, D. K. and Lennarz, W. J. (1980). The functions of saccharide lipids in synthesis of glycoproteins. In Lennarz, W. J. (ed.) *The Biochemistry of Glycoproteins and Proteoglycans,* pp. 35–83 (New York: Plenum Press)

28. Schachter, H. and Roseman, S. (1980). Mammalian glycosyltransferases: their role in the synthesis and function of complex carbohydrates and glycolipids. In Lennarz, W. J. (ed.) *The Biochemistry of Glycoproteins and Proteoglycans,* pp. 85–160 (New York: Plenum Press)

29. Robey, P. G. and Neufeld, E. F. (1982). Defective phosphorylation and

processing of β-hexosaminidase by intact cultured fibroblasts from patients with mucolipidosis III. *Arch. Biochem. Biophys.*, **213**, 251

30. Neufeld, E. F. (1981). Recognition and processing of lysosomal enzymes in cultured fibroblasts. In Callahan, J. W. and Lowden, J. A. (eds.) *Lysosomes and Lysosomal Storage Diseases*, p. 115 (New York: Raven Press)

31. Karson, E. M., Neufeld, E. F. and Sando, G. N. (1980). *p*-Isothiocyanatophenyl 6-phospho-α-D-mannopyranoside coupled to albumin. A model compound recognized by the fibroblast lysosomal enzyme uptake system. *Biochemistry*, **19**, 3856.

32. Rome, L. H. and Miller, J. (1980). Butanedione treatment reduces receptor binding of a lysosomal enzyme to cells and membranes. *Biochem. Biophys. Res. Commun.*, **92**, 986

33. Davis, B. D. and Tai, P. C. (1980). The mechanism of protein secretion across membranes. *Nature (London)*, **283**, 433

NOTE ADDED IN PROOF

The biosynthesis of the mannose-6-phosphate recognition marker occurs by transfer of *N*-acetylglucosamine-1-phosphate from UDPGlcNAc to high-mannose chains on the newly synthesized precursor enzyme, followed by removal of the *N*-acetylglucosamine by a specific diesterase[34-37]. Up to three mannose residues may be phosphorylated on a single oligosaccharide chain[38]. An almost total lack of phospho-*N*-acetylglucosamine transferase activity is associated with I-cell disease, and a partial deficiency with the milder disorder, pseudo-Hurler polydystrophy[34,39].

34. Hasilik, A., Waheed, A. and von Figura, K. (1981). Enzymatic phosphorylation of lysosomal enzymes in the presence of UDP-*N*-acetylglucosamine. Absence of the activity in I-cell fibroblasts. *Biochem. Biophys. Res. Commun.*, **98**, 761

35. Reitman, M. L. and Kornfeld, S. (1981). UDP-*N*-acetylglucosamine: glycoprotein *N*-acetylglucosamine-1-transferase. Proposed enzyme for the phosphorylation of the high mannose oligosaccharide units of lysosomal enzymes. *J. Biol. Chem.*, **256**, 4275

36. Varki, A. and Kornfeld, S. (1980). Identification of a rat liver α-*N*-acetylglucosaminyl phosphodiesterase capable of removing "blocking" α-*N*-acetylglucosamine residues from phosphorylated high mannose oligosaccharides of lysosomal enzymes. *J. Biol. Chem.*, **255**, 8398

37. Waheed, A., Hasilik, A. and von Figura, K. (1981). Processing of the phosphorylated recognition markers in lysosomal enzymes. Characterization and partial purification of a microsomal α-*N*-acetylglucosaminyl phosphodiesterase. *J. Biol. Chem.*, **256**, 5717

38. Varki, A. and Kornfeld, S. (1980). Structural studies of phosphorylated high mannose-type oligosaccharides. *J. Biol. Chem.*, **255**, 10847

39. Reitman, M. L., Varki, A. and Kornfeld, S. (1981). Fibroblasts from patients with I-cell disease and pseudo-Hurler polydystrophy are deficient in uridine 5'-diphosphate-*N*-acetylglucosamine: glycoprotein-*N*-acetylglucosaminyl phosphotransferase activity. *J. Clin. Invest.*, **67**, 1574

8

Enzyme substitution by fibroblast transplantation

M. F. Dean, H. Muir, P. F. Benson
and L. R. Button

INTRODUCTION

The first inborn error of metabolism to be recognized was alcaptonuria, described by Garrod in 1908[1]. He developed the concept that some diseases occur because an enzyme which controls a single metabolic step is entirely absent or has a greatly reduced activity. More than 330 such disorders have now been described[2], more than 30 of which are lysosomal storage diseases.

In many of these inherited deficiencies in lysosomal enzymes an inactive protein is present, which is sufficiently similar in structure to the normal enzyme to cross-react with it immunologically[3-5]. Enzyme replacement therapy by supplementation of deficient enzymes from an external source is, therefore, unlikely to provoke an immune response in the recipient and has thus prompted numerous attempts at enzyme substitution. Among these attempts at therapy have been infusions of fresh plasma[6-8], leukocyte transfusions[9, 10], administration of purified enzymes[11], enzymes encapsulated in liposomes[12], organ transplants[13, 14], skin grafts[15], and transplants of skin fibroblasts[16-18]. In all of these methods of treatment it is assumed that normal enzymes reach deficient cells and can then be taken up by adsorptive endocytosis, subsequently becoming localized within lysosomes together with accumulated storage products, as has been shown to take place with fibroblasts *in vitro*[19-22].

Among the inborn errors of lysosomal metabolism are included the mucopolysaccharidoses, a large group of related diseases in which a deficiency in one of a series of lysosomal enzymes leads to systemic accumulation of partially degraded glycosaminoglycans (GAG) which are major macromolecular constituents of connective tissues. GAG are composed primarily of alternating residues of uronic acid and hexosamine. The uronic-acid residues are sometimes O-sulphated, while the hexosamine residues are usually N-acetylated and O-sulphated but may also be N-sulphated.

Normal catabolism of GAG is a two-stage process, in which complete glycosaminoglycan chains are first degraded into smaller fragments of hexa- or tetrasaccharide size by the action of endoglycosidases, e.g. testicular hyaluronidase. Catabolism is then completed by the concerted action of a number of exoglycosidase and sulphatase enzymes, which remove one sugar or one sulphate group at a time from the non-reducing terminal end of the oligosaccharide chain. The GAG chains are thus broken down to their constituent monosaccharide subunits and free inorganic sulphate. A deficiency in any one of these enzymes interrupts the catabolic sequence, leading to massive intracellular accumulation of partially degraded GAG as lysosomal storage products and their excretion in very large amounts in urine.

Normal plasma is perhaps the most readily available source of lysosomal enzymes for replacement therapy. When large volumes of plasma were infused into patients with mucopolysaccharidosis type II (Hunter's disease)[8] and mucopolysaccharidosis type III[7] (Sanfilippo disease) specific changes consistent with those expected from increased catabolism of accumulated storage products were observed. Such changes were not seen when an equivalent volume of iso-osmotic dextran solution was subsequently infused into one of the patients with Sanfilippo syndrome[23]. However, the changes observed following plasma infusion were only transient, presumably because of the relatively short intracellular half-life of many of the enzymes involved in catabolism of GAG, which range from 2 to 14 days[19, 24-28].

Since Neufeld et al. had shown that normal fibroblasts are able to correct glycosaminoglycan accumulation in mutant fibroblasts cultured from patients with one or other type of mucopolysaccharidosis[29, 30], and since normal fibroblasts contain and can release all of the lysosomal enzymes necessary to correct each type of enzyme deficiency present in the mucopolysaccharidoses, skin fibroblasts themselves appear to be a useful source of enzyme for replacement therapy. Lysosomal enzymes released into tissue-culture medium by normal fibroblasts can be taken up into the lysosomes of defective fibroblasts and restore their ability to catabolize accumulated GAG[19, 24, 28, 31]. Fibroblasts can thus provide a more continuous source of enzymes when transplanted and have the potential ability to increase circulating enzyme acitivity and GAG catabolism over an extended period of time.

MATERIALS AND METHODS

Fibroblasts were transplanted into three patients with Sanfilippo type A disease (glucosamine-N-sulphatase deficiency) and three with Hunter's disease (α-L-idurono-2-sulphate sulphatase deficiency). In all patients, diagnoses were made on the basis of their typical clinical features[32] and confirmed by demonstration of a severe deficiency of either glucosamine-N-sulphatase[33] (Sanfilippo A patients) or α-L-idurono-2-sulphate sulphatase[34] (Hunter patients) in cultured fibroblasts. All patients were severely affected and at the time of grafting were all mentally sub-normal.

The donors gave no mixed leukocyte reaction against their respective recipient cells and were either HLA identical or had no HLA antigens other than those shared by the recipient. Before grafting, the ability of donor fibroblasts to correct abnormal [^{35}S]sulphate incorporation in the recipients' own cells was confirmed in culture. All patients were on an immunosuppressive regimen of 25 mg Imuran and 25 mg prednisolone given daily for four weeks before fibroblast transplant. This was continued for approximately five months after transplant in the case of the Sanfilippo patients and for periods ranging between 6 and 12 months in the Hunter patients. Fibroblast cultures were established as described previously[16] and after two passages were resuspended in 10 ml of phosphate buffered saline. Approximately 2×10^8 viable cells were injected into four sub-cutaneous dorsal sites.

Glycosaminoglycans and oligosaccharides were isolated from urine collections (24 h whenever possible) as described previously[16]. Oligosaccharides were fractionated on a column of Bio-Gel P2 (2.0 $\times$ 100 cm), loaded and eluted in 0.2 mmol/l sodium acetate, pH 6.8. Uronic acid was determined by the method of Bitter and Muir[35], hexosamine by the procedure of Kraan and Muir[36], total sulphate as described by Ginsberg and Di Ferrante[37] and sulphamino groups by the method of Lagunoff and Warren[38] following acetylation. Corrective factors were concentrated by precipitation from urine with ammonium sulphate and assayed as described previously[15] and α-L-idurono-2-sulphate sulphatase measured using a radio-labelled disulphated disaccharide substrate[39, 40].

RESULTS

The effectiveness of HLA compatible fibroblasts in enzyme replacement therapy was assessed in two ways: firstly by analysis of changes in the amount and composition of excreted GAG and the oligosaccharides derived from them; secondly by increases in the amounts of previously deficient lysosomal enzymes. Increases in excreted enzymes were measured either as urinary corrective factor[15] or directly in circulating leukocytes and serum using an appropriate substrate[39, 40].

Quantitative assay of GAG excretion, measured as total uronic acid output per 24 h in patients with Hunter's syndrome or as mg/g creatinine in the Sanfilippo type A patients, showed that there was an overall but fluctuating increase in mean excretion after transplant (Figures 8.1 and 8.2). This increase was observed in both GAG precipitated with 5-aminoacridine hydrochloride (actasaccharides and above) and in the lower molecular weight oligosaccharides derived from them (Tables 8.1 and 8.2).

The enzyme deficiency in Hunter's disease (α-L-idurono-2-sulphate sulphatase) leads to an accumulation of both heparan and dermatan sulphates but analysis of the GAG precipitated with 5-amino acridine showed that these were derived primarily from dermatan sulphate, since the predominant hexosamine was galactosamine (70–76%). Hexosamine analysis of the oligosaccharides, on the other hand, indicated that glucosamine accounted for more than 65% of the total and that most of this fraction was therefore presumably derived from catabolism of heparan sulphate. The glucosamine N-sulphatase deficiency in Sanfilippo A syndrome blocks catabolism of heparan sulphate alone, since these linkages are not found in dermatan sulphate and hence both GAG and low molecular weight fractions isolated from these patients contained predominantly glucosamine (80–90% of total hexosamine). There were no major changes in the hexosamine composition of either GAG or oligosaccharides after transplant.

The oligosaccharide fractions were examined further for evidence of qualitative changes following transplant. Those separated from the urine of Hunter patients were fractionated into four components by chromatography on Bio-Gel P2 (Figure 8.3), the largest of which (component I) was a little more retarded than tetrasaccharides produced by testicular hyaluronidase (EC 3.2.1.35) acting on chondroitin sulphate. The most retarded fraction (component IV) was eluted at a position equivalent to that of glucuronic acid and the intermediate fractions (components II and III) corresponded to the monosulphated and desulphated disaccharides

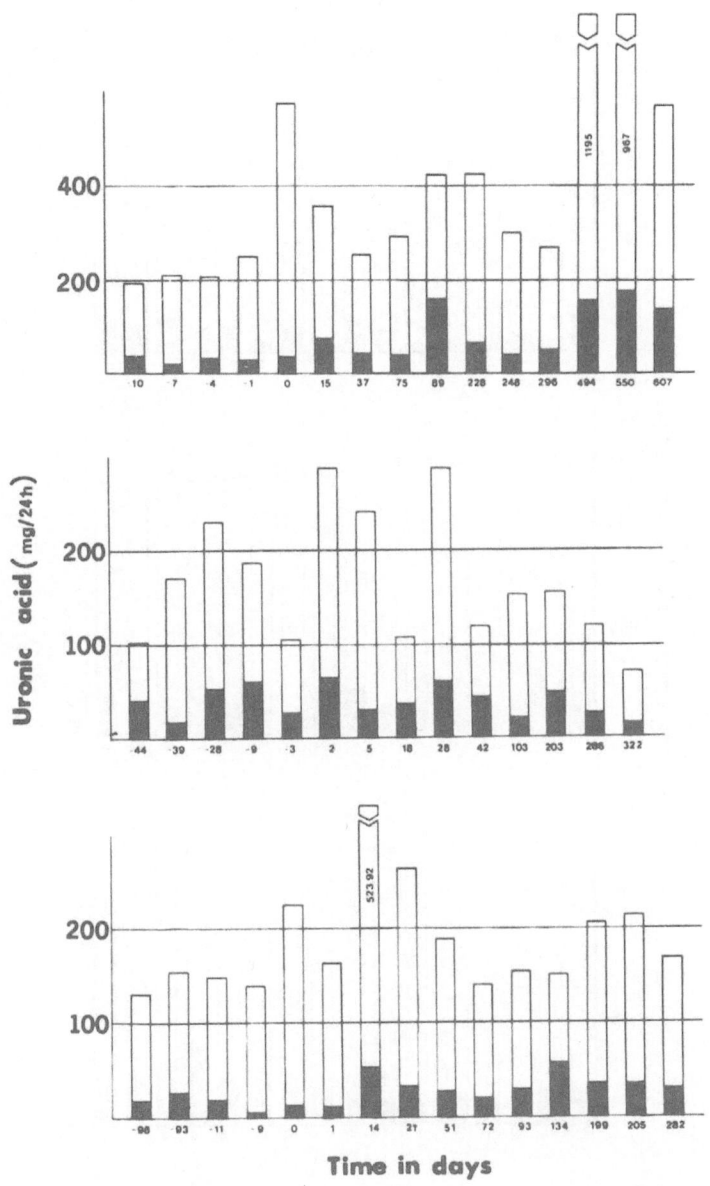

Figure 8.1 Total excretion (mg/24 h) of uronic acid in three patients with Hunter's syndrome before and after transplant. Days before transplant are indicated by negative numbers and after transplant by positive numbers

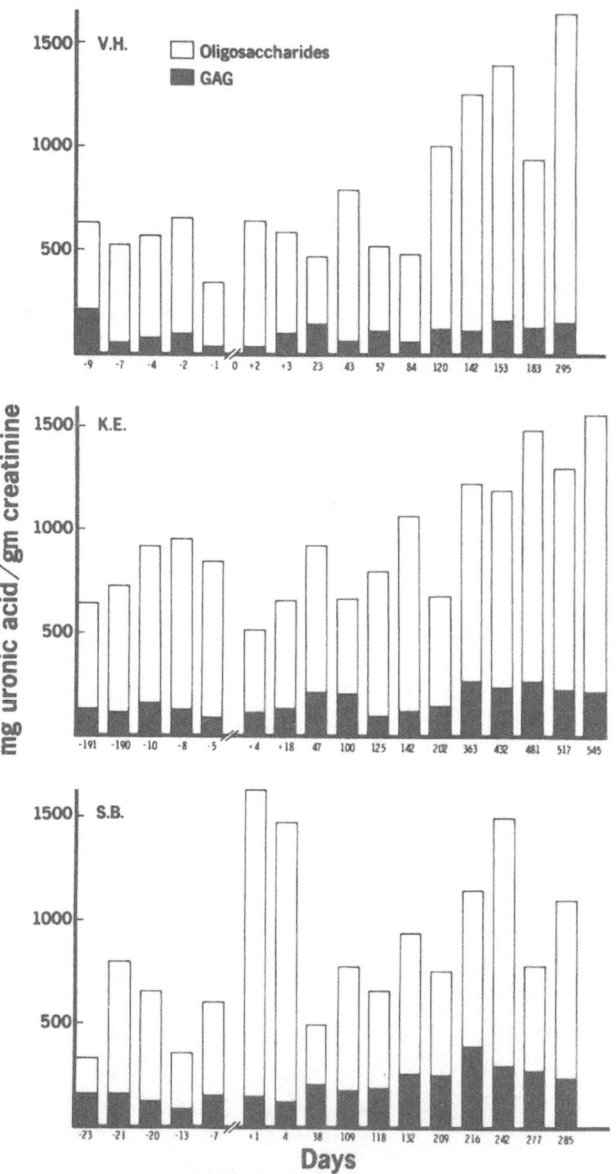

Figure 8.2 Total excretion (mg/g creatinine) of uronic acid in three patients with Sanfilippo A syndrome before and after transplant. Days before transplant are indicated by negative numbers and after transplant by positive numbers

TABLE 8.1 Excretion of uronic acid (mg/24 h) before and after transplant in three patients with Hunter's syndrome

Patient	Before transplant	After transplant	%Change
1	204 ± 31 (11)	350 ± 39 (44)	+72
2	203 ± 42 (6)	143 ± 20 (15)	−30
3	157 ± 8 (8)	186 ± 22 (22)	+19

Values are means ± SE. Number of analyses shown in parentheses

TABLE 8.2 Excretion of uronic acid (mg/g creatinine) before and after transplant in three patients with Sanfilippo A syndrome

Patient	Glycosaminoglycans			Oligosaccharides		
	Before transplant	After transplant	%Change	Before transplant	After transplant	%Change
1	80 ± 45 (6)	98 ± 11 (15)	+23	382 ± 82 (6)	701 ± 94 (15)	+84
2	137 ± 13 (8)	154 ± 10 (25)	+12	362 ± 48 (8)	648 ± 54 (34)	+ 3
3	122 ± 12 (10)	215 ± 18 (16)	+76	432 ± 126 (10)	713 ± 102 (14)	+65

Values are means ± SE. Number of analyses shown in parentheses

prepared from chondroitin sulphate after reaction with chondroitin ABC lyase (EC 4.2.2.4) followed by chondro-4-sulphatase (EC 3.1.6.9). In addition, a small excluded fraction was eluted with the void volume. Component I contained a higher proportion of glucosamine than the other fractions, amounting to some 75% of the total hexosamine present. Hexosamine analysis of components II and III showed that they contained 70 and 60% glucosamine, respectively, while fraction IV contained only trace amounts of hexosamine.

The elution profiles of oligosaccharides separated from samples taken prior to transplant contained a larger proportion of the higher molecular weight oligosaccharides than normal age-matched control urine. After transplant the relative proportions of higher molecular weight oligosaccharides decreased and the proportion of the monosaccharide fraction increased, so that the elution profiles of samples taken some 6–12 months after transplant closely resembled those of normal controls.

Oligosacharides from patients with Sanfilippo A disease were separated into five fractions by chromatography on Bio-Gel P2 (Figure 8.4) plus an unresolved component which eluted with the void volume. As with the

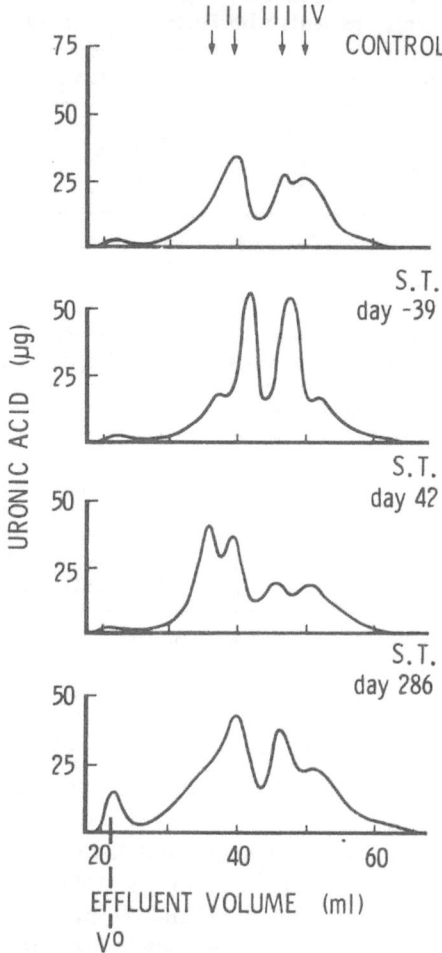

Figure 8.3 Typical elution profiles of oligosaccharides separated on Bio-Gel P-2 from urine samples of a patient with Hunter's syndrome. Samples taken before transplant, early and late post-transplant are shown with the profile of an age-matched control for comparison

Hunter patients, samples taken before transplant contained a much higher proportion of oligosaccharides of larger hydrodynamic size than those collected after treatment. When the peak areas of each fraction separated after transplant were expressed as a percentage of total uronic acid eluted

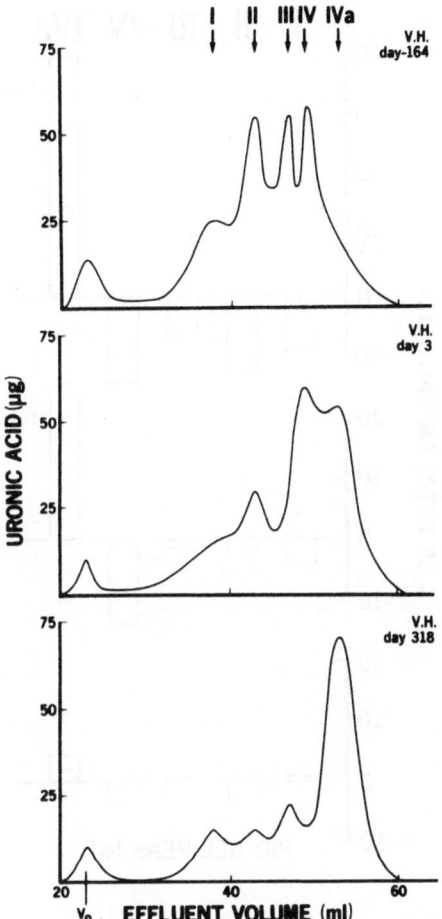

Figure 8.4 Typical elution profiles of oligosaccharides separated on Bio-Gel P-2 from urine samples of a patient with Sanifilippo A syndrome. A sample taken before transplant is shown with early and late post-transplant samples for comparison

and compared with the corresponding fractions eluted before transplant, a clear reduction in the relative proportions of fractions I–IV was visible with an accompanying marked increase in fraction IVa (Figure 8.5).

Since both Hunter and Sanfilippo A diseases are characterized by deficiences in sulphatase enzymes, the oligosaccharide fractions separated on Bio-Gel P2 were examined for changes in their sulphate contents subsequent to transplant. Preliminary analyses indicated that fraction I

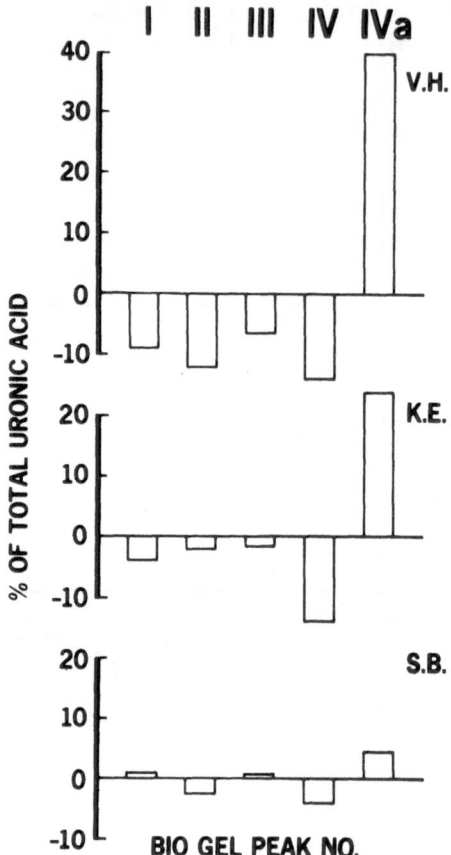

Figure 8.5 Mean percentage difference (uronic acid to total uronic acid) of oligosaccharide fractions eluted from Bio-Gel P-2 in three patients with Sanfillippo A syndrome

separated from Hunter patients before transplant was more heavily sulphated than the other fractions, and that this fraction became most heavily labelled when fibroblasts from Hunter patients were incubated with [^{35}S]-sulphate. Samples of fraction I, isolated from a number of different 24 h urine collections taken before and after transplant were, therefore, pooled and their sulphate to uronic-acid ratios determined. As can be seen from Table 8.4 mean ratios were double those of age matched controls before transplant, but decreased to normal levels after transplant in all three patients and were maintained at this lower level throughout the

TABLE 8.3 Sulphate to uronic acid molar ratios in samples of fraction I separated by chromatography on Bio-gel P-2 from three patients with Hunter's syndrome

Patient	Before transplant	After transplant
1	2.1 (3)	1.3 (7)
2	2.1 (3)	0.9 (2)
3	1.6 (6)	0.9 (4)
Control	1.0 (2)	—

Values are means $\pm$ SE. Number of analyses shown in parentheses

period of observation. Similarly, samples of fraction III separated from the urines of Sanfilippo A patients were pooled prior to determination of their sulphamino/hexosamine ratios, since the larger oligosaccharides in fractions I and II separated after transplant contained too little material for accurate analyses to be made. The sulphamino content of fraction III decreased in two of the three patients following transplant, but remained unchanged in the third case (Table 8.3).

TABLE 8.4 Sulphamino to hexosamine molar ratios in samples of fraction III separated by chromatography on Bio-gel P-2 from three patients with Sanfilippo A syndrome

Patient	Before transplant	After transplant
1	0.64	0.29
2	0.53	0.35
3	0.44	0.50

Four samples from each group were pooled prior to analysis

Urinary excretion of the previously deficient α-L-idurono-2-sulphate sulphatase and glucosamine-N-sulphatase enzymes was measured as 'corrective factors' by their ability to reduce [^{35}S]-sulphate incorporation in the patients' own fibroblasts (cultured before transplant) to normal levels. Very low levels of corrective-factor activity were present in the urine of the three Hunter patients before transplant (Figure 8.6), but after transplant fluctuating, although higher, levels continued to be recorded.

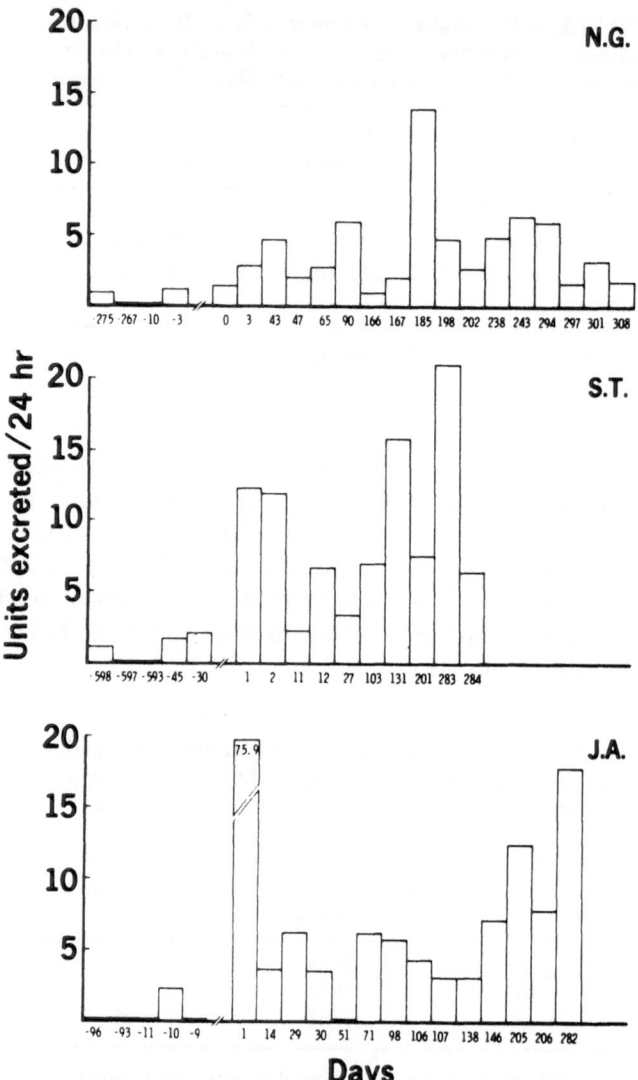

Figure 8.6   Amount of corrective factor (units/24 h) isolated from the urine of three patients with Hunter's syndrome before and after transplant. Samples taken before transplant are indicated by negative numbers and after transplant by positive numbers

Mean output of Hunter corrective factor rose from about 1 % of control levels before transplant to about 10 % afterwards (Table 8.5). Similarly, excretion of corrective factor in Sanfilippo patients rose from only 10 % of age-matched control values before treatment to average more than 50 % of normal following transplant (Figure 8.7, Table 8.6).

TABLE 8.5   Excretion of corrective factor (units/24 h) before and after transplant in three patients with Hunter's syndrome

Patient	Before transplant	After transplant	Control
1	0.5 ±0.1 (9)	4.0 ±0.8 (15)	45.1 (5)
2	0.5 ±0.2 (5)	5.0 ±1.6 (15)	49.0 (4)
3	0.5 ±0.2 (5)	6.3 ±1.3 (13)	59.8 (3)

Values are means ±SE. Number of analyses shown in parentheses

Direct measurements of the α-L-idurono-2-sulphate sulphatase activity in serum samples taken from each transplanted Hunter patient 2 years or more after treatment were made, using a disulphated disaccharide as substrate. Although mean activity in serum was very low, at a little over 1 % of control values, it was more than three times greater than the activity in sera from untreated Hunter patients (Table 8.7). Again when the α-L-idurono-2-sulphate sulphatase activity in leukocytes from two of the transplanted patients was determined, although it was only 4 % of control values, nevertheless activity was almost 10 times greater than that in leukocytes from untreated patients.

DISCUSSION

The elevated output of both Hunter and Sanfilippo type A corrective factors and the increase in the level of α-L-idurono-2-sulphate sulphatase measured directly in serum from Hunter patients suggests that transplanted fibroblasts can continue to release lysosomal enzymes over a period of many months. The increase in α-L-idurono-2-sulphate sulphatase in leukocytes from two of the transplanted patients indicates that at least some of this enzyme can be taken up by other cells.

Although the amounts of these deficient enzymes present in serum and leukocytes and excreted in urine after transplant amounted to only a small percentage of normal levels, they were sufficient to induce measureable change in mobilization and catabolism of stored GAG in both groups of patients. This was evidenced by the increased excretion of both GAG and oligosaccharides derived from them and by the reduction in the relative

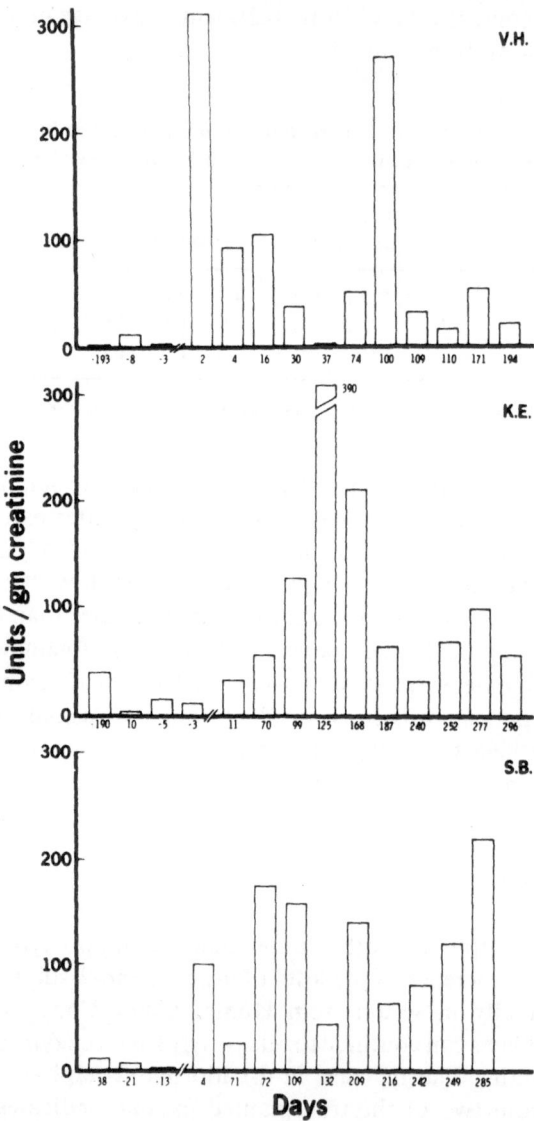

Figure 8.7 Amount of corrective factor (units/mg creatinine) isolated from the urines of 3 patients with Sanfilippo A syndrome before and after transplant. Samples taken before transplant are indicated by negative numbers and after transplant by positive numbers.

proportions of higher-molecular-weight oligosaccharides separated on Bio-Gel P2. Further direct evidence for an increase in catabolism after transplant was provided by the decrease in total sulphate content of the

TABLE 8.6   Excretion of corrective factor (units/g creatinine) before and after transplant in three patients with Sanfilippo A syndrome

Patient	Before transplant	After transplant
1	34 ±31 (4)	100 ±30 (12)
2	15 ± 8 (4)	86 ±25 (15)
3	5 ± 3 (3)	104 ±20 (11)
Control	178 ±31 (3)	—

Values are means ±SE. Number of analyses shown in parentheses

TABLE 8.7   The activity of iduronate-2-sulphate sulphatase in sera and leukocytes from transplanted Hunter patients, untreated patients and normal controls

	Untreated patients	Treated patients	Normal controls
Serum	0.11 ±0.01 (6)	0.37 ±0.04 (3)	27.1 ±2.6 (7)
Leukocytes	0.24 ±0.05 (2)	2.2 ±0 (2)	53.5 ±4.6 (6)

Values are means ±SE (nmol substrate hydrolysed/mg protein per h). Number of samples shown in parentheses. Final substrate concentration was 2 mmol/l.

oligosaccharide fractions from patients with Hunter syndrome and the N-sulphate content of oligosaccharides from patients with Sanfilippo A syndrome.

Since the patients and their donors were fully HLA histocompatible, and immunosuppressive therapy was continued for a considerable period after transplant, we can assume that the transplanted fibroblasts remained viable for many months or even years. During this time they could continue to function normally and to produce lysosomal enzymes. It is known that normal fibroblasts cultured *in vitro* release lysosomal enzymes which can be taken up by deficient fibroblasts and correct their abnormally high [^{35}S]-sulphate incorporation[19, 24, 41]. Furthermore, active endocytosis of externally added enzymes such as β-glucuronidase, α-L-iduronidase and α-N-acetyl hexosaminidase[21,42,43] by deficient fibroblasts is well documented. If the externally added enzyme contains sufficient of the so-called high uptake forms, then normal intracellular enzyme levels can be restored. For example, we have found (Dean *et al.*, unpublished) that β-glucuronidase released by some fibroblast cell lines contains a large proportion of high-uptake enzyme which can be actively endocytosed by β-glucuronidase deficient fibroblasts until their internal β-glucuronidase activity reaches normal levels. If enzyme release from transplanted cells and uptake by deficient cells continues *in vivo*, then this would explain the increases in catabolism of stored GAG that we observed.

Transfer of lysosomal enzymes from normal donor cells to deficient recipients is known to take place *in vivo* in other situations. For example Feder[44] has shown transfer of β-glucuronidase from normal to deficient cells in mosaic tissues from mice derived by fusion of normal and β-glucuronidase-deficient embryos. These include cells in the lymphatic system, nervous tissue and connective tissues. Again, transfer of α-mannosidase from normal to deficient lymphocytes has been demonstrated *in vivo* in chimeric twin calves[45]. It is assumed that this exchange takes place by release of enzyme from normal cells followed by uptake from the extracellular environment in a manner analogous to that seen *in vitro* and could also explain the higher levels of α-L-idurono-2-sulphate sulphatase activity seen in lymphocytes from Hunter patients who received fibroblast transplants than in untreated Hunter patients.

We do not know for how long HLA identical fibroblasts can survive in the host after transplantation, but the presence of increased urinary corrective factors and circulating enzyme for several years following a single transplant suggests that they can exist for at least this length at time. Although the increase in α-L-idurono-2-sulphate sulphatase seen after fibroblast transplant was small, this may be enough to have a disporportionately large effect on GAG catabolism, since in other types of mucopolysaccharidosis, e.g. Sanfilippo type B (α-*N*-acetyl glucosaminidase deficiency) a very small percentage increase in intracellular enzyme levels can produce a large decrease in the abnormally high $[^{35}S]$-sulphate incorporation[24]. Since normal fibroblasts can correct the abnormal catabolism in cells from patients with types of inherited enzyme deficiencies other than the mucopolysaccharidoses, e.g. metachromatic leuko-dystrophy[46] and α-mannosidosis[47], fibroblast transplantation may be of more general application in the treatment of a wide range of lysosomal deficiency diseases.

Acknowledgements

The authors gratefully acknowledge the technical assistance of Miss C. Östlund.

References

1. Garrod, A. E. (1908). Inborn errors of metabolism. Croonian Lectures. *Lancet*, **2**, 1
2. Stanbury, J. B., Wyngaarden, J. B. and Fredrickson, D. S. (1978). *The Metabolic Basis of Inherited Disease*, p. 14. (NewYork: McGraw Hill)
3. Neuwelt, E., Stumpf, D., Austin, J. and Kohler, P. (1971). A monospecific antibody to human sulphatase A. *Biochim. Biophys. Acta*, **236**, 333
4. Mersmann, G. and Buddecke, E. (1977). Evidence from mannosidosis fibroblasts cross reacting with anti-acidic α-mannosidase antibodies. *FEBS Lett.*, **73**, 123
5. Bell, C. E. Jr., Sly, W. S. and Brot, F. E. (1977). Human β-glucuronidase deficiency mucopolysaccharidosis: identification of cross-reactive antigen in cultured fibroblasts of deficient patients by primary enzyme immunoassay, *J. Clin. Invest.*, **59**, 97
6. Di Ferrante, N., Nichols, B., Donnelly, P. V., Neri, G., Hrgovcic, R. and Berglund, R. K. (1971). Induced degradation of glycosaminoglycans in Hurler's and Hunter's syndromes by plasma infusion. *Proc. Natl. Acad. Sci. USA*, **68**, 303
7. Dean, M. F., Benson, P. F. and Muir, H. (1973) Mobilisation of glycosaminoglycans by plasma infusions in mucopolysaccharidosis type III – Two types of response. *Nature (London) New Biol.*, **243**, 143.
8. Dean, M .F. Benson, P. F. and Muir, H. (1975). Differing patterns of glycosaminoglycan mobilisation in Sanfilippo and Hunter Syndromes following infusion of normal plasma. In *Proceedings of the 3rd International Congress for the Scientific Study of Mental Deficiency*, p. 270. (The Hague: International Association for the Scientific Study of Mental Deficiency)
9. Knudson, A. G., Di Ferrante, N. and Curtis, J. E. (1971). Effect of leucocyte transfusion in a child with type II mucopolysaccharidosis. *Proc. Natl. Acad. Sci. USA*, **68**, 1738
10. Moser, H. W., O'Brien, J. S., Atkins, L., Fuller, T. C., Keiman, A., Janowska, S., Russell, P. F., Bartsocas, C. S., Cosimi, B. and Dulaney, J. T. (1974). Infusion of normal HLA identical lymphocytes in Sanfilippo disease type B. *Arch. Neurol.*, **31**, 329
11. Brady, R. O., Tallman, J. F., Johnson, W. G., Gal, A. E., Leahy, W. R., Quick, J. M. and Dekaban, A. S. (1973). Replacement thrapy for inherited enzyme deficiency. Use of purified ceramidetrihexosidase in Fabry's disease. *N. Engl. J. Med.*, **289**, 9
12. Gregoriadis, G. (1979). Liposomes. In Gregoriadis, G. (ed.) *Drug Carriers in Biology and Medicine*, pp. 287–341 (London: Academic Press)
13. Clarke, J. T. R., Guttman, R. D., Wolfe, L. S., Beaudoin, J. G. and Morehouse, D. D. (1972). Enzyme replacement therapy by renal allotransplantation in Fabry's disease. *N. Engl. J. Med.*, **287**, 1215
14. Philippart, M., Franklin, S. S. and Gordon, A. (1972). Reversal of an inborn sphingolipidosis (Fabry's disease) by kidney transplantation. *Ann. Int. Med.*, **77**, 195
15. Dean, M. F., Muir, H. Benson, P. F., Button, L. R. Batchelor, J. P. and Bewick, M. (1975). Increased breakdown of glycosaminoglycans and in-

creased appearance of corrective enzyme after skin transplants in Hunter Syndrome. *Nature (London)*, **257**, 609

16. Dean, M. F., Stevens, R. L., Muir, H., Benson, P. F., Button, L. R., Anderson, R. L., Boylston, A. and Mowbray, J. (1979). Enzyme replacement therapy by fibroblast transplantation. Long-term biochemical study in 3 cases of Hunter's Syndrome. *J. Clin. Invest.*, **63**, 138

17. Dean, M. F., Muir, H., Benson, P. F., Button, L. R. (1980). Enzyme replacement therapy in the Mucopolysaccharidoses by fibroblast transplantation. In *Birth Defects*. Original Article Series Vol. XVI, No. 1, p. 445 (USA: March of Dimes Birth Defects Foundation)

18. Gibbs, D. A., Spellacy, E., Roberts, A. E. and Watts, R. W. E. (1980). The treatment of lysosomal storage diseases by fibroblast transplantation: Some preliminary observations. In *Birth Defects:* Original Article Series Vol. XVI, No. 1, p. 457 (USA: March of Dimes Birth Defects Foundation)

19. von Figura, K., and Kresse, H. (1974). Quantitative aspects of pinocytosis and the intracellular fate of *N*-acetyl-α-D-glucosaminidase in Sanfilippo B fibroblasts. *J. Clin. Invest.*, **53**, 85

20. Sando, G. N. and Neufeld, E. F. (1977). Recognition and receptor mediated uptake of a lysosomal enzyme, α-L-iduronidase by cultured human fibroblasts. *Cell*, **12**, 619

21. Ullrich, K., Mersmann, G., Weber, E. and von Figura, K. (1978). Evidence for lysosomal enzyme recognition by human fibroblasts via a phosphorylated carbohydrate moiety. *Biochem. J.*, **170**, 643

22. Rome, L. H., Garvin, A. J., Allietta, M. M. and Neufeld, E. F. (1979). Two species of lysosomal organelles in cultured human fibroblasts. *Cell*, **17**, 143

23. Dean, M. F., Benson, P. F. and Muir, H. (1975). The effect of dextran infusions on glycosaminoglycan excretion in the Sanfilippo Syndrome. *Devel. Med. Child. Neurol.*, **17**, 47

24. O'Brien, J. S., Miller, A. L., Loverde, A. W. and Veath, M. L. (1973). Sanfilippo disease type B: Enzyme replacement and metabolic correction in cultured fibroblasts. *Science*, **187**, 753

25. Barton, R. W. and Neufeld, E. F. (1971). The Hurler corrective factor: Purification and some properties. *J. Biol. Chem.*, **246**, 7773

26. Kresse, H. and Neufeld, E. F. (1972). The Sanfilippo A corrective factor: Purification and mode of action. *J. Biol Chem.*, **247**, 2164

27. Cantz, M., Chrambach, A., Bach, G. and Neufeld, E. F. (1i972). The Hunter corrective factor: Purification and preliminary characterisation. *J. Biol. Chem.*, **247**, 5456

28. Bach, G. and Liebmann-Eisenberg, A. (1979) Intracellular localization of exogenous β-glucuronidase in cultured skin fibroblasts. *Eur. J. Biochem.*, **96**, 613

29. Fratantoni, J. C., Hall, C. W. and Neufeld, E. F. (1968). Hurler and Hunter Syndromes. Mutual corrections of the defect in cultured fibroblasts. *Science (Wash.)*, **162**, 500

30. Fratantoni, J. C., Hall, C. W. and Neufeld, E. F. (1969). The defect in Hurler and Hunter Syndromes. II Deficiency of specific factors involved in mucopolysaccharide degradation. *Proc. Natl. Acad. Sci. USA*, **64**, 360

31. Rome, L. H., Garvin, A. J., Allietta, M. M. and Neufeld, E. F. (1979). Two species of lysosomal organelles in cultured human fibroblasts. *Cell*, **17**, 143

32. McKusick, V. A. (1972). *Heritable Disorders of Connective tissues*, p. 556. (St. Louis: Mosby)
33. Kresse, H. (1973). Mucopolysaccharidosis IIIA (Sanfilippo A Disease): A deficiency of a heparin sulphamidase in skin fibroblasts and leucocytes. *Biochem. Biophys. Res. Commun.*, **54**, 1111
34. Bach, G., Eisenberg, F. Jr., Cantz, M. and Neufeld, E. F (1973). The defect in the Hunter Syndrome: Deficiency of sulphoiduronate sulphatase. *Proc. Natl. Acad. Sci. USA*, **70**, 2134
35. Bitter, T. and Muir, H. (1962). A modified uronic acid carbazole reaction. *Anal. Biochem.*, **4**, 330
36. Kraan, J. and Muir, H. (1957). The determination of glucosamine. *Biochem. J.*, **66**, 55
37. Ginsberg, L. C. and Di Ferrante, N. (1977). Sensitive method for the determination of ester sulphate in biological systems. *Biochem. Med.*, **17**, 80
38. Lagunoff, D. and Warren, G. (1962). Determination of 2-deoxy-2-sulphaminohexose content of mucopolysaccharides. *Arch. Biochem. Biophys.*, **99**, 396
39. Lim, T. W., Leder, I. G., Bach, G. and Neufeld, E. F. (1974). Assay for iduronate sulphatase. *Carbohydr. Res.*, **37**, 103
40. Liebaers, I. and Neufeld, E. F. (1976). Iduronate sulphatase activity in serum, lymphocytes and fibroblasts – simplified diagnosis of the Hunter Syndrome, *Pediatr. Res.*, **10**, 733
41. Bach, G., Friedmann, R., Weismann, B. and Neufeld, E. F. (1972). The defect in Hurler and Scheie Syndromes. Deficiency of α-L-iduronidase. *Proc. Natl. Acad. Sci. USA*, **69**, 2084
42. Kaplan, A., Achord, D. T. and Sly, W. S. (1977). Phosphohexosyl components of a lysosomal enzyme are recognised by pinocytosis receptors on human fibroblasts. *Proc. Natl. Acad. Sci. USA.*, **74**, 2026
43. Sando, G. N. and Neufeld, E. F. (1977). Recognition and receptor mediated uptake of a lysosomal enzyme, α-L-iduronidase by cultured human fibroblasts. *Cell*, **12**, 619
44. Feder, N. (1976). Solitary cells and enzyme exchange in tetraparental mice. *Nature (London)*, **263**, 66
45. Jolly, R. D., Thompson, K. G., Murphy, C. E., Manktelow, B. W., Bruere, A. M. and Winchester, B. G. (1976). Enzyme replacement therapy – an experiment in nature in a clinical mannosidosis calf. *Pediatr. Res.*, **10**, 219
46. Kihara, H., Porter, M. and Fluharty, A. (1973). In *Birth Defects*, Original Article Series, Vol. 9, pp. 19 – 26, National Foundation March of Dimes. (New York: Williams and Wilkins)
47. Mersmann, G. and Buddecke, E. (1976). Storage of Mannose containing material in cultured human mannosidosis cells and metabolic correction by pig kidney α-mannosidase. *Hoppe-Seyler's Z. Physiol. Chem.*, **357**, 641

9

Artificial cell-encapsulated enzymes and adsorbents in congenital metabolic disorders
T. M. S. Chang

INTRODUCTION

The present status of artificial cell-encapsulated enzymes and adsorbents and the feasibility of using them for removing or converting accumulated metabolites will be discussed. For the present discussion it is convenient to divide congenital metabolic disorders[1,2] into two major groups: (1) those with extracellular or intracellular accumulation of metabolites, which might be helped by the removal of the metabolites from the extracellular fluid; and (2) those with intracellular accumulation of metabolites which cannot be removed by extracellular means.

PRINCIPLE OF ARTIFICIAL CELLS

Encapsulated enzymes and adsorbents are based on the principle of using artificial cells[3,4]. Artificial cells are designed to fulfil some of the simpler properties of biological cells. For instance, a spherical ultrathin membrane of cellular dimension could contain enzymes or adsorbents. The membrane could be designed in such a way that the enclosed enzymes or adsorbents do not leak out, but substrates and other metabolites can equilibrate rapidly across the membrane to be acted on by the enclosed enzyme or adsorbent. This would eliminate problems with immunological response to the encapsulated enzyme. In the case of adsorbent it would avoid problems of embolism and also problems of blood incompatibility with the adsorbent.

Encapsulated adsorbents

One of the encapsulated adsorbents which has been used extensively is activated charcoal. Activated charcoal itself is not blood compatible and results in adverse effects on blood cells, especially platelets. Furthermore, activated charcoal releases charcoal powder, resulting in emboli. By a process of direct coating with collodion followed by a second coating of human albumin, activated charcoal can be encapsulated within an ultrathin membrane, creating a blood compatible adsorbent system[5]. In this form the cellulose nitrate prevents charcoal powder from forming emboli and the human albumin coating results in a blood compatible surface. The albumin on the membrane also facilitates the transport of loosely albumin-bound molecules. A number of commercial modifications of this approach are available[6]. Most commercial models still have not reached the effectiveness and blood compatibility of the albumin–collodion laboratory model.

The encapsulated activated-charcoal system has been available for a number of years[7] and is now used in routine treatment of certain types of acute drug intoxication[6], including its recent use in the treatment of severe theophylline intoxication in children[8]. This approach has also been used for the treatment of patients with chronic renal failure[6]. It is effective in removing most of the uraemic metabolites and results in uraemic patients becoming symptom-free. By combining a small ultrafiltrator, water and salt can also be removed and with the development of a urea removal system, this approach may result in the most miniaturized artificial kidney available. It has also been shown that haemoperfusion resulted in the recovery of consciousness in grade IV hepatic coma patients[9,10]. Haemoperfusion has been used to remove phenols, mercaptans, peptides and amino acids from these patients. Although haemoperfusion resulted in recovery from grade IV hepatic coma, the effect on long-term recovery and survival in fulminant hepatic failure is not yet established. Animal studies have indicated that the timing of treatment is important, treatment given in the earlier grades of coma being statistically more effective[11]. Clinical trials are being continued with this early treatment approach.

Encapsulated enzymes

Enzyme has been enclosed within spherical ultrathin semipermeable membranes of cellular dimension[3,4]. The enzyme does not leak out to cause immunological or hypersensitivity reactions but substrate can diffuse rapidly across the membrane to be acted on by the enclosed enzyme. Protein and cells outside cannot enter the artificial cell to come into contact with the encapsulated enzyme. Studies have indicated that encapsulated enzymes are significantly more stable than free enzyme, both *in vitro* or *in vivo*[3,4,12]. A large number of synthetic membranes of nylon, cellulose nitrate, cellulose acetate, silicone rubber and other polymer membranes have been used to encapsulate the enzyme. Biological membranes which have been used include protein cross-linked, lipid, lipid–protein complex, lipid–polymer, liposome, and red blood-cell membranes. Biodegradable membranes used include the biological membranes mentioned and also synthetic membranes like polylactic-acid polymer membrane. Earlier studies show that encapsulated enzymes act effectively *in vivo*[3,4]. This has been demonstrated in substrate-dependent tumours using microencapsulated asparaginase[13], and in congenital acatalasaemia in mice using microencapsulated catalase[14,15].

For introduction into cells, studies have been carried out using liposome-[16,17] and erythrocyte-entrapped enzymes[18,19]. These will be discussed under 'Intracellular Actions'.

REMOVAL OF METABOLITES FROM EXTRACELLULAR COMPARTMENT

Metabolites accumulated through congenital metabolic disorders can sometimes be removed from the extracellular compartment[1,2]. The technology of encapsulated adsorbent haemoperfusion has been demonstrated to be effective in removing drugs and accumulated metabolites in patients with acute intoxication, uraemia, and liver failure[6,19–21]. Encapsulated enzymes have also been shown to be effective in laboratory studies involving model congenital metabolic disorders. However, these technologies have not yet been tried in congenital metabolic disorders in humans for removal of extracellular metabolites.

Encapsulated adsorbents for haemoperfusion

It has already been demonstrated that microencapsulated activated charcoal can effectively remove uric acid, phenolic compounds, some organic acids, galactose, mercaptans, some amino acids, various peptide molecules, and other metabolites[6,19-21]. Thus in studies of patients with chronic renal failure it has been demonstrated that after one pass through the column at a blood flow rate of 300 ml/min, nearly all uric acid in the blood had been removed[6,19]. Studies in animals using galactose have shown that haemoperfusion through the albumin–collodion activated charcoal column can remove a significant amount of galactose from the extracellular compartment[22]. Other studies also demonstrated effective removal of phenolic compounds[23], mercaptans[24], and some amino acids[25]. In some hereditary metabolic disorders the metabolites which require removal may accumulate in the extracellular space or may be present in the intracellular compartment but in equilibrium with the extracellular compartment. In such cases if these metabolites can be adsorbed by activated charcoal, then a technology is already available for immediate application. The use of artificial cells containing other types of adsorbents is being investigated, e.g. resins for the removal of bilirubin and other types of waste metabolites[20,21].

Use of encapsulated enzymes for acting on metabolities in the extracellular compartment

The first study demonstrating the use of microencapsulated enzymes for experimental therapy in congenital enzyme deficiencies involved the use of encapsulated catalase in acatalasaemic mice[14,15]. In this study it was shown that microencapsulated catalase effectively supplemented the defective enzyme in the acatalasaemic mice and protected the animals from peroxides. It was also demonstrated that repeated injection of microencapsulated catalase did not result in immunological reactions. The same amount of free enzyme injected repeatedly resulted in an immunological reaction and severe anaphalactic shock. Microencapsulated enzyme could either be injected, or retained in extracorporeal chambers perfused by peritoneal fluid or by blood. In the extracorporeal approach the artificial cells do not enter the body at any time and can be discarded when their function has been performed. Microencapsulation of uricase can be used for the conversion of uric acid[3]. Tyrosinase has also been microencapsulated and found to act effectively *in vitro* and *in vivo* on tyrosine[26,27]. Thus, microencapsulated tyrosinase acts effectively in an extracorporeal shunt system to lower blood tyrosine[27]. Further studies involve the use of multienzyme systems with sequential functions. For instance artificial cells, each containing a multienzyme system of glutamate dehydrogenase, glucose dehydrogenase, and glutamate-alanine transaminase have been studied[28,29]. In this way, ammonia can be converted into glutamic acid by glutamate dehydrogenase. The required cofactor NADH is recycled by the enclosed glucose dehydrogenase and glucose present in the blood. The glutamic acid formed can be changed into other amino acids by transaminase located in the same artificial cell. After transamination, the α-ketoglutarate formed can be recycled back to combine with ammonia. It should be possible to adapt into this multienzyme system various compounds which combine with glutamine or glycine to form compounds which can be excreted easily by the kidney[30].

INTRACELLULAR ACTION OF ENZYMES AND ADSORBENTS

The selective introduction of enzymes or other agents into the cell is a much more difficult problem. Unfortunately a large number of congenital metabolic disorders belong to the group[1,2] in which the accumulated metabolite is located intracellularly and in order to be effective the enzyme or other agent has to be introduced into the cell[31], e.g. the various types of storage disease. Liposome, which is a modification of the microencapsulated enzyme approach, has been used most extensively for introduction into cells[16,17]. Studies on liposome entrapment of enzymes have been carried out by a number of centres, and reviews on this topic are available[17,32].

Intravenously injected liposomes containing enzyme can be transported across cell membranes and into lysosomes[17,32]. There are indications that this results in enzymatic action on the accumulated substrates[32]. In a preliminary clinical trial, liposomes containing β-glucosidase were injected intravenously into patients with Gaucher's disease[33]. There was some initial decrease in liver size but the results are not yet conclusive. Liposome is an excellent adjuvant and studies seem to indicate that repeated injection can result in some forms of immunological reaction[34]. Another approach being tested is the use of erythrocyte-entrapped enzyme[18]. In this approach, by a process of reverse haemolysis, enzyme can be introduced into the red blood cell[18]. Theoretically, autologous erythrocytes carrying enzyme should be immunologically compatible and this method is the subject of current research[18]. Other studies being carried out involve the linkage of enzymes to different carrier molecules which allows them to be more selectively located[32]. Extensive research is being carried out, but as outlined in a number of reviews an acceptable system has not yet been developed[1,12,17,32,34].

SUMMARY

Encapsulated adsorbent, especially encapsulated charcoal, has already been used clinically in patients in the treatment of acute intoxication, uraemia, liver failure, and other conditions. This system has been demonstrated to function safely and effectively in removing certain drugs or waste metabolites from the circulation of the patient. It has also been demonstrated in laboratory studies that some metabolites which accumulate in certain congenital metabolic disorders can also be removed by the encapsulated charcoal system. Therefore this technology is now available, although clinical testing in patients with congenital metabolic disorders has not yet been carried out. Encapsulated enzymes have been tested and found to be effective in removing substrates from extracellular compartments in animal models of congenital metabolic disorders, e.g. acatalasaemia. Techniques for the introduction of enzymes or agents into the intracellular compartment or intracellular organelles are now being developed.

References

1. Scriver, C. R. (1977). A biomedical view of enzyme replacement strategies in genetic disease. In Chang, T. M. S. (ed.) *Biomedical Applications of Immobilized Enzymes and Proteins*, Vol. I, pp. 121–146. (New York: Plenum Press)
2. Desnick, R. J., Bernlohr, R. W. and Krivit, W. (1973). *Enzyme Therapy in Genetic Diseases*, p. 236. (Baltimore: Williams & Wilkins)
3. Chang, T. M. S. (1964). Semipermeable microcapsules. *Science*, **146**, 524
4. Chang, T. M. S. (1972). *Artificial Cells*, p. 212. (Springfield: Thomas)
5. Chang, T. M. S. (1969). Removal of endogenous and exogenous toxins by a microencapsulated absorbent. *Can. J. Physiol. Pharmacol.*, **47**, 1043
6. Chang, T. M. S. (1977). Criteria, evaluation, and perspectives of various microencapsulated charcoal hemoperfusion systems. *J. Dial. Transpl.*, **6**, 50
7. Chang, T. M. S., Coffey, J. F., Barre, P., Gonda, A., Dirks, J. H., Levy, M. and Lister, C. (1973). Microcapsule artificial kidney: Treatment of patients with acute drug intoxication. *Can. Med. Assoc. J.*, **108**, 429

8. Chang, T. M. S., Espinosa-Melendez, E., Francoeur, T. E. and Eade, N. (1980). Albumin-collodion activated charcoal hemoperfusion in the treatment of severe theophylline intoxication in a 3-year-old patient. *Pediatrics*, **65**, 811

9. Chang, T. M. S. (1972). Haemoperfusions over microencapsulated adsorbent in a patient with hepatic coma. *Lancet*, **2**, 1371

10. Gazzard, B. G., Weston, M. H., Murray-Lyon, I. M., Flax, H., Record, C. O., Portman, B., Langley, P. G., Dunlop, E. H., Mellon, P. J., Ward, M. D. and William, S. R. (1974). Charcoal hemoperfusion in the treatment of fulminating hepatic failure. *Lancet*, **1**, 1301

11. Chang, T. M. S., Lister, C., Chirito, E., O'Keefe, P. and Resurreccion, E. (1978). Effects of hemoperfusion rate and time of initiation of ACAC charcoal hemoperfusion on the survival of fulminant hepatic failure rats. *Trans. Am. Soc. Artif. Intern. Organs*, **24**, 243

12. Chang, T. M. S. (1977). *Biomedical Applications of Immobilized Enzymes and Proteins*. Vols. I and II, p. 415. (New York: Plenum Press)

13. Chang, T. M. S. (1971). The in vivo effects of semipermeable microcapsules containing L-asparaginase on 6C3HED lymphosarcoma. *Nature (London)*, **229**, 117

14. Chang, T. M. S. and Poznansky, M. J. (1968). Semipermeable microcapsules containing catalase for enzyme replacement in acatalasemic mice. *Nature (London)*, **218**, 243

15. Poznansky, M. J. and Chang, T. M. S. (1974). Comparison of the enzyme kinetics and immunological properties of catalase immobilized by microencapsulation and catalase in free solution for enzyme replacement. *Biochim. Biophys. Acta*, **334**, 103

16. Gregoriadis, G., Leathwood, P. D. and Ryman, B. E. (1971). Enzyme entrapment in liposomes. *FEBS Lett.*, **14**, 95

17. Gregoriadis, G. (1977). Liposomes as carriers of enzymes and proteins in medicine. In Chang, T. M. S. (ed.). *Biomedical Applications of Immobilized Enzymes and Proteins*, Vol. I, pp. 191–215. (New York: Plenum Press)

18. Ihler, G. and Glew, R. (1977). Enzyme-loaded erythrocytes. In Chang, T. M. S. (ed.) *Biomedical Applications of Immobilized Enzymes and Proteins*, Vol. I, pp. 219–226. (New York: Plenum Press)

19. Chang, T. M. S. (1976). Hemoperfusion alone and in series with ultrafiltration or dialysis for uremia, poisoning and liver failure. *Kidney Int.*, **10**, S305

20. Chang, T. M. S. (1978). *Artificial Kidney, Artificial Liver, and Artificial Cells*, p. 315. (New York: Plenum Press)

21. Sideman, S. and Chang, T. M. S. (1980). *Hemoperfusion: Part I – Artificial Kidney and Liver Support and Detoxification*, p. 473. (Washington: Hemisphere)

22. Nasielski, P. and Chang, T. M. S. (1978). Microencapsulated charcoal hemoperfusion for galactosemia. In Chang, T. M. S. (ed.) *Artificial Kidney, Artificial Liver, and Artificial Cells*, pp. 255–257. (New York: Plenum Press)

23. Kaziuka, E. N. and Chang, T. M. S. (1979). *In-vitro* assessment of the removal of phenols by ACAC hemoperfusion. *Int. J. Artif. Organs*, **2**, 215

24. Chang, T. M. S. and Lister, C. (1980). Analysis of possible toxins in hepatic coma including the removal of mercaptan by albumin-collodion charcoal. *Int. J. Artif. Organs*, **3**, 108

25. Odaka, M., Tabata, Y., Kobayashi, H., Nomura, Y., Soma, H., Hirasawa, H. and Sato, H. (1978). Clinical experience of bead-shaped charcoal hemoperfusion in chronic renal failure and fulminant hepatic failure. In Chang, T. M. S. (ed.). *Artificial Kidney, Artificial Liver, and Artificial Cells*, pp. 79–88. (New York: Plenum Press)

26. Shu, C. D. and Chang, T. M. S. (1980). Tyrosinase immobilized within artificial cells for detoxification in liver failure: I. Preparation and *in-vitro* studies. *Int. J. Artif. Organs*, **3**, 287

27. Shu, C. D. and Chang, T. M. S. (1981). Tyrosinase immobilized within artificial cells for detoxification in liver failure: II. *In-vivo* studies in fulminant hepatic failure rats. *Int. J. Artif. Organs*, **4**, 82

28. Chang, T. M. S. and Malouf, C. (1978). Artificial cells microencapsulated multienzyme system for converting urea and ammonia to amino acid using α-ketoglutarate and glucose as substrate. *Trans. Am. Soc. Artif. Intern. Organs*, **24**, 18

29. Chang, T. M. S., Malouf, C. and Resurreccion, E. (1979). Artificial cells containing multienzyme systems for the sequential conversion of urea into ammonia, glutamate and alanine. *Int. J. Artif. Organs*, **3**, (suppl.), 284

30. Brusilow, S., Tinker, J. and Batshaw, M. L. (1980). Amino acid acylation. *Science*, **207**, 659

31. William, S. L. Y. (1980). Saccharide traffic signals in receptor-mediated endocytosis and transport of acid hydrolases. In Svennerholm, L., Mandel, P., Dreyfus, H. and Urban, P. (eds.) *Structure and Function of the Gangliosides*, pp. 433–441. (New York: Plenum Press)

32. Gregoriadis, G. (1979). *Drug Carriers in Biology and Medicine*, p. 363. (New York: Academic Press)

33. Belchetz, P. E., Braidman, I. P., Crawley, J. C. W. and Gregoriadis, G. (1977). Treatment of Gaucher's disease with liposome-entrapped glucocerebroside: β-glucosidase. *Lancet*, **2**, 116

34. Desnick, R. J. (1980). *Enzyme Therapy in Genetic Diseases*. Vol. 2, p. 544. (New York: Liss)

10

Prospects for enzyme replacement therapy in heritable metabolic disorders

R. O. Brady, J. A. Barranger, P. G. Pentchev, F. S. Furbish and A. E. Gal

INTRODUCTION

Since the discovery that insufficient activity of lipid catabolizing enzymes formed the basis of heritable lipid-storage disorders, a number of therapeutic strategies have been suggested[1]. Approaches to the treatment of such disorders included:

(1) enzyme supplementation by implantation of normal or hybridized (corrected) patient cells;

(2) organ transplantation;

(3) administration of purified enzymes;

(4) activation of catalytically defective mutated enzymes by allosteric agents; and

(5) administration of appropriate messenger RNA or DNA cistrons[2].

It was realized that the implementation of some of these proposals was likely to be exceedingly difficult. Even now, 14 years later, only the first three of these possibilities have been undertaken in humans. The purpose of this chapter is to survey the results that have been obtained in these attempts, and to try to provide reasonable suggestions for improving the therapy of inherited metabolic disorders.

FIBROBLAST IMPLANTATION

Experiences in enzyme replacement through implantation of normal human fibroblasts are detailed by M. F. Dean in this volume[3]; accordingly, this topic will be discussed only briefly here. Several years ago, before procedures to obtain an adequate supply of enzyme for replacement trials in Gaucher's disease were developed, we were confronted with a patient with this disorder in a critical condition. We knew that cultured skin fibroblasts contained glucocerebrosidase, the enzyme that is lacking in patients with Gaucher's disease, in high specific activity[4]. In order to try to provide relief for this patient, we carried out the following assessment of the possible use of these cells in Gaucher's disease. We measured the intracellular glucocerebrosidase activity in skin fibroblasts and then determined the amount of enzymatic activity in the culture medium. Less than 1 % of the catalytic activity was released extracellularly. Our calculations indicated that an exorbitant number of cells would have to be used in order to anticipate any clinical effect. We concluded that fibroblast grafts would not be useful for the treatment of this disorder, and this approach has not been pursued for the treatment of sphingolipid storage diseases.

ORGAN TRANSPLANTATION

Spleen

High among the major sources of sphingolipids that accumulate in peripheral organs of patients with lipid-storage diseases are the glycolipids in the membranes of senescent leukocytes and erythrocytes[5]. Since the spleen is a principal site of erythro- and leukocytorrhexis, and it is a major depot for glucocerebroside that accumulates in patients with Gaucher's disease[6], it seemed logical to consider the possibility of spleen grafts in patients with this disorder. This procedure was performed by Groth and his associates in a patient with Type III Gaucher's disease[7]. No appreciable benefit was observed, and the patient died from a severe imcompatibility reaction several months after the operation.[8] This procedure has not been attempted in other Gaucher patients as far as we are aware.

Liver

This organ is also involved extensively in lipid-storage disorders such as Gaucher's disease[6] and Niemann–Pick disease[9]. Furthermore, it seemed reasonable to consider liver transplantation in Niemann–Pick disease, since this organ was found to have the highest level of sphingomyelinase in a survey of mammalian tissues[10]. This enzyme is lacking in patients with this condition. Liver transplantation has been performed in a patient with Type A Niemann–Pick disease, the classic infantile form of the disorder with central nervous system involvement[11]. The investigators reported that pupillary reflex to light appeared in one eye one month following transplantation, and six months later, the light reflexes became bilateral. There was a regression of 'lipidic infiltration' of the retina, increased facial mobility, disappearance of myoclonia, and increased vigour of the deglutition reflex. No accumulation of sphingomyelin was detected in the grafted organ. Serum sphingomyelinase activity increased and the level of this enzyme in cerebrospinal fluid was in the normal range. Interestingly, there was a progressive increase in sphingomyelinase activity in the grafted liver. One wonders whether this augmentation were due to induction of this enzyme by increased quantities of sphingomyelin presented to the liver for catabolism, as had been noted in earlier loading experiments[12]. Nevertheless, no clinical improvement occurred after the first six months following transplantation, and the patient died of septicaemia approximately two years afterwards.

Kidney

Gaucher's disease   Two attempts of kidney transplantation have been made in patients with Gaucher's disease. The first transplantation was performed on an infant with severe central nervous system involvement; no improvement of the patient's clinical condition was observed[13]. The second procedure, carried out more recently on a ten-year-old patient with a juvenile form of Gaucher's disease, also failed to exert a beneficial effect in the recipient[14]. These negative findings are of considerable significance, since it has been found that kidney tissue contains a fairly high level of glucocerebrosidase activity[15,16]. The inference may be drawn that the grafted kidney did not provide significant quantities of this enzyme to pathologically involved tissues, if in fact any enzyme were released into the circulation at all.

Fabry's disease   Kidney homografts are frequently employed as a life-saving measure in patients with renal destruction. Patients with Fabry's disease usually experience severe impairment of kidney function in their fourth and fifth decades, due to the accumulation of ceramidetrihexoside in this organ[17]. It therefore seemed reasonable to examine the effect of kidney transplantation in patients with this disorder. This procedure has been carried out in several patients and improvement of the signs and symptoms of uraemia has been reported[18, 19]. It is generally agreed that the transplanted kidney does not accumulate ceramidetrihexoside. However, most investigators believe that the accumulation of this metabolite elsewhere in the body is not reduced by kidney allografts[20, 21]. Conflicting reports have appeared concerning an increase of ceramidetrihexosidase activity in the circulation after kidney transplantation. Van den Bergh and coworkers[22] did not observe an increase in this enzyme in the blood of a kidney-graft patient, a finding we also noted in a patient whose course we monitored[23]. The Van den Bergh group made the further important observation that there was no increase of α-galactosidase activity (an indicator of ceramidetrihexosidase through assays with artificial substrates) in the liver of the grafted patient under their surveillance. This important finding provides further evidence that grafted kidneys do not appear to release lipid-catabolizing enzymes into the circulation. It was concluded from these trials that organ allografts provide only limited benefit to patients with heritable metabolic disorders and do not represent a feasible therapeutic approach to the management of these conditions.

ENZYME REPLACEMENT

Metachromatic leukodystrophy

The first investigations of direct enzyme replacement in human lipid-storage disorders were carried out in patients with metachromatic leuko-dystrophy. In the first trial, arylsulphatase A, the deficient enzyme, was partially purified from human urine and injected intrathecally[24]. The recipient had a moderately severe pyrogenic reaction and no clinical improvement was noted. A somewhat similar investigation was carried out by Greene and coworkers using a beef-brain arylsulphatase preparation[25]. Again, fever followed intrathecal injection and no clinical benefit was observed. Both groups of investigators made the relevant observation that intrathecally infused enzyme did not penetrate into the substance of the brain (this particular determination was carried out in pigs by Austin[24]). In both of the human trials, no antibody appeared to be elicited by the injected enzyme. Furthermore, Greene's group found much of the intravenously injected arylsulphatase in the patient's liver. It was concluded from these determinations that intrathecal and intravenous injection of enzyme was unlikely to be beneficial for the treatment of this genetic disorder.

Despite these negative trials, two groups of investigators subsequently reported that the addition of urinary arylsulphatase A to cultured skin fibroblasts corrected the defective degradation of sulphatide in these cells[26, 27]. This observation, plus the fact that neither Austin nor Greene's group detected sensitization of the recipients to the exogenous enzymes, seemed to indicate that trials of enzyme replacement might be worth investigating in other metabolic disorders. With regard to sensitization, it is particularly noteworthy that Greene and coworkers employed a non-human source for the exogenous enzyme used in their trial.

Tay-Sachs disease

The first experiment concerning enzyme replacement in a human ganglioside-storage disorder was carried out in 1971 in a patient with the Sandhoff-variant form of Tay–Sachs disease[28]. Although both major A and B isozymes of hexosaminidase are lacking in these patients, only hexosaminidase A is thought to catalyse the catabolism of accumulating ganglioside G_{M2}. Hexosaminidase A was isolated from human urine and aliquots of the enzyme were infused intravenously into the patient on two consecutive days. No improvement in the patient's clinical course was observed. This lack of response was not unexpected, since the preceding experiments with intravenous arylsulphatase A were unproductive and it is well known that macromolecules the size of these enzymes do not cross the blood–brain barrier. In fact, assays of hexosaminidase A activity in brain biopsies before and after infusion of enzyme indicated that it had not reached this organ. However, the *in vivo* administered enzyme apparently exerted catabolic activity on another lipid called globo-side, *N*-acetylgalactosaminyl-galactosyl-galactosyl-glucosylceramide. The quantity of this metabolite in the circulation had decreased 43 % by 4 h after injection of hexosaminidase A. It was known that hexosaminidase A can cleave the terminal aminosugar from this molecule *in vitro*, and this experiment demonstrated that an exogenous enzyme could catalyse the catabolism of an accumulating lipid *in vivo*. At the time this investigation was carried out, it was not clear where the catabolism of globoside had actually occurred. The clearance of the enzyme from the blood stream was extraordinarily rapid ($T_{1/2}$ of 7.5 min). The decrease of circulating globoside was noted 4 h after enzyme infusion; however, because a careful time course of the clearance of this lipid was not performed, no inference regarding the intravascular or cellular site of catabolism could be made. Because much of the injected enzyme activity was detected in the liver, it was presumed likely that considerable hydrolysis of globoside occurred there. Strong support for this deduction has recently been provided by Rattazzi et al.[29]. These investigators noted a virtually complete disappearance of hepatic globoside in a feline animal model of total hexosaminidase deficiency following injection of human placental hexosaminidase. Furthermore, they report an apparent decrease in hepatic G_{M2} in the hexosaminidase-treated animals. Both of these deductions were made by comparing the level of globoside and G_{M2} in the liver of the infused animals with that in untreated homozygous cats. The authors make the reservation that strict comparison of pre- and post-enzyme infusion globoside and G_{M2} levels has not yet been carried out, although the magnitude of the change in globoside makes it appear likely that the effect was due to the administered hexosaminidase.

Less encouraging results have been obtained in recent trials in humans[30, 31]. Human placental hexosaminidase was injected intracisternally and intrathecally into two[31] patients with the conventional form of Tay–Sachs disease. The preparation used was a mixture of free and polyvinylpyrrolidone-bound hexosaminidase A. The infusions were complicated by pyrogenic reactions on several occasions (cf. Refs. 24 and 25), but by and large, the procedure was well tolerated. There was no apparent improvement in the clinical course of the recipients. Two interesting ancillary observations were made in the course of these investigations.

(1) No immune response at the humoral level was detected.
(2) There appeared to be a dramatic drop in the concentration of G_{M2} in the serum of one of the patients from 24.9 and 28.8 µg/ml to < 1 µg/ml shortly after the enzyme had been infused.

The investigators made the interesting comment that it was not clear whether this effect took place in vivo or in vitro. The patient on whom this critical determination was made received free hexosaminidase A and the serum sample was obtained 2 h after injection. Since the investigators reported that no exogenous free hexosaminidase could be detected in the serum 20–40 min after infusion, the possibility of in vitro degradation seems unlikely. The magnitude and rapidity of the reduction of G_{M2} seems most compatible with extracellular catabolism. It is extraordinarily difficult to reconcile this deduction with the pH optimum of 4.2 for purified hexosaminidase A and the fact that virtually no catalytic activity can be detected above pH 5.3[32]. However, a dilemma of this sort is encountered again in the section on Fabry's disease.

From the results obtained by the various groups cited above who have attempted enzyme replacement in metachromatic leukodystrophy and in Tay–Sachs disease, it was concluded that enzyme replacement is likely to be ineffectual for disorders such as those involving the central nervous system, unless a procedure is developed for more effective delivery of exogenous enzymes to the sites of accumulation in the brain. We therefore began a series of experiments to determine whether, by increasing the permeability of the blood–brain barrier, enzymes could gain access to the central nervous system. This study seemed particularly desirable since it was learned that neuronal cells had high affinity receptors on their plasma-cell membrane for hexosaminidase A[33, 34]. We found that careful infusion of hyperosmolar solutions of mannitol or arabinose caused temporary shrinking of the endothelial cells that form the blood–brain barrier, so that exogenous enzymes could reach the brain[35 – 37]. Furthermore, a portion of the endocytosed enzyme ultimately becomes associated with subcellular organelles (lysosomes), at exactly the intracellular localization of the accumulating lipid[38]. The experiments have been extended, and it has been shown that repeated blood–brain barrier alteration did not cause pathological changes in primates[39]. Furthermore, successful barrier modification has been carried out in humans[40]. These findings, coupled with the presence of high affinity receptors for hexosaminidase A on neuronal cells, suggest that enzyme replacement may eventually prove useful for Tay–Sachs disease. The sharply decreasing turnover of gangliosides in the postnatal period and the presence of an alternate (salvage) pathway for G_{M2} catabolism initiated by a neuraminidase in normal individuals and patients with the conventional form of Tay–Sachs disease[41, 42], provide a continuing impetus for further investigation of enzyme replacement as a potentially effective therapeutic procedure in this disorder.

Fabry's disease

As a consequence of the inability to deliver exogenous enzymes to the nervous system in the preceding trials, practical consideration dictated that successful enzyme replacement would be more likely in disorders in which the brain was not involved in the pathological process. The two lipid-storage disorders that were potentially available for such trials were Fabry's disease and Type I Gaucher's disease. Accordingly, we undertook the isolation of ceramidetrihexosidase and glucocerebrosidase from human placental tissue for enzyme replacement trials in these conditions. Human placental ceramidetrihexosidase was the first of these enzymes to become available in sufficient purity for human administration[43]. When relatively small quantities of this enzyme were infused into two patients with Fabry's disease, a significant decrease in the elevated level of plasma ceramidetrihexoside was observed[44]. Because this lowering occurred within 1 h following administration of the enzyme, the site of catabolism was again unclear. However, for the following reasons it was deduced that the ceramidetrihexoside had been hydrolysed within tissue stores such as the liver:

(1) The maximal decrease in plasma ceramidetrihexoside occurred shortly after the enzyme had been completely cleared from the circulation.
(2) The enzyme is catalytically inactive at pH 7 and above.
(3) There was no evidence of an increase of ceramidelactoside, the immediate product of the reaction in the plasma of the recipients.

Although the organ(s) involved in the enzymatic breakdown of ceramidetrihexoside have not been identified, the fact that liver had increased ceramidetrihexosidase activity following enzyme infusion suggests that this tissue may have been a primary site of catabolism of this glycolipid.

Several additional observations made during these trials are important.

(1) The recipients experienced no untoward reaction to the exogenous enzyme.
(2) There was no indication of sensitization to the placental protein when they were challenged with intradermal injection a year after infusion of the enzyme[45].
(3) Plasma ceramidetrihexoside returned to the preinfusion level between 48 and 72 h following infusion of enzyme.
(4) There was no noticeable change in the patient's clinical status.
(5) Further replacement trials in Fabry patients with placental enzyme have been delayed by the presence of pyrogenic material in the larger quantities of enzyme that will apparently be required to effect a prolonged decrease in plasma (? and tissue) ceramidetrihexoside.

A rather similar study has been performed recently by Desnick and collaborators using ceramidetrihexosidase derived from human spleen or plasma[46, 47]. These investigators infused enzyme preparations that were < 2% pure on repeated occasions into two Fabry patients. The splenic enzyme was cleared from the circulation with a $T_{1/2}$ of 10.5 min. A decrease of plasma ceramidetrihexoside of about 50 % of the preinfusion level was observed 15 min following injection of the enzyme. The lipid returned to the pre-injection figure by 2 h after infusion. This observation again raises the possibility that the enzyme exerted its catalytic effect in the circulation. A more prolonged reduction of plasma ceramidetrihexoside was observed in the second patient who received enzyme derived from human plasma. The enzyme was presumed to contain more sialic-acid residues and its $T_{1/2}$ in the circulation was 70 min. This enzyme preparation caused a 25-fold greater clearance of plasma ceramidetrihexoside than that obtained with the splenic preparation. It seems difficult to reconcile the extended persistence of the enzyme in the circulation and its greater effect on accumulating lipid if the proposed extracirculatory site of its catalytic activity is correct[47]. A potential solution to this dilemma would be more effective intracellular packaging of the slowly removed plasma enzyme preparation compared with the rapidly cleared spleen preparation. It is conceivable that the effectiveness of the splenic enzyme preparation is reduced because the majority of this material is destroyed by intracellular proteases before incorporation into a lysosomal compartment with limited capacity for enzyme uptake. A further point in this regard may be made by comparing the effectiveness of the placental ceramidetrihexosidase used in the earlier study with the plasma-derived enzyme. Infusion of 11 000 units of placenta-derived α-galactosidase (a measure of catalytic effectiveness using 4-methylumbelliferyl-α-D-galactopyranoside as substrate) reduced plasma ceramidetrihexoside to normal, whereas 180 000 units of plasma enzyme were required to achieve a similar reduction. Since the $T_{1/2}$ of the placental enzyme in the circulation was 12 min, it might be argued that its greater catalytic effect was due to its more efficient endocytosis and lysosomal packaging in cells that are involved in homeostatic regulation of this lipid in the circulation. This deduction seems contradictory to the argument proposed to explain the relative ineffectiveness of the splenic enzyme and, for practical purposes, merely reflects the fact that we simply need to carry out a more precise evaluation of the disposition and site of function of such exogenous enzymes. This conclusion is heightened by the fact that again in the more recent trial, no detectable improvement in the patient's clinical status could be attributed to the exogenous enzyme. On the positive side, it appears that preparations even as inhomogeneous as those used in the recent study did not evoke an immunological reaction in the patients injected intravenously on six occasions over a period of 117 days[47]. Additional investigation is certainly required to reach a decision concerning the future effectiveness of enzyme replacement in the management of Fabry's disease.

Gaucher's disease

The most extensive trials of enzyme replacement for a human metabolic disorder have been carried out in patients with Gaucher's disease. In the initial study, it was reported that intravenous injection of human placental glucocerebrosidase caused a reduction in the quantity of stored glucocerebroside in the liver and in the quantity of this material associated with erythrocytes in the circulation[48]. The decrease of glucocerebroside in the blood occurred gradually during a three day period following infusion of the enzyme, suggesting a redistribution of glucocerebroside from sites of tissue storage such as the liver. Furthermore, the reduction of red cell-associated glucocerebroside appeared to persist over a comparatively long period of time[45, 49]. A subsequent trial showed considerably less reduction in hepatic glucocerebroside, and in this patient, no change in the elevated circulating lipid was observed[50].

At this point, it became apparent that it would be necessary to infuse much larger quantites of enzyme. The placental preparation obtained by conventional enzyme purification methods[51] appeared to clear 0.4 nmol of glucocerebroside from hepatic stores per unit of enzyme activity infused[50] (one unit catalysed the hydrolysis of 1 nmol of glucocerebroside *in vitro*). Because the isolation procedure could not be scaled up, a novel purification method was developed that provided highly-enriched placental glucocerebrosidase in good yield and free of pyrogenic material[52]. Clinical trials with this enzyme provided the following information. The enzyme is cleared from the circulation with a $T_{1/2}$ of 20 min, which is precisely the same as the rate observed in the previous trials. However, catabolism of stored glucocerebroside in the liver has not been observed to be consistent. Encouraging results were obtained in two young boys with Type I Gaucher's disease in whom there was a 12% and 15% reduction of liver glucocerebroside, respectively, following infusion of enzyme[53]. Some lowering of the circulating glucocerebroside was also noted. Because of the possibility that repeated infusions of enzyme might exert more benefit than single replacement episodes, we began a prospective trial of enzyme infusion on a bimonthly basis in four young male patients. It is our impression, and it is shared by the paediatricians providing primary care for these recipients, that: (i) their general health is improved, (ii) the progression of their organomegaly has been arrested, and (iii) there has been stabilization of the blood platelet counts[54]. Because of these observations, we have begun a similar regimen in additional patients.

We had less satisfactory results in four adults with Type I Gaucher's disease where no reduction of hepatic or circulating glucocerebroside was detected after infusion of this enzyme[53]. In an attempt to improve the effectiveness of exogenous enzyme in patients in this age group, we pretreated several patients with prednisone prior to infusion of the enzyme. The initial responses to this combination seemed encouraging[53] and we are presently evaluating this approach with a more extended clinical trial.

FUTURE STRATEGIES

We have long been aware of the fact that replacement of an enzyme by intravenous infusion of an exogenous catalyst is an unphysiological undertaking. Each tissue in the body appears to synthesize its own requirement of enzymes. The amount of a particular catabolic enzyme produced in an organ appears to vary with the load of substrate that it is required to degrade[12]. Thus, delivery of enzyme to an organ that accumulates a metabolite in a patient with a heritable metabolic disorder might be fortuitous, at best. Initially we were encouraged by the fact that Wakim and others had shown that enzymes were removed from the circulation by cells of the reticuloendothelial system[55], precisely the site of accumulating glycolipids in sphingolipid-storage diseases. We were disappointed to discover that most of the injected placental glucocerebrosidase was not taken up by these cells in the liver, but it was preferentially concentrated in hepatocytes[56, 57]. It became apparent that the oligosaccharide portion of placental glucocerebrosidase contained the 'complex' carbohydrate oligosaccharide configuration, namely N-acetylneuraminyl-galactosyl$-N$-acetylglucosaminyl-(fucosyl)-mannosyl-X, where X is the link to the polypeptide backbone. Thus, when the terminal molecule of N-acetyl-neuraminic acid was removed, even more enzyme appeared in hepatocytes in experimental animals, presumably because of the galactose receptor on the membranes of these cells[56]. Subsequent removal of galactose resulted in increased uptake by Kupffer cells[58]; cleaving fucose reduced the quantity of hepatocyte glucocerebrosidase[59]. Cleavage of N-acetylglucosamine (and fucose) yielded an enzyme that was five-fold more effectively endocytosed by Kupffer cells than native placental enzyme[60]. Accordingly, we plan to examine the clinical effectiveness of the mannose terminated enzyme when sufficient quantities of this material become available.

We have begun an alternative approach to carbohydrate directed uptake of enzyme by Kupffer cells. We are attempting to link mannose and mannose oligosaccharides to placental glucocerebrosidase. We shall determine whether the uptake of enzyme altered in this fashion is also enhanced in Kupffer and other reticuloendothelial cells. If the results of these studies are sufficiently encouraging, we expect that clinical trials with this preparation will be undertaken. Although we[61] and others[62, 63] have convincingly demonstrated that infusion of placental glucocerebrosidase does not elicit antibody formation, careful monitoring of patients will certainly be necessary with the carbohydrate modified preparations.

CONCLUDING REMARKS

A decision concerning the ultimate effectiveness of enzyme replacement therapy is not possible, as yet. We and others[29, 47, 62, 63] believe that further investigation of enzyme replacement therapy is clearly warranted. Certainly this approach will be strengthened if the responses that appear to have occurred in the young Gaucher patients can be confirmed. The success of such therapy appears to hinge upon effective delivery of the enzyme to the storage sites. Careful attention must be paid to the experiments of other investigators delineating cellular specificity and the subcellular fate of proteins, as these parameters are influenced by their oligosaccharide residues[64]. We are also mindful that the effects of more complicated polypeptide 'signals' may have to be taken into consideration[65]. Finally, we believe we are justified in presuming that proper application of the expanding knowledge of the genesis, processing, and physiological disposition of enzymes seems likely to provide means for effective treatment of heritable metabolic diseases.

References

1. Brady, R. O. (1966). The sphingolipidoses. *N. Engl. J. Med.*, **275**, 312
2. Brady, R. O. (1973). The abnormal biochemistry of inherited disorders of lipid metabolism. *Fed. Proc.*, **32**, 1660
3. Dean, M. F., Muir, H., Benson, P. F. and Button, L. R. (1982). This volume, chapter 8
4. Brady, R. O., Johnson, W. G. and Uhlendorf, B. W. (1971). Identification of heterozygous carriers of lipid storage diseases. *Am. J. Med.*, **51**, 423
5. Kattlove, H. E., Williams, J. C., Gaynor, E., Spivack, M., Bradley, R. M., and Brady, R. O. (1969). Gaucher cells in chronic myelocytic leukemia: an acquired abnormality. *Blood*, **33**, 379
6. Brady R. O. (1978). Glucosyl ceramide lipidoses: Gaucher's disease. In Stanbury, J. B., Wyngaarden, J. B. and Fredrickson, D. S. (eds.) *The Metabolic Basis of Inherited Disease.* 4th Edn., pp. 731–746. (New York: McGraw-Hill)

7. Groth, C. G., Hagenfeldt, L., Dreborg, S., Löfström, B., Öckerman, P. A., Samuelsson, K., Svennerholm, L., Werner, B. and Westberg, G. (1971). Splenic transplantation in a case of Gaucher's disease. *Lancet*, **1**, 1260

8. Groth, C. G., Berström, K., Collste, L., Egberg, N., Högman, C., Holm, G. amd Möller, E. (1972), Immunologic and plasma protein studies in a splenic homograft recipient. *Clin. Exp. Immunol.*, **10**, 359

9. Brady, R. O. (1978). Sphingomyelin lipidoses: Niemann–Pick disease. In Stanbury, J. B., Wyngaarden, J. B. and Fredrickson, D. S. (eds.) *The Metabolic Basis of Inherited Disease*. 4th Edn., pp. 718–730. (New York: McGraw-Hill)

10. Kanfer, J. N., Young, O. M., Shapiro, D. and Brady, R. O. (1966). The metabolism of sphingomyelin. I. Purification and properties of a sphingomyelin- cleaving enzyme from rat liver tissue. *J. Biol. Chem.*, **241**, 1081

11. Daloze, P., Delvin, E. E., Glorieux, F. H., Corman, J. L., Bettez, P., and Toussi, T. (1977). Replacement therapy for inherited enzyme deficiency: liver orthotopic transplantation in Niemann–Pick disease Type A. *Am. J. Med. Genet.*, **1**, 22

12. Kampine, J. P., Kanfer, J. N., Gal, A. E., Bradley, R. M. and Brady, R. O. (1967). Response of sphingolipid hydrolases in spleen and liver to increased erythrocytorrhexis. *Biochim. Biophys. Acta*, **137**, 135

13. Desnick, S. J., Desnick, R. J., Brady, R. O., Pentchev, P. G., Simmons, R. L., Najarian, J. S., Swaiman, K., Sharp, H. L. and Krivit, W. (1973). Renal transplantation in Type 2 Gaucher's disease. In Desnick, R. J., Bernlohr, R. W. and Krivit, W., (eds.) *Enzyme Therapy in Genetic Diseases*, pp. 109–119 (Baltimore: Williams and Wilkins).

14. Groth, C. G., Collste, H., Dreborg, S., Håkansson, G., Lundgren, G. and Svennerholm, L. (1979). Attempt at enzyme replacement in Gaucher disease by renal transplantation. *Acta Paediatr. Scand.*, **68**, 475

15. Groth, C. G., Collste, H., Dreborg, S., Håkansson, G., Lundgren, G. and Svennerholm, L. (1980). Attempt at enzyme replacement in Gaucher disease by renal transplantation. *Enzyme Therapy in Genetic Disease*, Vol. 2, pp. 475–490. (New York: Liss)

16. Freese, A., Brady, R. O. and Gal, A. E. (1980). A β-glucosidase in feline kidney that hydrolyzes amygdalin (Laetrile). *Arch. Biochem. Biophys.*, **201**, 363

17. Desnick, R. J., Klionsky, B. and Sweeley, C. C. (1978). Fabry's disease (α-galactosidase A deficiency). In Stanbury, J. B., Wyngaarden, J. B., and Fredrickson, D. S. (eds.) *The Metabolic Basis of Inherited Disease*. 4th Edn., pp. 810–840. (New York: McGraw-Hill)

18. Desnick, R. L., Simmons, R. C., Allen, K. Y., Woods, L. E., Anderson, C. F., Najarian, J. S. and Krivit, W. (1972). Correction of enzymatic deficiencies by renal transplantation: Fabry's disease. *Surgery*, **72**, 203

19. Philippart, M., Franklin, S. S. and Gordon, A. (1972). Reversal of an inborn sphingolipidosis (Fabry's disease) by kidney transplantation. *Ann. Intern. Med.*, **77**, 195

20. Clarke, J. T. R., Guttmann, R. D., Wolfe, L. S., Beaudoin, J. G. and Morehouse, D. D. (1972). Enzyme replacement therapy by renal allo-transplantation in Fabry's disease. *N. Engl. J. Med.*, **287**, 1215

21. Spence, M. W., MacKinnon, K. E., Burgees, J. K., d'Entremont, D. M.,

Belitsky, P., Lannon, S. G. and MacDonald, A. S. (1976). Failure to correct the metabolic defect by reneal allotransplantation in Fabry's disease. *Ann. Intern. Med.*, **84**, 13

22. Van den Bergh F. A. J. T. M., Rietra, P. J. G. M., Kolk-Vegter, A. J., Bosch, E. and Tager, J. M. (1976). Therapeutic implications of renal transplantation in a patient with Fabry disease. *Acta Med. Scand.*, **200**, 249

23. Brady, R. O. (1978). Elucidation of clinical lysosome deficiencies. In Berlin, R., Herrmann, H., Lepow, I. H. and Tanzer, J. (eds.) *Molecular Basis of Biological Degradative Processes*, pp. 39–64 (New York: Academic Press)

24. Austin, J. H. (1967). Some recent findings in leukodystrophies and in gargoylism. In Aronson, S. M. and Volk, B. W. (eds.) *Inborn Disorders of Sphingolipid Metabolism*, pp. 359–387. (New York: Pergamon Press)

25. Greene, H. L., Hug, G. and Schubert, W. K. (1969). Metachromatic leukodystrophy. Treatment with arylsulfatase A. *Arch. Neurol.*, **20**, 147

26. Porter, M. T., Fluharty, A. L. and Kihara, H. (1971). Correction of abnormal cerebroside sulfate metabolism in cultured metachromatic leukodystrophy fibroblasts. *Science*, **172**, 1263

27. Wiesmann, U. N., Rossi, E. E. and Herschkowitz, N. N. (1972). Correction of the defective sulfatide degradation in cultured fibroblasts from patients with metachromatic leukodystrophy. *Acta Paediatr Scand.*, **61**, 296

28. Johnson, W. G., Desnick, R. L., Long, D. M., Sharp, H. L., Krivit, W., Brady, B. and Brady, R. O. (1973). Intravenous injection of purified hexosaminidase A into a patient with Tay–Sachs disease. In Desnick, R. L., Bernlohr, R. W. and Krivit, W. (eds.) *Enzyme Therapy in Genetic Diseases*, pp. 120–124 (Baltimore: Williams and Witkins).

29. Rattazzi, M. C., Appel, A. M. and Baker, J. H. (1980). Enzyme replacement in feline G_{M2} gangliosidosis: reduction of glycolipid storage in visceral organs. Presented at the *31st Meeting of the Am. Soc. Hum. Genet.*, September 24–27, New York, NY

30. von Specht, B. U., Geiger, B., Arnon, R., Passwell, J., Keren, G., Goldman, B. and Padeh, B. (1979). Enzyme replacement in Tay–Sachs disease. *Neurology*, **29**, 848

31. Godel, V., Blumenthal, M., Goldman, B., Keren, G. and Padeh, B. (1978). Visual functions in Tay–Sachs diseased patients following enzyme replacement therapy. *Metab. Ophthalmol.*, **2**, 27

32. Tallman, J. F., Brady, R. O., Quirk, J. M., Villalba, M. and Gal, A. E. (1974). Isolation and relationship of human hexosaminidases. *J. Biol. Chem.*, **249**, 3489

33. Kusiak, J. W., Toney, J. H., Quirk, J. M. and Brady, R. O. (1979). Specific binding of ^{125}I-β-hexosaminidase A to rat brain synaptosomes. *Proc. Natl. Acad. Sci. USA*, **76**, 982

34. Kusiak, J. W., Quirk, J. M. and Brady, R. O. (1980). Specific binding of β-hexosaminidase A to rat brain synaptic plasma membranes. In Desnick, R. J. (ed.) *Enzyme Therapy in Genetic Diseases*, Vol. 2, pp. 93–102 (New York: Liss)

35. Barranger, J. A., Pentchev, P. G., Rapoport, S. I. and Brady, R. O. (1977). Augmentation of a brain lysosomal enzyme activity following enzyme infusion with concomitant alteration of the blood–brain barrier. *Trans. Am. Neurol. Assoc.*, **102**, 10

36. Barranger, J. A., Rapoport, S. D., Fredericks, W. R., Pentchev, P. G., MacDermot, K. D., Steusing, J. K. and Brady, R. O. (1979). Modification of the blood–brain barrier: increased concentration and fate of enzymes entering the brain. *Proc. Natl. Acad. Sci. USA*, **76**, 481

37. Barranger, J. A., Rapoport, S. I. and Brady, R. O. (1980). Access of enzymes to the brain following osmotic alteration of the blood–brain barrier. In Desnick, R. J. (ed.) *Enzyme Therapy in Genetic Diseases*, Vol. 2, pp. 195–205 (New York: Liss)

38. Tallman, J. F., Jr., Brady, R. O. and Suzuki, K. (1971). Enzymic activities associated with membranous cytoplasmic bodies and isolated brain lysosomes. *J. Neurochem.*, **18**, 1975

39. Smith, M. T., Girton, M., Rapoport, S. I., Brady, R. O. and Barranger, J. A. (1980). Pathology of reversible blood–brain barrier opening. *J. Neuropathol. Exp. Neurol.*, **39**, 389

40. Neuwelt, E. A., Frenkel, E. P., Diehl, J., Vu, L. H., Rapoport, S. and Hill, S. (1980). Reversible osmotic blood–brain barrier disruption in man: implications for chemotherapy of malignant brain tumours, *Neurosurgery*, **7**, 44

41. Brady, R. O. and Kolodny, E. H. (1972). Disorders of ganglioside metabolism. In Steinberg, A. G. and Bearn, A. G. (eds.) *Progress in Medical Genetics*, Vol. VIII, pp. 225–214 (New York: Grune and Stratton).

42. Brady, R. O. and Barranger, J. A. (1981). Inborn lysosomal enzyme deficiencies. In Davison, A. N. and Thompson, R. H. S. (eds) *The Molecular Basis of Neuropathology*, pp. 188–220. (London: Edward Arnold)

43. Johnson, W. G. and Brady, R. O. Ceramidetrihexosidase from human placenta (1972). *Meth. Enzymol.* **XXVIII**, 849–856.

44. Brady, R. O., Tallman, J. F., Johnson, W. G., Gal, A. E., Leahy, W. E., Quirk, J. M. and Dekaban, A. S. (1973). Replacement therapy for inherited enzyme deficiency: use of purified ceramidetrihexosidase in Fabry's disease. *N. Engl. J. Med.*, **289**, 9

45. Brady, R. O. Heritable catabolic and anabolic disorders of lipid metabolism. *Metabolism*, **26**, 329

46. Desnick, R. J., Dean, K. J., Grabowski, G. A., Bishop, D. F. and Sweeley, C. C. (1979). Enzyme therapy in Fabry's disease: differential *in vivo* plasma clearance and metabolic effectiveness of plasma and splenic α-galactosidase A isozymes. *Proc. Natl. Acad. Sci. USA*, **76**, 5326

47 Desnick, R. J., Dean, K. J., Grabowski, G. A., Bishop D. F. and Sweeley, C. C. (1980). Enzyme therapy XVII: metabolic and immunologic evaluation α-galactosidase A replacement in Fabry disease. In Desnick, R. J. (ed.) *Enzyme Therapy in Genetic Diseases*, Vol. 2, pp. 393–413 (New York: Liss)

48. Brady, R. O., Pentchev, P. G., Gal, A. E., Hibbert, S. R. and Dekaban, A. S. (1974). Replacement therapy for inherited enzyme deficiency: use of purified glucocerebrosidase in Gaucher's disease. *N. Engl. J. Med.*, **291**, 989.

49. Pentchev, P. G., Brady, R. O., Gal, A. E. and Hibbert, S. R. (1975). Replacement therapy for inherited enzyme deficiency: sustained clearance of accumulated glucocerebroside in Gaucher's disease following infusion of purified glucocerebrosidase. *J. Molec. Med.*, **1**, 73

50. Brady, R. O., Pentchev, P. G., Gal, A. E., Hibbert, S. R., Quirk, J. M., Mook, G. E., Kusiak, J. W., Tallman, J. F. and Dekaban, A. S. (1976). Enzyme replacement therapy for the sphingolipidoses. In Volk, B. W. and Schneck, L.

(eds.) *Current Trends in the Sphingolipidoses and Allied Disorders,* pp. 523–532, (New York: Plenum Press)

51. Pentchev, P. G., Brady, R. O., Hibbert, S. R., Gal, A. E. and Shapiro, D. (1973). Isolation and characterization of glucocerebrosidase from human placenta. *J. Biol. Chem.,* **248,** 5256

52. Furbish, F. S., Blair, H. E., Shiloach, J., Pentchev, P. G. and Brady, R. O. (1977). Enzyme replacement therapy in Gaucher's disease: large-scale purification of glucocerebrosidase suitable for human administration. *Proc. Natl. Acad. Sci. USA,* **74,** 3560

53. Brady, R. O., Barranger, J. A., Gal, A. E., Pentchev, P. G. and Furbish, F. S. (1980). Status of enzyme replacement therapy for Gaucher disease. In Desnick, R. J. (ed.) *Enzyme Therapy in Genetic Diseases,* Vol. 2, pp. 361–368 (New Tork: Liss)

54. Brady, R. O., Barranger, J. A., Furbish, F. S. and Stownes, D. W. Effect of long term enzyme replacement in young patients with Type I Gaucher's disease. (In preparation)

55. Wakim, K. G. and Fleisher, G. A. (1963). Fate of enzymes in body fluids–experimental study. IV. Relationship of reticuloendothetical system to activities and disappearance rates of various enzymes. *J. Lab. Clin. Med.,* **61,** 107

56. Furbish, F. S., Steer, C. J., Barranger, J. A., Jones, E. A. and Brady, R. O. (1978). The uptake of native and desialylated glucocerebrosidase by rat hepatocytes and Kupffer cells. *Biochem. Biophys. Res. Commun.,* **81,** 1047

57. Morrone, S., Pentchev, P. G., Thorpe, S. and Baynes, J. (1981). Studies *in vivo* of the tissue uptake cellular distribution, and catabolic turnover of exogeneous glucocerebrosidase in rat. *Biochem.,* **194,** 733

58. Steer, C. J., Furbish, F. S., Barranger, J. A., Brady, R. O. and Jones, E. A. (1978). The uptake of agalacto-glucocerebrosidase by rat hepatocytes and Kupffer cells. *FEBS Lett.,* **9,** 202

59. Furbish, F. S., Krett, N. L., Barranger, J. A. and Brady, R. O. (1980) Fucose plays a role in the clearance and uptake of glucocerebrosidase by rat liver cells. *Biochem. Biophys. Res. Commun.,* **95,** 1768.

60. Furbish, F. S., Steer, C. J., Krett, N. L. and Barranger, J. A. (1981). Targeting of a lysosomal enzyme: uptake and distribution of placental glucocerebrosidase in rat heptic cells and effects on sequential deglycosylation. *Biochim. Biophys. Acta,* **673,** 425

61. Britton, D. E., Leinikki, P. O., Barranger, J. A. and Brady, R. O. (1978). Gaucher's disease: lack of antibody response to intravenous glucocerebrosidase. *Life Sci.,* **23,** 2517

62. Beutler, E., Dale, G. L. and Kuhl, W. (1980). Replacement therapy in Gaucher's diease. In Desnick, R. J. (ed.) *Enzyme Therapy in Genetic Diseases,* Vol. 2, pp. 369–381 (New York: Liss)

63. Gregoriades, G., Neerunjun, D., Meade, T. W., Goolamali, S. K. Weereratne H. and Bull, G. (1980). Experiences after long-term treatment of a Type I Gaucher disease patient with liposome-entrapped glucocerebroside: β-glucosidase. In Desnick, R. J. (ed.) *Enzyme Therapy in Genetic Diseases,* Vol. 2, pp. 383–392 (New York: Liss)

64. Neufeld, E. F. (1982). This volume, chapter 7

65. Blobel, G. (1980). Intracellular protein topogenesis. *Proc. Natl. Acad. Sci. USA.,* **77,** 1496

SECTION THREE

Inborn Errors of Metabolism affecting Brain Development (Animal Models)

11

Inborn errors of metabolism affecting brain development – Introduction

N. Herschkowitz

To my knowledge, no complete pathogenetic chain leading from the abnormal enzyme activity to an abnormal function has been shown for any inborn error of metabolism (IEM) affecting brain development. Many steps are known; for example, the abnormal enzyme activity, which may be due to an abnormal structure of the enzyme protein or to a reduced amount of enzyme. Abnormal metabolites may be present, or normal metabolites accumulate in the cells. Sometimes the cellular localization of the defect is known, as well as the brain structures which are affected by the abnormal metabolism. But this still does not explain completely the abnormal function which is frequently observed in IEM. The difficulty lies in determining the hierarchy of causes, distinguishing between cause and effect and in relating structure and function.

Animal models of human IEM may be of great help in studying pathogenetic mechanisms. No animal model can completely mimic a human disease, but it can help us to understand at least *some* aspects of the human disease. This can be on the level of the enzymatic defect, the abnormal metabolites, the subcellular localization, the organelle structure or of some basic functions of the nervous system.

The main problem is to ask the right question using the right animal, taking into account the specific metabolic problem and the specific development of the nervous system, e.g. with respect to birth.

The great advantage of animal models is the possibility of investigating 'individuals' with a common genetic background, to compare mutants with normals which differ only in the mutant locus and thus eliminate many secondary and tertiary factors. Animal models offer the opportunity to study pathogenetic mechanisms in a comprehensive way, using all available disciplines. The study can be carried out during development, in the early stages of a disease, and not only in a terminal 'burned out' stage.

Many aspects of metabolism can also be studied *in vivo*. Tissue levels of metabolites can be compared with concentrations in the extracellular compartments. Of special importance is the opportunity given to rigidly standardize and manipulate the entire environment.

The ideal animal model of a human disease would correspond at all levels to the human disorder – from enzyme defect to abnormal behaviour (Table 11.1). However, it is particularly with respect to behaviour that an animal model can seldom be compared to the human disease. Good models exist on isolated levels, for example, in the organ system involved (Table 11.2), the metabolites affected (Table 11.3) or the enzymatic or structural protein (Table 11.4).

In the future, more attention must be paid to studying pathogenetic mechanisms in depth, even if the animal model does not correspond on all

TABLE 11.1 Animal models of inborn errors of metabolism – level of defect

1. Enzyme protein, structural protein
2. Metabolites
3. Organ system
4. Physiological functions
5. Behaviour

TABLE 11.2   Animal models of inborn errors of metabolism – organ system

Nervous system
Hypertension
Cardiomyopathy
Megaoesophagus
Diabetes mellitus
Muscular dystrophy
Arthrogryposis
Hydronephrosis
Retinal degeneration
Cochleosaccular degeneration

TABLE 11.3   Animal models of human inborn errors of
metabolism – metabolites

Niemann–Pick's disease
Gaucher's disease
Metachromatic leukodystrophy(?)
Hyperprolinaemia
Kinky hair disease
Neuronal ceroid-lipofuscinosis

TABLE 11.4   Animal models of inborn errors of
metabolism – enzyme, structural protein

GM_1 gangliosidosis
GM_2 gangliosidosis
Krabbe's disease
Mannosidosis
Maroteaux–Lamy syndrome
Galactosaemia
Glycogenosis IA; VIA
Histidinaemia
Acatalasaemia
Haemolytic anaemia
Crigler–Najjar syndrome
Swiss type combined immunodeficiency
Ehlers–Danlos syndrome
Hypothyroidism

levels to the human disease, as long as it provides favourable conditions for investigating the linking mechanisms from the enzymatic defect to the clinical manifestations.

In this section, we shall start with a review of mouse models affecting the nervous system (N. Baumann), followed by IEM affecting mainly myelin (J.-M. Matthieu). We shall then discuss the possibility of imitating an IEM, phenylketonuria, by chemically inducing the defect (F. A. Hommes). To conclude, we will concentrate on one mutation affecting myelin: the *Jimpy* mutant (L. Bologa-Sandru). Beside discussing the advantages of the animal models we shall point to the limitations and possible pitfalls. I would like to mention two recent excellent reviews which deal with the problem of animal models for human disease, by Hommes[1] and Andrew et al.[2].

References

1. Hommes, F. A. (ed.) (1979). *Models for the Study of Inborn Errors of Metabolism.* (Amsterdam: Elsevier)
2. Andrew, F. J., Ward, B. C. and Altman, N. H. (eds.) (1979). *Spontaneous Animal Models of Human Disease I, Vol. II.* (London: Academic Press)

12

Mutations in mice affecting brain development and their correlations with human diseases

N. Baumann, F. Lachapelle and J.-C. Turpin

In the human, many genetic diseases of brain development are manifest during the last trimester of fetal life and the first postnatal year, when glial multiplication and myelination, outgrowth of dendrites and axons, and establishment of neuronal connections occur. Mice appear to be particularly useful for studying hereditary inborn errors of brain metabolism and differentiation. In mice, these processes occur postnatally during a short span of the animal's life. About a hundred mutations have been identified involving the nervous system or the sensory organs (see References 1–4 for reviews). For many years, they have interested only the geneticist, but since the pioneer work of Sidman and colleagues, they have become an increasingly valuable tool as genetically derived pathology in mice may have clinical analogues in man. Some of these mutations are clearly identical or closely related to human genetic diseases, others could possibly act as models for as yet undetected human disorders as there are many similarities in the genetic constitutions of mice and man. Most genetic defects in rodents are identified and collected in specialized centres where they are available to the scientific community (see *Mouse News Letters*, February 1980). Although each mutant is potentially valuable and deserves preservation, at least until it has been adequately characterized, some of them have been lost or their whereabouts is unknown. Surprisingly, many of them have not yet had a complete neuropathological examination.

It is important to consider the genetic background which may affect the expressivity of a neurological mutation when trying to understand the pathology of human or animal genetic disease. Mutant identification and care should be standardized as much as possible so that observations made in different laboratories can be meaningfully compared. Genetic variations may be responsible for significant differences in chemical composition or enzymatic activities and these differences may confuse the results and lead to incorrect interpretations. Some of the established mice strains, e.g. the C57 BL/6 and the BALB/c present genetically determined differences in noradrenergic input to the brain cortex[5]; in comparison to other strains, ICR mice exhibit delayed myelination. It is important to differentiate between differences due to the strain and those due to the pleiotropic effect of a gene. Once such factors have been taken into account, these mutants represent an invaluable tool for the understanding of human diseases. They have been discovered because of gross malformations of the nervous system, or because of an abnormal gait and tremor. They consist mainly of dysraphic disorders, hydrocephalus, cerebellar abnormalities and defects of myelin formation. Others have been identified because of convulsions.

Dysraphic disorders in man consist mostly of anencephaly and spina bifida. Although recessive cases for anencephaly (2055) and spina bifida cystica (2566) occur, it has been suggested that the genetic basis is multifactorial for these open neural tube defects, the appearance of the malformation being determined by as yet undetermined environmental factors. In mice, many mutations (Table 12.1) involving these malformations are monogenic; several have a spectrum of anomalies which are similar to human disorders and syndromes. Through studies before and during the process of neurulation in the embryo[6], they may help to determine the specific cellular and molecular steps involved in the pathological development. Recently, the concept of genetic and environmental factors affecting the teratogenic threshold has been highlighted in studies on the *Curly-tail* (*ct*) mouse. The expression of the recessive gene for spina bifida and anencephaly could be considerably modified by the maternal genetic background. In this mutant, as in the human, the expression of anencephaly, but not of spina bifida, is strongly sex-linked, although the mutation is autosomal. In this mutant, excess vitamin A, a well known teratogen in the human, can affect neural tube closure when administered before or during the period of neurulation. These facts give more validity to the model[7].

TABLE 12.1 Dysraphic disorders

Symbol	Name	Genetics Chr	DR	FS	V	LSl	Neurological disorders	Other organs	Model for genetic human disease	Availability
my	Blebs	3	R (VP)			L	pseudencephaly	acrania, malformations eye, skull, skin, kidney		JAX
Cd	Crooked	6	1/2D (VP)	F		L	pseudencephaly, exencephaly or anencephaly	crooked tail, defects in other organs		LUC, MON
Ds	Disorganization	14	1/2D (VP)			L	exencephaly, pseudencephaly, anencephaly	cranioschisis		JAX, PAS
ct	Curly-tail	?	R (VP)			Sl	lumbosacral spina bifida, sometimes anencephaly	curly or kinky tail, skeletal abnormalities	spina bifida	Embury et al.[7]
Fu	Fused	17	1/2D			L	cord malformations (folding, duplication, overgrowth)	malformations tail, vertebrae, urogenital tracts		JAX, PAS
Fu^{Ki}	Kinky	17	1/2D			L	cord malformations (folding, duplication, overgrowth)	malformations tail, vertebrae, urogenital tracts		ALB, PAS
Lp	Loop-tail	1	1/2D			L	open neural plate	abnormalities skin, axial skeleton	spina bifida	JAX, NIJ
Sp	Splotch	1	1/2D			L	spina bifida, cranial hernia, myeloschisis (overgrowth neural tissue)	rachischisis, abnormal pigmentation	spina bifida aperta	HAR, JAX

Abbreviations: Chr: chromosome; R: recessive; D: dominant; V: viable; L: lethal; Sl: sublethal; VP: variable penetrance; F: fertile; ALB: Albert Einstein; HAR: Harwell; JAX: Jackson Laboratory; LUC: London University College; MON: Montreal, McGill University; NIJ: Nijmegen; PAS: Institut Pasteur

Hydrocephalus can be classified as communicating and non-communicating. In the latter type, the cerebrospinal fluid does not enter the subarachnoid space due to obliteration or stenosis of the aqueduct or foramina. Genetic hydrocephalus in man can be due to congenital stenosis of the aqueduct of Sylvius (3062, 2288), to atresia of foramen of Magendie (2288, 2254) and of Luschka (2154). A genetic human hydrocephalus has been found to be associated with polycystic kidneys and polydactyly (2504). Some of the mice mutants (Table 12.2) also involve one or the other of these abnormalities associated with hydrocephalus. Although they are of the communicating type, unlike most children with congenital hydrocephalus, they may give some insight into the specific biological mechanisms involved in cerebrospinal fluid resorption, and possibly into the aetiology of congenital hydrocephalus in man.

Several mutations (Table 12.3) involve cerebellar development[1,8,9]. Two cause massive degeneration of granule cells: *Staggerer* and *Weaver*. In *Staggerer*, this may be related to a defect in Purkinje cell dendrites which fail to establish synapses with granule cell axons, i.e. parallel fibres[10,11] giving rise to a trans-synaptic degeneration. The mutant *Weaver* has an absence of granule cells (internal layer) due to the fact that the cells of the external granule layer fail to migrate and die; as a consequence, this mutant offers a situation where a single category of neurons is absent, allowing the study of the development of the cerebellar circuitry in a well-defined and deficient cellular milieu[12]. In another mutant, *Purkinje cell degeneration*, there is rapid degeneration of this cell type and slow degeneration of mitral cells in the olfactory bulb and photoreceptors. Degeneration of Purkinje cells is also observed in the *Nervous* and *Lurcher* mutants. In the human, several genetic cerebellar malformations have been observed[13] and can be compared with these mutations: congenital cerebellar atrophy of granular layer type[14] (in which there is likelihood of familial incidence), and congenital cerebellar atrophy with loss of Purkinje cell. In the latter, other neuronal cell types should be examined, especially photoreceptors, in relation to what is seen in animal models. Another human disease is characterized by an absence of most of the vermis (2617) which defect is observed in the *Swaying* mutation of the mouse. Thus, several mutants appear to be true models of human cerebellar congenital malformations. Although others appear not to be identical to the human genetic diseases, they can give some insight into cerebellar maturation and into the specific systems which may be involved in genetic diseases of late onset such as, late cortical cerebellar atrophy (1153)[15].

Mutations giving rise to the epileptic seizures occur in the mouse. Mice appear to be more prone to convulsions than the human species. For instance, epileptic fits are seldom observed in myelin deficiencies in man

TABLE 12.2 Hydrocephalus

Sym-bol	Name	Genetics				Neurological disorders	Other organs	Model for genetic human disease	Availability
		Chr	DR	FS	VLSI				
cb	Cerebral degeneration	?	R	S	SI	hydrocephalus at birth; white matter degeneration in the cerebral hemispheres			LUC
hpy	Hydrocephaly, polydactyly	6	R	S	SI	hydrocephalus	polydactyly		CIN
ch	Congenital hydrocephalus	13	R		L	hydrocephalus with retarded development of the subarachnoid space	urogenital system		JAX
hy³	Hydrocephalus-3	8	R		L	hydrocephalus with atrophy of meninges			JAX

Abbreviations: CIN: Cincinnati University; LUC: London University College. For other abbreviations: see Table 12.1

TABLE 12.3 Cerebellar malformations

Symbol	Name	Genetics Chr	DR	FS	V/LSI	Neurological disorders	Other organs	Model for genetic human disease	Availability
sg	Staggerer	9	R		SI	granular cell degeneration by defect in Purkinje cell dendrites			JAX, PAS
wv	Weaver	16	R	S	SI	absence granular cells (defect in migration from the external layer)		congenital cerebellar atrophy of granular layer type[14]	JAX, PAS
pcd	Purkinje cell degeneration	13	R	S	V	Purkinje cell degeneration, of mitral cells of the olfactory bulb and of photoreceptors	structural abnormalities in spermatozoa		JAX
nr	Nervous	8	R		L	Purkinje cell degeneration, and photoreceptor degenerations		congenital cerebral atrophy with loss of Purkinje cell?	JAX, PAS
sw	Swaying	15	R			absence of most of the anterior part of the vermis		agenesis of vermis of cerebellum (2617)*	JAX
rl	Reeler	5	R	S		abnormal migration of neurons in cerebral and cerebellar cortex			JAX, PAS
Lr	Lurcher	6	1/2D		L	absence of Purkinje cells, reduced width of molecular and granular layers			HAR

For abbreviations see Table 12.1. * According to McKusick[19]

although they are known to occur at late stages of demyelinating states. In the mouse, all neurological mutants involving myelination in the central nervous system are known to convulse, including the *Dilute-lethal* mutant which involves a deficiency of phenylalanine catabolism (Table 12.4). It is not known, as yet, whether these manifestations are due to pleiotropic effect of the mutated genes, or a direct result of the myelin defect in the mouse. Another possibility would be a secondary effect on the neurons or the glial cells such as the gliosis known to occur in human epileptic foci. The *Quaking* dysmyelinating mutant presents tonic and clonic seizures and sometimes EEG spike and waves[16]; a protective action of drugs enhancing noradrenergic activity has been demonstrated[17]. Recent observations indicate that a noradrenergic system with α-adrenergic receptors is involved. Various investigations have implicated noradrenalin in convulsive phenomena. Preliminary results indicate that this mutant may provide an original approach for the study of anti-epileptic drugs. Audiogenic seizures which were thought to be a general characteristic of the DBA/2 strain has been mapped to a single gene (asp)[18]. As in man, several mutations giving rise to epilepsy, do not show evidence of neuropathological lesions. Such different mutants may be useful tools in the categorization at the cellular and molecular level, of this heterogeneous group.

Other neurological disorders such as Werdnig–Hoffmann, Friedreich's ataxia have animal models (Table 12.5).

As analogues, models of disease, or genetic tools for molecular dissection, the importance of mutations in laboratory rodents in the study of neurological disorders in man is obvious. These inherited abnormalities offer the advantage of being stable, stereotyped, thus allowing repeated morphological and biochemical investigations. Unlike human clinical material, the animals can be obtained in reasonably large quantities, and can be raised under strictly controlled environmental conditions which favour the investigations. In man, the early stages of a pathological process are often missed; in a mutant strain, the fate of the animal being predictable, investigations can start before the onset of the clinical disease and before the occurrence of secondary reactions which obscure our understanding of the underlying primary disorder.

References

1. Sidman, R. L., Green, M. C. and Appel, S. (1965). Catalog of the neurological mutants of the mouse. (Cambridge: Harvard University Press)
2. Green, E. L. (1966). *Biology of the Laboratory Mouse*. pp. 87–150. (New York: McGraw Hill)

TABLE 12.4 Epileptic seizures

Sym-bol	Name	Genetics				Neurological disorders	Other organs	Model for genetic human disease	Availability
		Chr	DR	FS	VLSl				
ji	Jittery	10	R		Sl	tonic–clonic, jerks, polycystic alterations of white matter			JAX
lh	Lethargic	2	R	F	V	focal clonic and/or tonic seizures, sometimes typical Jacksonian march, no pathological examination			JAX
asp	Audiogenic seizure prone	4	R	F	V	no pathological examination			Collins and Fuller[18]
tg	Tottering	8	R	F	V	spike-waves and focal motor seizures, no light microscopic lesions		centralopathic epilepsy (1148)	JAX
tg^la	Leaner	8	R	F	V	spike-waves and focal motor seizures, no light microscopic lesions + Purkinje cell loss			
d^l	Dilute-lethal	9	R		L	clonic convulsions abnormal behaviour myelin degeneration	dilute coat colour, increased phenylalanine in blood, low phenyl-hydroxylase activity	phenylketonuria (2493)*	HAR, JAX
du	Ducky	9	R		Sl	seizures, spinocerebellar degeneration			JAX
jp	Jimpy	X	R		Sl	hypertonic seizures, severe myelin deficiency			HAR, JAX
qk	Quaking	17	R	S	V	tonic and tonico-clonic seizures, myelin deficiency			JAX, ORL

shi	Shiverer	?	R	F	SI	severe hypertonic seizures, myelin deficiency, lack of immunodetectable CNS basic protein	HVD, SALP
shi^mld	myelin deficient	?	R	F	SI	severe hypertonic seizures, myelin deficiency, lack of immunodetectable CNS basic protein	HVD, SALP
wl	wabbler-lethal	14	R		L	tonic–clonic seizures, myelin degeneration	JAX, PAS

Abbreviations: ORL: Orleans. HVD: Harvard Medical School; SALP: Salpetriere. For other abbreviations see Table 12.1. *According to McKusick[19]

TABLE 12.5 Other neurological mutants

Sym-bol	Name	Genetics				Neurological disorders	Other organs	Model for genetic human disease	Availability
		Chr	DR	FS	VLSI				
wr	Wobbler	?	R (VP)	S	V	motor neuron disease of brain-stem and spinal cord	.	muscular atrophy infantile; Werdnig–Hoffmann (2422)*	LNH
spa	Spastic	3	R	F	V	spastic, no pathological examination		familial spastic paraplegia of Strümpell–Lorrain?	JAX, PAS
du	Ducky	9	R	F	V	spino-cerebellar degeneration		Friedreich's ataxia (1318)*	JAX

Abbreviations: LNH: London National Hospital. For other abbreviations see Table 12.1. *According to McKusick[19]

3. Benirschke, K., Garner, S. M. and Jones, T. C. (1978). *Pathology of Laboratory Animals*. Vol. 1, pp. 1983–1993 (New York: Springer)
4. Cummings, J. F. (1979). Nervous system. In Andrews, E. J., Ward, B. C. and Altman, N. H. (eds.) *Spontaneous animal models of human diseases*. Vol. 2, pp. 108–178. (New York: Academic Press)
5. Berger, B., Hervé, D., Dolphin, A., Barthelemy, C., Gay, M. and Tassin, J. P. (1979). Genetically determined differences in noradrenergic input to the brain cortex: a histochemical and biochemical study in two inbred strains of mice. *Neuroscience*, **5**, 877
6. Wilson, D. B. and Finta, I. A. (1979). Junctional vesicle in the neural tube of the splotch mutant mouse. *Teratology*, **19**
7. Embury, S., Seller, M. J., Adinolfi, M. and Polani, P. E. (1979). Neural tube defects in *curly-tail* mice. 1. Incidence, expression and similarity to the human condition. *Proc. R. Soc. Lond. B* **206**, 85
8. Caviness, V. S. and Rakic. P. (1978). Mechanisms of cortical development: a view from mutations in mice. *Annu. Rev. Neurosci.*, **1**, 297
9. Quinn, W. G. and Gould, J. L. (1979). Nerves and genes. *Nature* (London), **278**, 19
10. Landis, D. and Sidman, R. L. (1974). Cerebellar cortical development in the staggerer mouse. *J. Neuropathol. Exp. Neurol.*, **33**, 180
11. Sotelo, C. and Changeux, J. P. (1974). Transsynaptic degeneration 'en cascade' in the cerebellar cortex of staggerer mutant mice. *Brain Res.*, **67**, 519
12. Sotelo, C. and Privat, A. (1978). Synaptic remodeling of the cerebellar circuitry in mutant mice and experimental cerebellar malformations. *Acta Neuropathol. (Berl.)*, **43**, 19
13. Blackwood, W. and Corsellis, J. A. N. (eds.) (1976). *Greenfield's Neuropathology*, pp. 401–409. London: Edward Arnold
14. Norman, R. M. (1940). Primary degeneration of the granular layer of the cerebellum: an unusual form of cerebellar atrophy occurring in early life. *Brain*, **63**, 365
15. Pratt, R. T. C. (1967). *The Genetics of Neurological Disorders*. (London: Oxford University Press)
16. Chauvel, P., Louvel, J., Kurcewicz, I. and Debono, M. (1980). Epileptic seizures of the quaking mouse: electro-clinical correlations. In Baumann N., (ed.) *Mutations Affecting Myelination*, pp. 513–516. (North-Holland: Elsevier-North Holland)
17. Chermat, R., Lachapelle, F., Baumann, N. and Simon, P. (1979). Anticonvulsant effect of yohimbine and prazosine. *Life Sci.*, **25**, 1471
18. Collins, R. L. and Fuller, J. L. (1968). Audiogenic seizure prone (asp): a gene affecting behavior in Linkage Group VIII of the mouse. *Science*, **162**, 1137
19. McKusick, V. (1968). *Mendelian Inheritance in Man*. (Baltimore: Johns Hopkins Press)

13

Murine mutations affecting myelination: models to study myelin diseases in the human

J.-M. Matthieu

INTRODUCTION

General introduction on myelin

The myelin sheath (Figure 13.1) is a modified and highly specialized plasma membrane which is wrapped around a portion of the axon like a spiral. The myelin membrane is an extension of the oligodendrocyte plasma membrane in the central nervous system (CNS) and of the Schwann-cell plasma membrane in the peripheral nervous system (PNS). During the process of myelin formation, the cytoplasm is extruded and the cellular leaflets are fused to form the major dense line (Figure 13.2). The external surfaces come together and form the myelin intraperiod line (also called minor dense line, Figure 13.2).

In the human brain, myelination starts at the 26th week of gestation and is still very active until the age of 2 years. In contrast, myelination in the mouse is a postnatal event which starts between days 5 and 10 and reaches a plateau at day 60. Myelin acts as an insulator and is responsible for the saltatory conduction which is a major evolutionary breakthrough.

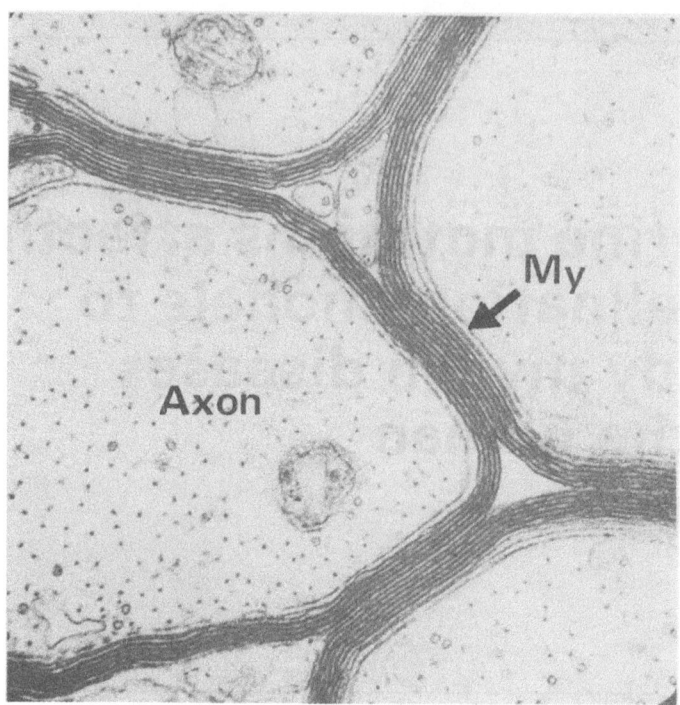

Figure 13.1 Electron micrograph of a cross-section through four myelinated axons. The multilamellar structure of the myelin sheath (My) is easy to recognize. In the CNS, the myelin sheath is not surrounded by the cytoplasm of the glial cell as in the PNS. Therefore, the myelin sheath from two adjacent axons can make direct contact. On this micrograph only the major dense line of myelin can be observed. Magnification *ca.* × 90,000 (Courtesy of Dr. H. deF. Webster)

Saltatory conduction allows action potentials to propagate faster in smaller axons which is an important step toward a miniaturized nervous network. Furthermore, saltatory conduction requires only a fraction of the energy necessary for a continuous sequential depolarization.

Myelin can be isolated from other cellular particles by ultracentrifugation of tissue homogenates on a sucrose gradient. Because of their high lipid content, myelin fragments have the lowest intrinsic density of any membrane fraction of the nervous system and can be isolated as a highly purified fraction[1]. In CNS myelin, the lipids represent 80 % of the solids and proteins the remaining 20 %. The lipid composition of myelin includes 25 % cholesterol, 30 % galactosphingolipids (mainly cerebrosides and

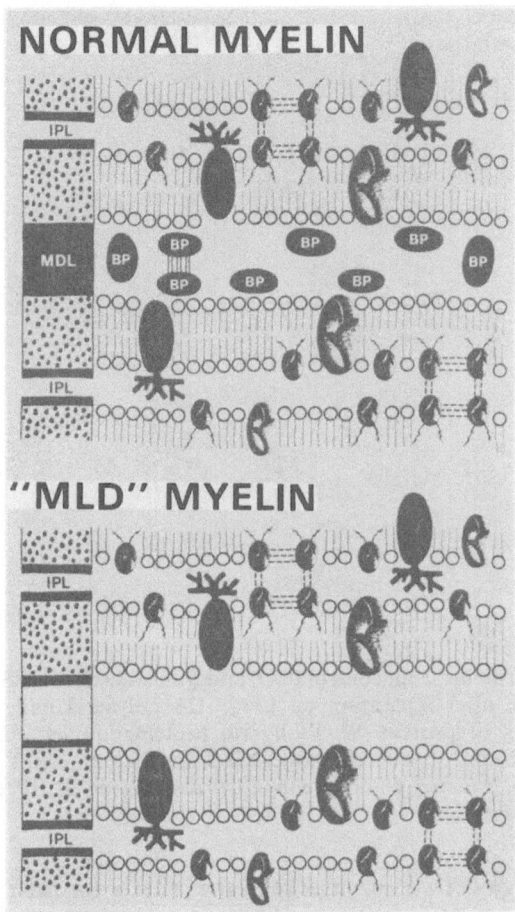

Figure 13.2 Schematic representation at the molecular level of a myelin lamella in normal and *mld* CNS. To the left of the figure, a schematic enlargement of the myelin lamella is presented. Myelin basic protein (BP) forms the major dense line. Several myelin proteins (dark ovoids) are inserted into the lipid bilayer (open circles). In *mld*, myelin basic proteins and the major dense line (MDL) are practically absent. IPL, intraperiod line. The molecular organization of the myelin membrane was inspired from P. E. Braun (In Morell, P. (ed.) (1977). *Myelin*, p. 110 Plenum Press)

sulphatides) and 45 % phospholipids (mainly ethanolamine phosphatides). PNS myelin has less galactolipids and more sphingomyelin than CNS myelin. The protein composition of myelin is shown in Figures 13.3–13.5. In contrast to other plasma membranes, myelin contains relatively little

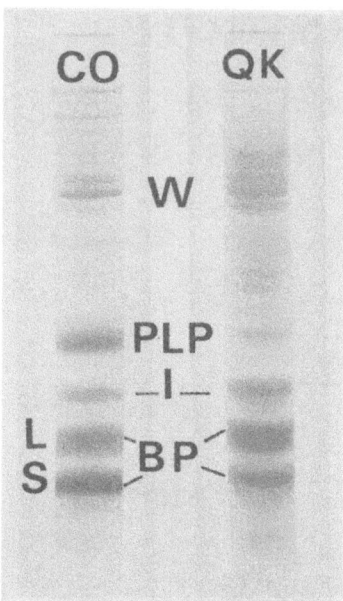

Figure 13.3   Proteins from control (CO) and *Quaking* (QK) CNS myelin stained with Fast Green after separation on 15% SDS–polyacrylamide gels. Each gel contained 150 µg of protein. W, Wolfgram protein doublet; PLP, proteolipid protein; I, intermediate protein; L, large and S, small components of myelin basic protein (BP). In *Quaking* CNS myelin, PLP and the small BP component are drastically decreased

enzymatic activity. Two enzymes fulfil the criteria for their being 'myelin specific'. One is 2′, 3′-cyclic nucleotide 3′-phosphodiesterase (EC 3.1.4.37; CNP) and the other, neutral cholesterol ester hydrolase (EC 3.1.1.13)[2]. Thirteen other enzymes have been detected in myelin, but the evidence for their localization in myelin in still speculative. These potentially myelin-localized enzymes include carbonic anhydrase (EC 4.2.1.1), UDP-galactose: ceramide galactosyltransferase (EC 2.4.1.62), 5′-nucleotidase (EC 3.1.3.5), Na^+–K^+-ATPase (EC 3.6.1.3) and two enzymes concerned with the last steps of phosphatidylcholine and phosphatidylethanolamine synthesis. In comparison with other plasma membranes, myelin has great metabolic stability and the replacement rate of its constituents is slow. This relative inertness can be explained, at least partially, by the enormous ratio of membrane to cytoplasm and the paucity of enzymatic activity.

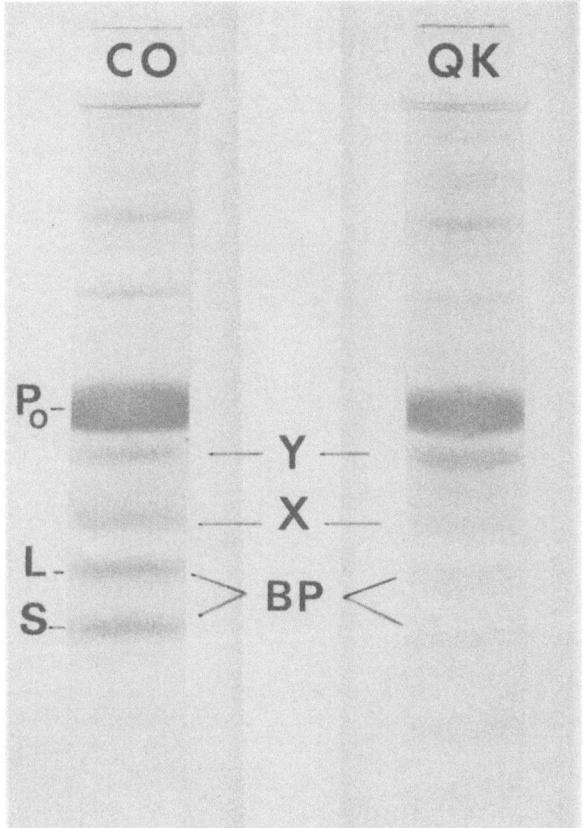

Figure 13.4 Proteins from control (CO) and *Quaking* (QK) PNS myelin stained and electrophoresed as described in Figure 13.3. P_0, major PNS myelin protein; Y and X, minor PNS myelin proteins. In control PNS L, large and S, small components of myelin basic protein (BP) are present. In *Quaking* PNS myelin, P_0 is practically normal, both BP components are decreased

Introductory remarks on myelin-deficient mutants

The development and organization of a complex structure like the myelin sheath must result from a progressive and sequential process in which the interaction between the axon, the oligodendrocyte (Schwann cell in PNS) and the environment modulates the expression of a basic genetic programme. In the human, inherited neurological disorders reveal that several

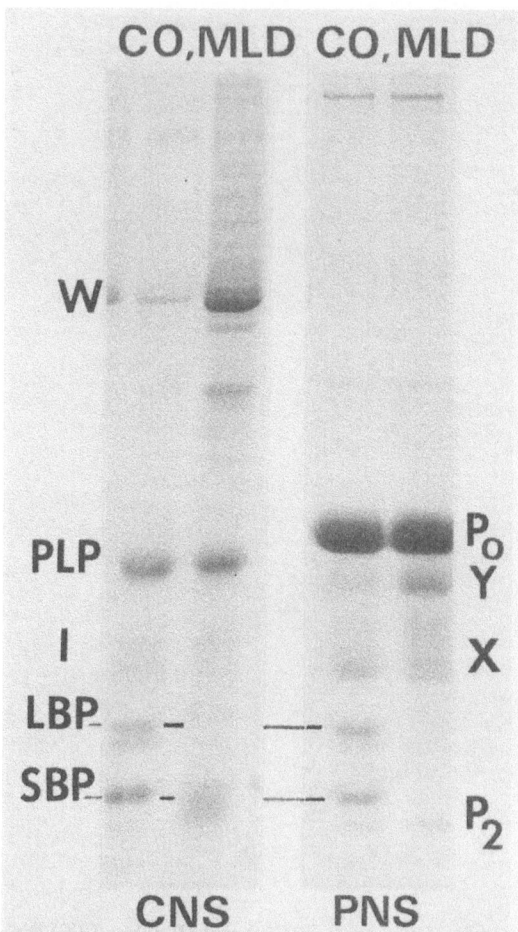

Figure 13.5 Proteins from control (CO) and *mld* CNS and PNS myelin stained with Fast Green after separation on a 12.5% SDS–polyacrylamide slab gel. Each column contained 100 μg of protein. The different protein bands are labelled as in Figures 13.3 and 13.4. P_2, specific PNS myelin basic protein, present in small amounts in mice. In *mld* myelin, both BP components are virtually absent. In the CNS, a broad band of a small molecular weight peptide (degradation product?) is apparent in the *mld* sample

genes are essential for normal myelin formation of central and peripheral nerves. Therefore, the study of mutations affecting myelination should provide improved understanding of the assembly and maintenance of myelin, and, in the case of identity or similitude with human diseases (Table

TABLE 13.1   Correlation between mouse mutations and human diseases affecting myelination

Mouse mutation	Human disease
Cribriform degeneration	Inherited spongy degeneration
Jimpy, msd	Pelizaeus–Merzbacher, sudanophilic leukodystrophy
Mottled (variant brindled)	Menkes' steely-hair syndrome
Trembler	Charcot–Marie–Tooth neuropathy, Dejerine–Sottas neuropathy
Twitcher	Globoid-cell leukodystrophy (Krabbe's disease)
Wobbler	Werdnig–Hoffmann, juvenile proximal spinal muscular atrophy (Kugelberg–Welander)

13.1), a direct insight into the pathophysiology of the diseases. Murine mutants, unlike human disorders have an homogeneous genetic background and can be studied in a controlled environment. Since a great number of animals can be bred readily, sequential analyses allow an examination of the dynamic processes of myelination.

Since the pioneer work of Sidman and coworkers[3] who first used mouse mutants to study myelinogenesis, new mutations affecting myelin have been reported almost every year (for reviews see Hogan[4] and Baumann[5]). In this short review murine mutations with genetic defects involving myelin (some of them discovered recently) will be presented and discussed in relation to human disorders.

MUTATIONS AFFECTING MYELINATION AS A PRIMARY EFFECT

Jimpy mutation

The *Jimpy* mouse, first described by Philips in 1954, is an X-linked recessive mutation (Table 13.2) resulting in a myelin deficiency in the CNS[3]. It was proposed as an analogue of human sudanophilic leukodystrophy, but it is more accurate to consider the *Jimpy* mutation as a model of Pelizaeus–Merzbacher disease[6] since the myelin dysplasia results from malformation of the oligodendrocytes[7, 8]. Merzbacher conceived the disorder he described to be the result of a congenital aplasia of myelin sheaths. In *Jimpy*, the histology is that of an almost total lack of myelin in the entire CNS, but PNS myelin appears normal. *Jimpy* cultures do not produce adequate myelin and mixed cultures of mutant and control tissue do not show cross-influences, indicating that the disorder is intrinsic to the CNS. Several anomalies involving the lipid and protein metabolism of myelin in *Jimpy* mice have been reported[4, 9]. Recently, Barbarese and colleagues presented evidence that the mutation blocks the conversion of precursor membranes into myelin[10]. This is consistent with the accumulation of membranous material within *Jimpy* oligodendroglia observed by Meier and Bischoff[6] and with the lack of transfer of myelin basic protein from the cytosol to myelin[11]. In addition to its value as a model for Pelizaeus–Merzbacher disease, the *Jimpy* mouse has contributed greatly to the understanding of myelin biochemistry by making it possible to evaluate whether a given component is a true myelin constituent.

Msd mutation

Although not studied in as much detail as the *Jimpy* mutation, the *myelin synthesis deficiency*, mutants (*msd*) are affected by a lack of myelin very similar to that described in *Jimpy* mice. It is likely that the *msd* gene is allelic to the *jp* locus[12].

Quaking mutation

The *Quaking* mutation is transmitted as an autosomal recessive trait (Table 13.2). The myelinated axons in the CNS show a marked reduction in number of myelin lamellae with a lack of compaction of the myelin sheaths. In the PNS, myelin is also thinner than in controls. Together with the *Jimpy* mutation, the *Quaking* mice have been the most widely studied mutation from a morphological and biochemical point of view. Several anomalies involving the metabolism of myelin related lipids, proteins and glyco-proteins have been reported[4, 5, 9]. The many alterations found in the nervous system of the *Quaking* mutant seem most consistent with a failure in maturation of the myelin sheath[13] which can also be termed an arrest of myelinogenesis[14–16]. This hypothesis is supported by morphological and biochemical studies showing that the myelin deficit is greatest in those regions in which myelination starts latest. This could suggest the influence of some extrinsic factors at a precise moment during brain development. This theory seems unlikely, since studies with primary cultures of *Quaking* cerebellar cells showed very poor myelination and the addition of the conditioned culture medium from *Quaking* to the culture of the control

TABLE 13.2 Seven mutations in mice with primary demyelination or dysmyelination: genetics and clinical features

Feature	Mutation				
	Jimpy, MSD*	Quaking	Shiverer, MLD*	Trembler	Dystrophic
Genetics	X-linked	autosomal recess.	autosomal recess.	autosomal domin.	autosomal recess.
Clinical symptoms	onset at 10–12 d	onset at 10–12 d	onset at 12 d	onset at 10–12 d	onset at 3½ weeks
Tremor	++	++	++	+++	++
Ataxia	+	+	+	+	+
Paralysis	0–+	0	0–+	+	++
Convulsions	+++	+	++	only in young animals	0
Mortality	100% at 30 d	slight increase	95% before 3 mo.	many between 15–30 d	few live longer than 6 mo.
Myelin content % of controls in CNS	5%	7–17%	3–4%	normal	normal
in PNS	normal	50%	80%†	3%	65%

* Msd and MLD are probably alleles of Jimpy and Shiverer, respectively
† Result obtained from MLD sciatic nerves.

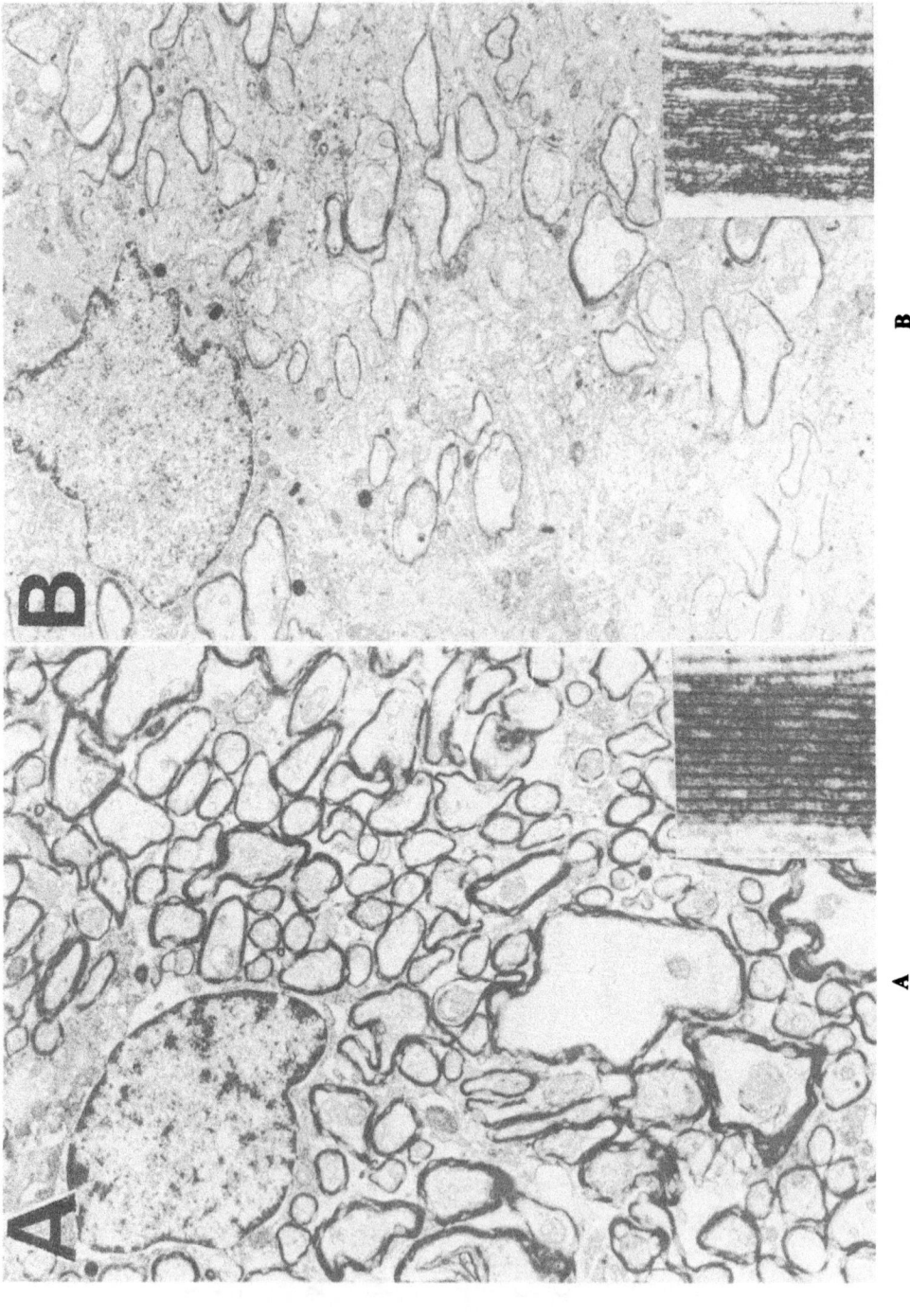

cerebellum did not interfere with myelination[17]. Furthermore, anomalies of long-chain fatty acid synthesis[18-20], and of myelin proteins (Figures 13.3 and 13.4) and glycoproteins never resembled those found in immature animals[21]. These observations suggest that the *Quaking* mutation is a dysmyelinating disorder rather than a hypomyelinating disease[21]. Recently there have been indications of a possible defect in the mechanism of final myelin assembly rather than abnormal synthesis of myelin components[22]. Obviously more work has to be done in order to understand the basic molecular defect in this mutation.

Shiverer mutation

The *Shiverer* mouse carries an autosomal recessive mutation that results in a severe myelin deficit in the CNS (Table 13.2). In the CNS of *Shiverer* mice, the major dense line of myelin is missing[23] and less than 3 % of the normal content of myelin basic protein is recovered from *Shiverer* brain homogenates[24]. In *Shiverer* PNS, the myelin sheath seems intact at the electron microscopic level, although it also lacks myelin basic proteins[25]. The specific activities of the myelin specific enzyme CNP in different regions of the *Shiverer* brain were not different from controls[26]. Purified myelin from *Shiverer* brains had an absence of myelin basic proteins, a low proteolipid protein content and high amounts of Wolfgram proteins[26].

Myelin deficient mutation (*mld*)

Myelin deficient mice are affected by an autosomal recessive mutant gene causing rapid trembling of the hind limbs and of the caudal trunk during locomotion. Brain, brain stem, optic nerves and spinal cord show a dramatic lack of myelination. In CNS myelin from *mld* mice, the two myelin basic components are virtually absent, whereas CNP and the Wolfgram proteins are increased (Figure 13.5). Electron microscopy shows that the major dense line of myelin is absent[27] (Figure 13.6). The yield of

Figure 13.6 Electron micrographs of (A) control and (B) *mld* optic nerves (33 days). Cross-sectioned axons of different diameters are surrounded by a dark ring, the myelin sheath. In *mld* optic nerves, very few axons are myelinated and the myelin sheath appears very thin. Inserts: high power magnification of control and *mld* myelin. In control myelin, the sheath is well compacted and the major and minor dense lines are easily identified. In contrast, *mld* myelin is poorly compacted and only the minor dense line seems present. Magnifications (A) × 8400 and (B) × 125 000

myelin isolated from *mld* sciatic nerves was not significantly different from controls. In spite of a normal electron microscopic appearance, PNS myelin had no myelin basic proteins[28]. Striking similarities between *Shiverer* and *mld* suggest that the two mutants could be alleles. Cross breeding between *Shiverer* and *mld* gave 50% offsprings exhibiting the neurological symptoms observed in *Shiverer* or *mld*[29] but the position of the two genes relative to one another still has to be determined in order to demonstrate the allelism between these two genes[29]. *Shiverer* and *mld* mutations present a striking confirmation of previous investigations, indicating that myelin basic proteins are located on the inner surfaces of the membrane bilayer (Figure 13.2) corresponding to the major dense line of the myelin sheath. In contrast, in PNS myelin, it is possible that myelin basic proteins are not important for the molecular organization of the myelin sheath and that the major PNS myelin protein P_0 could be responsible for the compaction of the multilamellar structure[25].

Dystrophic mutation

This autosomal recessive mutation (Table 13.2) was at first erroneously named *muscular dystrophy*. Its neurogenic origin was recognized when authors found a severe abnormality in lumbosacral spinal roots, characterized by a large number of normal axons totally devoid of myelin sheaths and a lack of Schwann cells. The basal lamina secreted by *Dystrophic* Schwann cells presents important defects[30, 31]. In normal conditions, neuron-related Schwann cells in the absence of fibroblasts generate a number of extracellular matrix components, including basal lamina and thin collagenous fibrils but not the larger fibrils typical of endoneurium[32]. Thus, the complex axon–myelin–Schwann cell is isolated from the surroundings by the basal lamina.

In long-term tissue cultures of dorsal root ganglia from dystrophic mice, Okada and colleagues found, as *in vivo*, discontinuity in the basal lamina and regions of incomplete ensheathment of unmyelinated fibers[31]. However, the substantial ensheathment failure present in certain *Dystrophic* nerve roots *in vivo* was not expressed in cultures; myelination and Schwann cell numbers were similar to those found in control cultures. *Dystrophic* Schwann cells related to normal axons showed basal lamina defects, whereas normal Schwann cells ensheathing *Dystrophic* axons did not. Since normal Schwann cell differentiation appears to require contact not only with an axon but also with certain extracellular matrix components[32], Okada and coworkers propose that *Dystrophic* mice are affected by an abnormality of the extracellular matrix of the peripheral nerve tissues.[31] In this mutation, the protein composition of myelin is normal[33].

Trembler mutation

Trembler mice (Table 13.2), a spontaneous mutation, are affected by a dominantly inherited neuropathy. The main morphological findings are hypomyelination, segmental demyelination and onion bulb formation, a picture almost identical to that of hypertrophic interstitial neuropathy in man (Dejerine–Sottas disease)[34]. Aguayo and colleagues have shown with nerve transplantation (including the transplantation of human nerve biopsy specimens into immuno-suppressed mice) that Schwann cells from *Trembler* mice or from patients with Charcot–Marie–Tooth disease express their characteristic abnormality with normal mouse axons.[35]

The yield of myelin isolated from *Trembler* nerves is extremely low and all the typical PNS myelin proteins are depressed[36]. These findings are similar to those found in animals after Wallerian degeneration and are consistent with marked demyelination. Lipid analysis of *Trembler* nerves showed that both cerebrosides and sulphatides are decreased[37]. Recently, we found an increased *in vivo* sulphate and galactose incorporation into non-lipid material which could reflect the overproduction of endoneurial and perineurial connective tissue, whereas the high turnover rate of sulphatides could be correlated with intense demyelination and remyelination observed in *Trembler* PNS. Since cerebroside sulphotransferase (EC 2.8.2.11, CST), the enzyme responsible for the synthesis of sulphatides, is increased in *Trembler* PNS, it would be of interest to measure it in human neuropathies to see whether this test could be of help in sorting out the different forms.[38].

MUTATIONS AFFECTING MYELINATION AS A SECONDARY EFFECT

In these mutations, the primary defect does not seem to directly affect the genetic control of myelin formation, but influences it as a secondary phenomenon.

Dwarf mutation

The homozygous, recessive mutants of Snell's dwarf strain of mice are affected by underdevelopment of the anterior pituitary, thyroid, thymus, adrenals, pancreas and gonads[39]. Low levels of thyroid-stimulating hormone, growth hormone and prolactin along with secondary hypothyroidism have been reported[40]. In 19-day-old hypopituitary Snell's dwarf mice, the number of myelinated axons in the corticospinal tract and anterior commissure is significantly decreased[41]. The yield of isolated myelin is decreased by 56% in the *Dwarf* mouse. The composition of proteins[41, 42], glycoproteins[41], and CNP activity[41, 42] in purified myelin from *Dwarf* mice is nearly equivalent to that of control myelin. The metabolism of oligodendrocytes does not seem to be disabled. These findings agree with the observation that thyroid and growth-hormone deficiencies impair myelinogenesis in the CNS.

Mottled mutation

The X-linked *Mottled* mouse mutants (Table 13.1) are homologous to the human congenital copper-deficiency disease Menkes' steely-hair syndrome, and can be used in elucidating the pathogenesis of the human[43-45]. The mottled locus contains five allelic genes and we studied myelination in the brain of *blotchy* whose affected males survive to beyond the age at which myelination is usually complete, and of *brindled* males which is lethal at an earlier stage of brain development than the human disease (Danks and Matthieu, unpublished results). In *blotchy* mice, myelination was not affected. In *brindled* males, Yajima and Suzuki noted widespread neuronal degeneration in the cerebral cortex and thalamic nuclei after the 12th postnatal day[46]. These authors did not find obvious abnormalities in the white matter of male hemizygotes. In 14-day-old brains, myelin was isolated in decreased amounts, but its protein and lipid composition was normal (Danks and Matthieu, unpublished results).

Crinkled mutation

The possibility of an abnormal copper metabolism was suggested[47] but Mann and co-workers (*Biol. Trace Element Res.*, 1981, **3**, 117) did not find any evidence to support this contention. In these mice, myelin disruption seems secondary to axonal degeneration[47].

Twitcher mutation

This newly discovered mutation is transmitted as an autosomal recessive trait. Clinical abnormalities including low body weight, progressive wasting, tremor and muscular weakness appear at about the 15th day and death occurs before 3 months[48]. Important demyelination affects the CNS. In the PNS both demyelination and remyelination are observed. In both CNS and PNS, globoid cells are present[48]. Biochemical analyses show the identity between Twitcher and human globoid cell leukodystrophy (Krabbe's disease); in both conditions galactosylceramidase is deficient[49].

Wobbler mutation

Wobbler is transmitted in an autosomal recessive manner. The primary defect involves degeneration of motor nerve cells in the brain stem and spinal cord with a progressive motor denervation of skeletal muscles[50]. Peripheral nerve involvement is mainly due to Wallerian degeneration with secondary demyelination. Spinal and brain stem motor neurons are vacuolized. The mice die at about one year. Wobbler mutants offer a model in mice for hereditary motor nerve cell diseases in man like Werdnig–Hoffmann disease or juvenile proximal spinal muscular atrophy (Kugelberg–Welander).

Tabby mutation

This X-linked mutation is 20 crossing-over units apart from the Jimpy locus. Abnormalities of the coat and vibrissae have been used as a genetic marker in cross-breeding experiments to identify Jimpy hemizygotes prior to the onset of symptoms. Growth is often retarded in Tabby mutants. Deficient myelination observed in vitro[51] as well as reduced activity of cerebroside sulphotransferase [52] are probably secondary phenomena.

Miscellaneous mutations

Cribriform degeneration is an autosomal recessive mutation. Homozygotes present a small body size, weakness and ataxic behaviour beginning at about 3 weeks of age. Affected mutants show severe vacuolar degeneration in white and grey matter of the spinal cord and brain stem, normocytic anaemia at birth decreasing in severity with age, and abnormalities of electrolyte distribution presenting some analogy to cystic fibrosis[53]. Focal damage of myelin sheaths and axons is suggestive of secondary Wallerian degeneration. The mode of inheritance and the neuropathological characteristics are similar to those of inherited spongy degeneration in man.

Ducky mutants are affected by spinomedullocerebellar dysgenesis. The reduction of tissue cerebroside in the brain stem and spinal cord indicates a myelin deficit secondary to axonal dystrophy and loss of Purkinje cells.[54] Similar focal hypomyelination or demyelination occur in *Ataxia* or *Paralytic* mutants[55], and in the *Teetering* mutation[56].

In the autosomal recessive mutation *Dilute lethal*, the reduced cerebroside synthesis (a major myelin lipid) reflects a reduced growth rate caused by poorer nutrition in the affected mice[57]. *Wabbler lethal* mice are affected by a disorder of the vestibulocerebellar and spinocerebellar tracts. Although not extensively studied, this mutation also presents a limited deficit of myelin. Using a cerebellar tissue culture of these two mutants, Hamburgh and Bornstein showed that *in vitro*, myelin is synthetized and maintained just as well as in the control cultures.[58] This indicates that the defect in these two autosomal recessive mutations is probably extrinsic and not specific to the oligodendrocyte[58]. *Sprawling* is a dominantly transmitted mutation. The affected animals have ataxia and defective position sense chiefly affecting the hind limbs. Duchen found a failure in the maturation and myelination of sensory axons[59]. Sensory ganglion cells show marked chromatolysis in the absence of axonal degeneration or regeneration. Two peripheral neuropathies, *Shambling*[60] and *Dystonia Musculorum*[61] present possible secondary myelin defects but little information is available on these two mutations.

CONCLUSION

In this review I have briefly presented 22 mutations which affect mice myelination directly or indirectly. Some of these mutations are analogous to human disorders and an understanding of the molecular defects in the human diseases can be achieved using these animal models. Moreover, these mutations should also be valuable for therapeutic studies. Although in many cases the mutations do not seem to have their counterpart in the human (yet), a great deal of our knowledge about the localization of myelin-specific components within the myelin membrane and about the mechanisms of their insertion into the membrane has been obtained with myelin-deficient mutants. I am confident that these genetic experiments of nature have still more to reveal about the mechanisms of myelinogenesis, which is, with synaptogenesis, the most important event of nervous system development.

Acknowledgments

The author wishes to thank Prof. E. Gautier for his continued interest and Ms. Betty Thorpe for reading the manuscript.

Supported, in part, by the Swiss National Science Foundation (Grant 3.446.79) and the Multiple Sclerosis Society of Switzerland.

References

1. Norton, W. T. (1977) Isolation and characterization of myelin. In Morell, P. (ed.) *Myelin*, pp. 161–199. (New York: Plenum Press)
2. Suzuki, K. (1980) Myelin-associated enzymes. In Baumann, N. (ed.) *Neurological Mutations Affecting Myelination*, pp. 333–347. (Amsterdam: Elsevier-North Holland Biomedical)
3. Sidman, R. L., Dickie, M. M. and Appel, S. H. (1964). Mutant mice (*Quaking* and *Jimpy*) with deficient myelination in the central nervous system. *Science*, **144**, 309
4. Hogan, E. L. (1977). Animal models of genetic disorders of myelin. In Morell, P. (ed.) *Myelin*. pp. 489–520. (New York: Plenum Press)
5. Baumann, N. (1980). Mutations affecting myelination in the central nervous system: research tools in neurobiology. *Trends Neurosci.*, **3**, 82
6. Meier, C. and Bischoff, A. (1974). Dysmyelination in 'Jimpy' mouse. Electron microscopic study. *J. Neuropath. Exp. Neurol.*, **33**, 343
7. Torii, J., Adachi, M. and Volk, B. W. (1971). Histochemical and ultrastructural studies of inherited leukodystrophy in mice. *J. Neuropathol. Exp. Neurol.*, **30**, 278
8. Meier, C., Herschkowitz, N. and Bischoff, A. (1974). Morphological and biochemical observations in the Jimpy spinal cord. *Acta Neuropathol. (Berl.)*, **27**, 349
9. Matthieu, J.-M. (1980). Biosynthesis of myelin proteins and glycoproteins. In Baumann, N. (ed.) *Neurological Mutations Affecting Myelination*, pp. 275–298 (Amsterdam: Elsevier-North Holland Biomedical)
10. Barbarese, E., Carson, J. H. and Braun, P. E. (1979). Subcellular distribution and structural polymorphism of myelin basic protein in normal and Jimpy mouse brain. *J. Neurochem.*, **32**, 1437
11. Zimmerman, T. R. Jr. and Cohen, S. R. (1979). The distribution of myelin basic protein in subcellular fractions of developing jimpy mouse brain. *J. Neurochem.*, **32**, 817
12. Eicher, E. M. and Hoppe, P. C. (1973). Use of chimeras to transmit lethal genes in the mouse and to demonstrate allelism of the two X-linked male lethal genes JP and MSD. *J. Exp. Zool.*, **183**, 181

13. Hogan, E. L. and Joseph, K. C. (1970). Composition of cerebral lipids in murine leukodystrophy: the Quaking mutant. *J. Neurochem.*, **17**, 1209

14. Wisniewski, H. and Morell, P. (1971). Quaking mouse: ultrastructural evidence for arrest of myelinogenesis. *Brain Res.*, **29**, 63

15. Singh, H., Spritz, N. and Geyer, B. (1971) Studies of brain myelin in the 'quaking mouse'. *J. Lipid Res.*, **12**, 473

16. Greenfield, S., Norton, W. T. and Morell, P. (1971). Quaking mouse: isolation and characterization of myelin protein. *J. Neurochem.*, **18**, 2119

17. Mikoshiba, K., Nagaike, K., Aoki, E. and Tsukada, Y. (1979). Biochemical and immunohistochemical studies on dysmyelination of Quaking mutant mice *in vivo* and *in vitro*. *Brain Res.*, **177**, 287

18. Baumann, N. A., Harpin, M. L. and Bourre, J.-M. (1970). Long chain fatty acid formation: key step in myelination studied in mutant mice. *Nature* (London), **227**, 960

19. Kishimoto, Y. (1971). Abnormality in sphingolipid fatty acids from sciatic nerve and brain of Quaking mice. *J. Neurochem.*, **18**, 1365

20. Bourre, J.-M., Daudu, O. L. and Baumann, N. A. (1975). Fatty acid biosynthesis in mice brain and kidney microsomes: comparison between Quaking mutant and control. *J. Neurochem.*, **24**, 1095

21. Matthieu, J.-M., Koellreutter, B. and Joyet, M.-L. (1978). Protein and glycoprotein of myelin subfractions from brains of 'Quaking' mice. *J. Neurochem.*, **30**, 783

22. Greenfield, S., Williams, N. I., White, M., Brostoff, S. W. and Hogan, E. L. (1979). Proteolipid protein: synthesis and assembly into Quaking mouse myelin. *J. Neurochem.*, **32**, 1647

23. Privat, A., Jacque, C., Bourre, J.-M., Dupouey, P. and Baumann, N. (1979). Absence of the major dense line in myelin of the mutant mouse 'Shiverer'. *Neurosci. Lett.*, **12**, 107

24. Dupouey, P., Jacque, C., Bourre, J.-M., Cesselin, F., Privat, A. and Baumann, N. (1979). Immunochemical studies of a myelin basic protein in Shiverer mouse devoid of major dense line of myelin. *Neurosci. Lett.*, **12**, 113

25. Kirschner, D. A. and Ganser, A. L. (1980). Compact myelin exists in the absence of basic protein in the shiverer mutant mouse. *Nature (London)*, **283**, 207

26. Mikoshiba, K., Aoki, E. and Tsukada, Y. (1980). 2′, 3′-Cyclic nucleotide 3′-phosphohydrolase activity in the central nervous system of a myelin deficient mutant (Shiverer). *Brain Res.*, **192**, 195

27. Matthieu, J.-M., Ginalski, H., Friede, R. L., Cohen, S. R. and Doolittle, D. P. (1980a) Absence of myelin basic protein and major dense line in CNS myelin of the mld mutant mouse. *Brain Res.*, **191**, 278

28. Matthieu, J.-M., Ginalski, H., Friede, R. L. and Cohen, S. R. (1980b). Low myelin basic protein levels and 'normal' myelin in peripheral nerves of myelin deficient mutant mice (mld). *Neuroscience*, **5**, 2315

29. Lachapelle, F., de Baecque, C., Jacque, C., Bourre, J.-M., Delassalle, A., Doolittle, D., Hauw, J. J. and Baumann, N. (1980). Comparison of morphological and biochemical defects of two probably allelic mutations of the mouse myelin deficient (mld) and shiverer (shi). In Baumann, N. (ed.) *Neurological Mutations Affecting Myelination*, pp. 27–32. (Amsterdam: Elsevier-North Holland Biomedical)

30. Jaros, E. and Bradley, W. G. (1979). Atypical axon–Schwann cell relationships in the common peroneal nerve of the dystrophic mouse: an ultrastructural study. *Neuropathol. Appl. Neurobiol.*, **5**, 133

31. Okada, E., Bunge, R. P. and Bunge, M. B. (1980). Abnormalities expressed in long-term cultures of dorsal root ganglia from the dystrophic mouse. *Brain Res.*, **194**, 455

32. Bunge, M. B., Williams, A. K., Wood, P. M., Uitto, J. and Jeffrey, J. J. (1980). Comparison of nerve cell and nerve cell plus Schwann cell cultures, with particular emphasis on basal lamina and collagen formation. *J. Cell. Biol.*, **84**, 184

33. Wiggins, R. C. and Morell, P. (1978). Myelin of the peripheral nerve of the dystrophic mouse. *J. Neurochem.*, **31**, 1101

34. Ayers, M. M. and Anderson, R. McD. (1973). Onion bulb neuropathy in the Trembler mouse: a model of hypertrophic interstitial neuropathy (Dejerine–Sottas) in man. *Acta Neuropathol. (Berl.)*, **25**, 54

35. Aguayo, A. J., Bray, G. M., Perkins, C. S. and Duncan, I. D. (1979). Axon-sheath cell interactions in peripheral and central nervous system transplants. *Soc. Neurosci. Symp.*, **4**, 361

36. Matthieu, J.-M., Fagg, G. E., Darriet, D., Larrouquère-Régnier, S., Cassagne, C. and Bourre, J.-M. (1979). Abnormal myelin protein distribution in a hereditary demyelinating neuropathy. *Proc. Int. Soc. Neurochem.*, **7**, 475

37. Larrouquère-Régnier, S., Boiron, F., Darriet, D., Cassagne, C. and Bourre, J.-M. (1979). Lipid composition of sciatic nerve from dysmyelinating Trembler mouse. *Neurosci. Lett.*, **15**, 135

38. Matthieu, J.-M., Reigner, J., Costantino-Ceccarini, E., Bourre, J.-M. and Rütti, M. (1980). Abnormal sulfate metabolism in a hereditary demyelinating neuropathy. *Brain Res.*, **200**, 457

39. Bartke, A. (1967). Prolactin deficiency in genetically sterile dwarf mice. *Mem. Soc. Endocrinol.*, **15**, 193

40. Reier, P. J., Froelich, J. S., Sawchak, J. A. and Hughes, A. F. W. (1974). Maturation of nonmyelinated fiber bundles in a strain of Dwarf (Snell's) mice. *Anat. Rec.*, **178**, 103

41. Reier, P. J., Matthieu, J.-M. and Zimmerman, A. W. (1975). Myelin deficiency in heridtary pituitary dwarfism: a biochemical and morphological study. *J. Neuropathol. Exp. Neurol.*, **34**, 465

42. Lees, A., Sarliève, L. L., Neskovic, N. M., Wintzerith, M. and Mandel, P. (1977). Changes in brain components during the development of mice homozygous for the locus "Dwarf" (dw). *Neurochem. Res.*, **2**, 11

43. Hunt, D. M. (1974). Primary defect in copper transport underlies mottled mutants in the mouse. *Nature (London)*. **249**, 852

44. Danks, D. M. (1977). Copper transport and utilisation in Menkes' syndrome and in mottled mice. *Inorg. Perspect. Biol. Med.*, **1**, 73

45. Mann, J. R., Camakaris, J. and Danks, D. M. (1980). Copper metabolism in Mottled mouse mutants. Defective placental transfer of ^{64}Cu to foetal brindled (Mo^{br}) mice. *Biochem. J.*, **186**, 629

46. Yajima, K. and Suzuki, K. (1979). Neuronal degeneration in the brain of the brindled mouse – a light microscope study. *J. Neuropath. Exp. Neurol.*, **38**, 35

47. Theriault, L. L., Dungan, D. D., Simons, S., Keen, C. L. and Hurley, L. S.

(1977) Lipid and myelin abnormalities of brain in the crinkled mouse. *Proc. Soc. Exp. Biol. Med.*, **155**, 549

48. Duchen, L. W., Eicher, E. M., Jacobs, J. M., Scarvilli, F. and Teixeira, F. (1980). A globoid cell type of leukodystrophy in the mouse: the new mutant *Twitcher*. In Baumann, N. (ed.) *Neurological Mutations Affecting Myelination*, pp. 107–114. (Amsterdam: Elsevier-North Holland Biomedical)

49. Kobayashi, T. and Suzuki, K. (1980). Biochemistry of twitcher mouse: an authentic murine model of human globoid cell leukodystrophy. In Baumann, N. (ed.) *Neurological Mutations Affecting Myelination*, pp. 253–256. (Amsterdam: Elsevier-North Holland Biomedical)

50. Duchen, L. W. and Strich, S. J. (1968). An hereditary motor neurone disease with progressive denervation of muscle in the mouse: the mutant 'wobbler'. *J. Neurol. Neurosurg. Psychiat.*, **31**, 535

51. Wolf, M. K. and Holden, A. B. (1969). Tissue culture analysis of the inherited defect of central nervous system myelination in Jimpy mice. *J. Neuropathol. Exp. Neurol.*, **28**, 195

52. Matthieu, J.-M. and Herschkowitz, N. (1973). Effect on 'Tabby' locus, on brain [^{35}S]sulfatide synthesis. *Neurobiology*, **3**, 39

53. Green, M. C., Sidman, R. L. and Pivetta, O. H. (1972). Cribriform degeneration (cri): a new recessive neurological mutation in the mouse. *Science*, **176**, 800

54. Meier, H. and Macpike, A. D. (1970). A neurological mutation (MSD) of the mouse causing a deficiency of myelin synthesis. *Exp. Brain Res.*, **10**, 512

55. D'Amato, C. J. and Hicks, S. P. (1965). Neuropathologic alterations in the ataxia (paralytic) mouse. *Arch. Pathol.*, **80**, 604

56. Meier, H. (1967a). The neuropathy of teetering, a neurological mutation in the mouse. *Arch. Neurol.*, **16**, 59

57. Winterbourn, C. C., Woolf, F. and Woolf, L. I. (1971). Brain lipids of mice homozygous for the gene "dilute lethal" (d^1). *J. Neurochem.*, **18**, 1077

58. Hamburgh, M. and Bornstein, M. K. (1970). Myelin synthesis in two demyelinating mutations in mice. *Exp. Neurol.*, **28**, 471

59. Duchen, L. W. (1975). 'Sprawling': a new mutant mouse with failure of myelination of sensory axons and a deficiency of muscle spindles. *Neuropathol., Appl. Neurobiol.*, **1**, 89

60. Meier, H. (1967b). Pathological findings in shambling, a hereditary neuropathy of mice. *J. Neuropath. Exp. Neurol.*, **26**, 620

61. Duchen, L. W. and Strich, S. J. (1964). Clinical and pathological studies of an hereditary neuropathy in mice (Dystonia Musculorum). *Brain*, **87**, 367

14

The effect of phenylalanine on myelin metabolism in adolescent rats

F. A. Hommes, A. G. Eller
and E. H. Taylor

A true genetic animal model for phenylketonuria (PKU) does not exist. The technique developed by Mintz could bring about generation of such a model[1]. However, the phenylalanine-4-mono-oxygenase is not expressed in teratocarcinoma cells (S. Molenaar and F. A. Hommes, unpublished observation), so it will be difficult, although not impossible, to search for the appropriate mutant cell line. Therefore, chemically-induced models have to be used. Presently, two such models are under investigation, namely those induced by the addition of extra phenylalanine to the diet in combination with an inhibitor of the phenylalanine-4-mono-oxygenase, the difference between the two models being the inhibitor: p-chloro-phenylalanine[2] or α-methylphenylalanine[3].

The question arises as to whether these models approach the human PKU condition sufficiently well. Classical PKU is characterized by symptoms, such as EEG abnormalities and irritability, which can be reversed by decreasing the blood phenylalanine level, and by a permanent effect (mental retardation) which is irreversible once it has become manifest. At the biochemical level, the only long-lasting effect of classical, untreated PKU, which has been well documented, is a deficiency of myelin in the central nervous system (CNS)[4-6]. Although myelin deficiencies in experimental hyperphenylalaninaemia have been described[7-10], such studies, as pointed out by Kaufman[11], suffer from the disadvantage of being initiated in newborn rats whose brain maturation is comparable to that of the human fetus of around 18 weeks of gestation[12]. The hyperphenylalaninaemic condition was thus induced at a stage where glial proliferation had still to take place. It is mainly for this reason that we chose to induce the hyperphenylalaninaemic condition in rats of 25 days of age[13,14]. This allowed us to evaluate the validity of the termination of dietary treatment – at least as far as some biochemical parameters were concerned – of PKU patients aged 5–8 years, because as far as brain maturation is concerned the rat of 25 days of age is roughly equivalent to a child of 8 years.

To evaluate the interference which an increased blood phenylalanine level has on myelin metabolism, both the rate of myelin synthesis and myelin turnover were measured in rats placed on the hyperphenylalaninaemia-inducing diet (normal laboratory chow supplemented with 3% L-phenylalanine and 0.12% DL-p-chloro-phenylalanine) at the age of 25 days (*HyPhe* rats). Rats of the same age, with unlimited access to normal food (C rats), with limited access to normal food so as to match the weights of the *HyPhe* rats (WMC rats), and with unlimited access to normal food containing 0.12% DL-p-chlorophenylalanine (*p*Cl rats), served as controls. Experimental procedures have been previously described[14]. Myelin was subfractionated according to the methods of Matthieu and coworkers[15]. Myelin proteins were separated by SDS–gel electrophoresis[16].

Previous experiments had demonstrated a striking difference in the turnover between myelin of C rats and of *HyPhe* rats[13,14]. In the C rats part of the myelin is degraded with a half life of 13 days (corrected for the metabolically stable compound), while in the *HyPhe* rats 50% of the incorporated radioactivity is lost within two days. After that the radioactivity remains stable for about 50 days, while a third phase can be distinguished, with a half life of about 65 days. The turnover of myelin in the *HyPhe* rats is therefore qualitativity and quantitively different from that in C rats, particularly in the fast component[17,18].

The initial phase of myelin turnover was therefore studied in more detail. These experiments were carried out for a total of 20 days on dietary treatment, which meant that the slow components of myelin and myelin proteins of the controls could not be measured[17]. For this reason all half-life values given have not been corrected for the slow components. Maximum labelling in the basic proteins of the controls increased slowly,

TABLE 14.1 Body and brain weights of C, HyPhe, WMC and pCl rats placed on one of four diets at 25 days of age

Days on diet	C rats		HyPhe rats		WMC rats		pCl rats	
	Body	Brain	Body	Brain	Body	Brain	Body	Brain
3	79.5 ± 2.6	1.47 ± 0.01	60.0 ± 2.5	1.46 ± 0.02	60.8 ± 7.4	1.38 ± 0.05	74.3 ± 6.2	1.40 ± 0.02
4	84.6 ± 1.7	1.41 ± 0.04	55.5 ± 1.5	1.99 ± 0.02	58.2 ± 7.0	1.38 ± 0.10	77.2 ± 5.5	1.57 ± 0.07
5	90.3 ± 2.0	1.53 ± 0.01	55.7 ± 1.5	1.49 ± 0.03	68.8 ± 8.2	1.49 ± 0.01	80.4 ± 6.0	1.53 ± 0.07
6	96.7 ± 2.5	1.57 ± 0.04	57.6 ± 1.8	1.45 ± 0.01	59.4 ± 6.3	1.44 ± 0.09	82.2 ± 6.8	1.47 ± 0.09
7	101.1 ± 2.5	1.52 ± 0.02	59.0 ± 1.9	1.49 ± 0.01	62.4 ± 7.1	1.42 ± 0.10	87.7 ± 5.6	1.46 ± 0.06
10	120.6 ± 3.3	1.56 ± 0.03	64.1 ± 1.8	—	75.8 ± 7.3	1.37 ± 0.18	101.3 ± 6.7	1.56 ± 0.05
11	127.9 ± 5.6	—	66.3 ± 1.9	1.44 ± 0.02	70.9 ± 8.5	—	—	—
12	130.2 ± 6.1	1.61 ± 0.01	67.8 ± 2.3	—	75.6 ± 7.4	1.41 ± 0.07	108.5 ± 6.2	1.52 ± 0.08
13	137.1 ± 6.0	—	68.6 ± 2.5	1.39 ± 0.09	76.6 ± 6.6	—	116.0 ± 7.5	1.61 ± 0.15
14	143.8 ± 5.8	1.65 ± 0.02	71.4 ± 3.3	—	78.4 ± 6.7	1.43 ± 0.09	—	—
17	161.1 ± 4.2	—	79.8 ± 8.4	1.45 ± 0.04	86.2 ± 7.2	—	128.5 ± 8.1	1.64 ± 0.05
20	184.5 ± 5.3	1.67 ± 0.02	88.4 ± 7.1	1.43 ± 0.07	88.2 ± 8.4	1.51 ± 0.04	139.6 ± 12.0	1.63 ± 0.06

Results are expressed in g ± SD. The number of rats in each group was 40 at the start of the experiment, decreasing to four for the last measurement, for body weight. The brain weights are the mean brain weight of four rats

so that an estimate of the half-life could not be made during this short period of investigation. The body and brain weights of the rats on the four diets are given in Table 14.1. The body weights of the WMC rats were within 5 % of those of the *HyPhe* rats, while the brain weights of the WMC rats were the same, within experimental error, as those of the *HyPhe* rats. The brain weights of the *p*Cl rats did not differ significantly from those of the C rats.

Table 14.2 summarizes the studies on myelin turnover. Myelin turnover in the *HyPhe* rats is considerably increased compared to that of controls. This increased turnover is due, only to a small degree, to the slowing down of growth, since the myelin turnover in WMC rats is somewhat increased relative to that of the controls, but not at all comparable to that observed in the *HyPhe* rats. It is known that postnatal nutritional deprivation leads to inhibition of myelin synthesis[19,20] and that the turnover of myelin is higher in the very young brain than in the more mature brain[21]. Since a slightly higher turnover of myelin has been observed in the present study in the nutritionally deprived rats – the dietary regimen starting at the age of 25 days – nutritional deprivation in the newborn rat may lead to increased turnover of myelin, contrary to the interpretation of Wiggins *et al.*[22]

The *p*Cl rats similarly showed a slightly increased turnover of myelin, but as with the WMC rats this was not at all comparable to that observed in the *HyPhe* rats. The values for the half-lives as given in Table 14.2 do not necessarily represent absolute values, because the data are uncorrected for the more stable compounds and utilization of the injected precursor was not taken into account. The data for the C-rats are, however, in agreement

TABLE 14.2   Summary of half lives (in days) of fast/slow components of myelin and myelin proteins in normal (C), hyperphenylalaninaemic (*HyPhe*), weight matched controls (WMC) and *p*-chlorophenylalanine-fed rats (pCl)*

	C rats	WMC rats	pCl rats	HyPhe rats
Whole myelin	37/n.d.[†]	30	33	2/n.d.
Small basic protein	—	—	—	9/n.d.
Large basic protein	—	—	—	3/16
DM-20	57/n.d.	—	—	9/60
Proteolipid protein	33/n.d.	—	—	2/16
Wolfgram protein	43/n.d.	—	—	5/76

* The specific diets were given to rats of 25 days of age, at which age [³H] lysine (1 µ Ci/g b.w.) was injected intravenously via the tail vein
[†] n.d.: not determined

with those reported by Sabri et al.[17]. In that study rats of the same age were used, and the same route for administration of the precursor was followed. The data for myelin turnover in the rats on the four diets can be compared with each other to evaluate the effect specifically due to the hyper-phenylalaninaemic condition. Since neither the WMC rats, nor the p-Cl rats showed an increase in myelin turnover comparable to that observed in the *HyPhe* rats, it can be concluded that the decreased half-lives for myelin in the *HyPhe* rats is indeed due to the hyperphenylalaninaemic condition.

Rates of myelin synthesis were measured during the first 20 days in rats on the diets. The results are summarized in Table 14.3. The rate of

TABLE 14.3   Myelin synthesis in C rats and in HyPhe rats*

Days on diet	C	HyPhe
3	654 ± 66	376 ± 77
4	457 ± 47	253 ± 24
5	347 ± 35	272 ± 31
6	330 ± 62	268 ± 76
7		246 ± 54
10	362 ± 22	338 ± 25
11		182 ± 29
12	402 ± 56	146 ± 38
13		221 ± 53
14	308 ± 35	
18	242 ± 31	
20	270 ± 59	257 ± 32

* [4, 5-³H] Lysine (1 μ Ci/g body w.) was injected via the tail vein 1 h prior to sacrifice. Results are expressed as dpm/mg protein ± SD (n = 4)

incorporation of label into myelin proteins in the *HyPhe* rats was considerably lower than that in C rats, especially during the early phase of the dietary regimen, in agreement with earlier observations[13,14]. Fractionation of myelin into the light, medium and heavy fractions[15] revealed a 40% decreased incorporation of label into the light fraction, a 50% decreased incorporation into the medium fraction and a 30% decreased incorporation into the heavy fraction.

Experimental hyperphenylalaninaemia induced by adding p-chlorophenylalanine and phenylalanine to the diet results, therefore, in an increased turnover of myelin and in a decreased rate of myelin synthesis. The ultimate result of both these processes is a decrease in total myelin in the brain. In this respect the experimental model mimics the human PKU condition, as far as a long lasting biochemical effect of this disease is concerned. It should be pointed out that these studies have been carried out in rats where the hyperphenylalaninaemic condition was initiated when the rats were 25 days of age, after they had grown up under normal conditions. The implication is that even at this relatively mature stage of brain development, myelin is still vulnerable to increased levels of phenylalanine. Since the effects are due to the hyperphenylalaninaemic condition and not due to the inhibitor used or to the retardation in growth, the observations may have some relevance to the termination of the dietary treatment of PKU patients at a relatively young age. Although the difference between the hyperphenylalaninaemia in the *HyPhe* rats with blood phenylalanine levels of 1–1.5 mmol/l and an older PKU patient on a limited protein intake should be recognized, the experiments described above provide sufficient evidence for extreme care in terminating the dietary treatment of PKU patients.

References

1. Mintz, B. (1979). Teratocarcinoma cells as tools for production of mouse models of human genetic diseases. In Hommes, F. A. (ed.) *Models for the Study of Inborn Errors of Metabolism*, pp. 343–354. (Amsterdam: Elsevier/North Holland Biomedical Press)
2. Berry, H. K., Butcher, R. E., Kasmaier, K. and Poncet, J. B. (1975). Biochemical effects of induced phenylketonuria in rats. *Biol. Neonat.*, **26,** 88
3. Del Valle, J. A., Diemel, G. and Greengard, O. (1978). Comparison of α-methylphenylalanine and *p*-chlorophenylalanine as inducers of chronic hyperphenylalaninemia in developing rats. *Biochem. J.*, **170,** 449
4. Alvord, E. C., Stevenson, L. D., Vogel, F. S. and Engle, R. L. (1950). Neuropathological findings in phenylpyruvic oligophrenia (phenyl-ketonuria). *J. Neuropathol. Exp. Neurol.* **9,** 298
5. Crome, L., Thymms, V. and Woolf, L. I. (1962). A chemical investigation of the defects of myelination in phenylketonuria, *J. Neurol. Neurosurg. Psychiat.*, **25,** 143
6. Shah, S. N., Peterson, N. A. and McKean, C. M. (1972). Lipid composition of human cerebral white matter and myelin in phenylketonuria. *J. Neurochem.*, **19,** 2369
7. Shah, S. N., Peterson, N. A. and McKean, C. M. (1972). Impaired myelin formation in experimental hyperphenylalaninemia. *J. Neurochem.*, **19,** 479
8. Loo, Y. G., Scotto, J. and Wisniewski, H. (1978). Myelin deficiency in experimental phenylketonuria. Contribution of the aromatic metabolites of phenylalanine. *Adv. Exp. Med. Biol.*, **100,** 453
9. Lane, J. D., Schöne, B., Langenbeck, U. and Neuhoff, V. (1979). Characterization of experimental phenylketonuria. In Hommes, F. A. (ed.)

Models for the Study of Inborn Errors of Metabolism, pp. 141–148. (Amsterdam: Elsevier/North Holland Biomedical Press)

10. Lane, J. D., Schöne, B., Langenbeck, U. and Neuhoff, V. (1980). Characteristics of experimental phenylketonuria. Augmentation of hyperphenylalaninemia with α-methylphenylalanine and p-chlorophenylalanine. *Biochim. Biophys. Acta*, **627**, 144

11. Kaufman, S. (1977) Phenylketonuria: biochemical mechanisms. *Adv. Neurochem.*, **2**, 1

12. Dobbing, J. (1975) Prenatal nutrition and neurological development. In Buchwald, N. A. and Brasier, M. A. B. (eds.) *Brain Mechanisms in Mental Retardation*. pp. 401–420. (New York: Academic Press)

13. Berger, R., Springer, J. and Hommes, F. A. (1977). Impairment of myelin metabolism in experimental phenylketonuria. *Hum. Hered.*, **27**, 165

14. Berger, R., Springer, J. and Hommes, F. A. (1980). Brain protein and myelin metabolism in young hyperphenylalaninemic rats. *Mol. Cell Biol.*, **26**, 31–36

15. Matthieu, J. M., Quarles, R. H., Brady, R. O. and DeF. Webster, H. (1973). Variation of proteins, enzyme markers and gangliosides in myelin subfractions. *Biochim. Biophys. Acta*, **329**, 305

16. Agrawal, H. C., Burton, R. M., Fishman, M. A., Mitchell, R. F. and Prensky, A. L. (1972). Partial characterization of a new myelin compound. *J. Neurochem.*, **19**, 2083

17. Sabri, M. T., Bone, A. H. and Davison, A. N. (1977). Turnover of myelin and other structural proteins in the developing rat brain. *Biochem. J.*, **142**, 499

18. Singh, H. and Jungalwala, F. B. (1979). The turnover of myelin proteins in adult rat brain. *Int. J. Neurosci.*, **9**, 123

19. Fishman, M. A., Madyastha, P. and Prensky, A. L. (1971). The effect of undernutrition on the development of myelin in the rat central nervous system. *Lipids*, **6**, 458

20. Nakhasi, H. L., Toenes, A. D. and Horrocks, L. A. (1975). Effects of a postnatal protein deficiency on the content and composition of myelin from brains of weanling rats. *Brain Res.*, **83**, 176

21. Lajtha, A., Toth, J., Fujimato, K. and Agrawal, H. C. (1977). Turnover of myelin proteins in mouse brain. *Biochem. J.*, **164**, 323

22. Wiggins, R. C., Miller, S. L., Benjamins, J. A., Krigman, M. R. and Morell, P. (1976). Myelin synthesis during postnatal nutritional deprivation and subsequent rehabilitation. *Brain Res.*, **107**, 257

15

Abnormal oligodendrocyte differentiation in a mouse mutant with defect in myelination

L. Bologa-Sandru, H.-P. Siegrist,
A. Z'graggen, U. Wiesmann
and N. Herschkowitz

INTRODUCTION

Animal mutants with myelination defects, particularly those showing a similarity with human diseases, are useful models for the study of inherited neurological disorders.

A mutant which shows a decreased amount of myelin in the central nervous system is the *Jimpy* mouse. This was discovered in 1954 due to its particular behaviour. Briefly, at 12 days of age it shows ataxia and tremor, at 18 days tonic convulsions, and death occurs between days 21 and 30. This mutant is considered to be a model for Pelizeaus–Merzbacher disease[1].

The *Jimpy* mouse has been the subject of many morphological[2-5] and biochemical[6-9] studies. With one exception[10] these studies were not made in culture. However, the analysis of the in-culture situation is very useful, since here the extrinsic factors can be avoided.

In our report we analyse, in *Jimpy* brain cell cultures, the development of oligodendrocytes[7]; these are key cells for the myelination in the central nervous system. Because of conflicting reports concerning the aspect of astrocytes in *Jimpy* mouse brain, *Jimpy* astrocytes in culture were also observed[11-13]. This task was facilitated by publications which reported galactocerebroside (GC) as a membrane marker for oligodendrocytes[14], myelin basic protein (MBP) as an internal marker for oligodendrocytes[15] and glial fibrillary acidic protein (GFAP) as an internal marker for astrocytes[16]. We used both GC and MBP to identify oligodendrocytes, since in previous work we had shown that in normal cultures there are two oligodendrocyte subpopulations: one which exhibits only GC, and a more differentiated subpopulation exhibiting both GC and MBP[17].

MATERIALS AND METHODS

Animals

Three-day-old *Jimpy* mice (C57 bl/6J-W A-J) and their normal litter mates were used.

Cultures

Mechanically dissociated brain cells (15×10^6), suspended in 10 ml Minimum Essential Medium Eagle Dulbecco modified containing 10% fetal calf serum, were cultivated on glass coverslips (60×24 mm) in 10 cm diameter petri dishes, at 37°C in a 5% CO_2 and 80% humid atmosphere. They were analysed after 7, 14 and 18 days.

Antisera

The production and the specificity of rabbit and mouse anti-GC, and rabbit anti-MBP sera used are previously described[17]. The rabbit anti-GFAP serum was a gift from Dr. Doris Dahl (Boston, USA).

Indirect immunofluorescence technique

This was done by applying an established technique to our experimental conditions[17,18]. None of the pre-immunization sera stained brain cultures and, furthermore, none of the antisera stained mouse fibroblasts. Preparations were microscopically examined and stained cells were counted in a Wild Leitz Orthoplan microscope.

RESULTS

Quantitative estimations are presented in Table 15.1. In *normal* mouse-brain cell cultures the GC^+ oligodendrocytes were small, round, and situated in the upper layer of the culture. Although not numerous, they were clearly visible in 7-day-old cultures. On the 14th day, there was a significant ($p < 0.01$) increase in their number. Then a steady stage was reached, and at 18 days the number of GC^+ oligodendrocytes was the same as that observed at 14 days. MBP^+ oligodendrocytes were absent in 7-day-old normal cultures. At day 14, only a few, isolated MBP^+ cells were observed, and their number increased significantly ($p < 0.01$) to the 18th day. At this time, more than 50% of them were grouped in clusters (8–12 clusters per coverslip) of 7–55 cells, and sometimes long MBP^+ processes were seen between the cells of a cluster. MBP^+ cells were larger than GC^+ cells.

When cultures were double stained to reveal GC and MBP simultaneously, two types of oligodendrocyte were visible: one of small, round, phase dark cells which were GC^+ and MBP^-, and another of large, GC^+, MBP^+ cells. The GC^+, MBP^- oligodendrocytes were much more numerous than those which were both GC and MBP positive.

$GFAP^+$ astrocytes were present in the cultures from the earliest stage, and from the moment when the cultures were confluent, no apparent changes were observed in their number and shape.

In 7, 14 and 18-day-old *Jimpy* cultures, the GC staining pattern was similar to that obtained in normal cultures. In contrast to this, the staining with the anti-MBP serum revealed in *Jimpy* cultures a situation that was different from the normal (Figure 15.1). No MBP^+ cells were observed in 14-day-old *Jimpy* cultures. At 18 days, a few MBP^+ cells appeared, their number being only about 5% that of normal. Moreover, these MBP^+ cells had no long processes, were less brilliant and were not grouped in clusters.

$GFAP^+$ astrocytes in *Jimpy* cultures had a similar aspect to that of astrocytes from normal cultures.

DISCUSSION

The development of oligodendrocytes was compared in *Jimpy* and normal mouse dissociated brain-cell cultures. The expression of two markers of

TABLE 15.1 Numerical estimation of GC^+, MBP^- and GC^+, MBP^+ oligodendrocytes in normal and *Jimpy* dissociated brain-cell cultures during development

Days in culture	Normal cultures			Jimpy cultures		
	GC^+, MBP^- cells	GC^+, MBP^+ cells	$^\circ/_{\circ\circ}$ MBP^+ cells of GC^+ cells	GC^+, MBP^- cells	GC^+, MBP^+ cells	$^\circ/_{\circ\circ}$ MBP^+ cells of GC^+ cells
7	37×10^3 $\pm 8 \times 10^3$	0	0	36.5×10^3 $\pm 9 \times 10^3$	0	0
14	335×10^3 $\pm 21 \times 10^3$	38 ± 4	0.11	334×10^3 $\pm 18 \times 10^3$	0	0
18	332×10^3 $\pm 15 \times 10^3$	532 ± 20	1.60	335×10^3 $\pm 20 \times 10^3$	25 ± 5	0.07

Numbers are given per coverslip (1440 mm²). Results are expressed as mean values ± SEM of eight determinations.

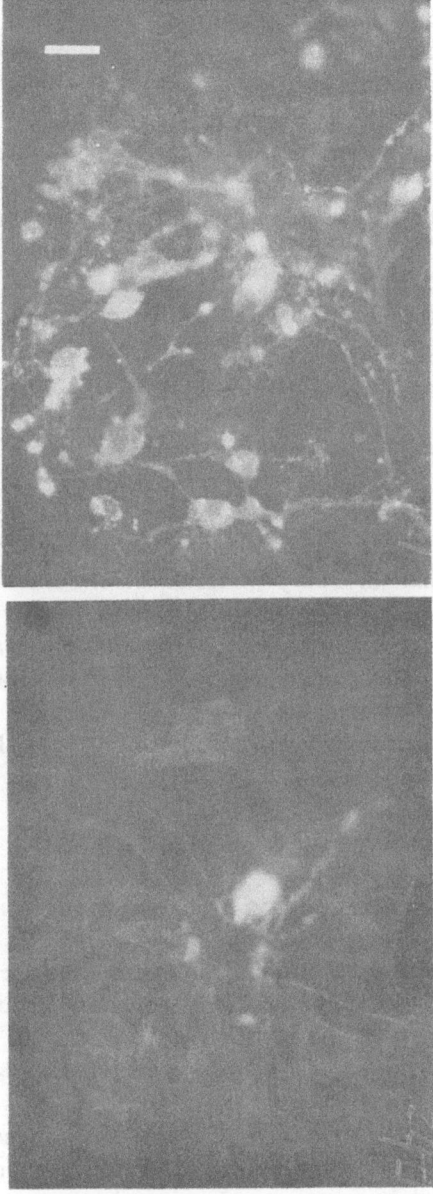

Figure 15.1 Immunofluorescence staining of 18-day-old fixed brain-cell cultures with the rabbit anti-MBP serum. (a) normal culture, (b) *Jimpy* culture. Bar represents 22 μm

oligodendrocytes – GC and MBP – was observed by indirect immuno-fluorescence. Results in normal cultures showed the presence of two oligodendrocyte subpopulations, one which expresses GC only, and another which expresses both the GC and MBP. Oligodendrocytes which are both GC$^+$ and MBP$^+$ represent at 18 days only $1.6^o/_{oo}$ of the number of GC$^+$, MBP$^-$ oligodendrocytes. They appear in culture later than GC$^+$ MBP$^-$ oligodendrocytes and seem to represent a more differentiated subpopulation. These results concerning dissociated brain-cell culture of the C57 B1/6J-W A-J normal litter mates are similar to previous data obtained with cultures from Jack River mice[17].

The aspect and the number of GC$^+$, MBP$^-$ oligodendrocytes was similar in normal and *Jimpy* cultures. In contrast, the GC$^+$, MBP$^+$ oligoden-drocyte showed a striking difference between the normal and the *Jimpy* cultures.

In *Jimpy* cultures, the more differentiated GC$^+$, MBP$^+$ oligodendrocyte subpopulation is only 5% that of the normal value. The presence of young, GC$^+$ MBP$^-$ oligodendrocytes in normal number, and the dramatic decrease of the GC$^+$, MBP$^+$ oligodendrocytes is in agreement with a recent report showing that the *Jimpy* mutation blocks the conversion of pre-cursors into myelin[19]. No apparent changes were observed in the expression of GFAP, suggesting that the abnormalities observed in astrocytes *in vivo* may be a secondary phenomenon[13]. These data suggest that in the *Jimpy* mutant the differentiation of oligodendrocytes which are GC$^+$, MBP$^-$ to oligodendrocytes which are both GC$^+$, MBP$^+$, is defective.

SUMMARY

The development of oligodendrocytes and astrocytes was studied in both normal and *Jimpy* (a mutant with defect in myelination) mouse dissociated brain-cell cultures by the indirect immunofluorescence double-staining technique. The expression of two oligodendrocyte markers – galactocerebroside and myelin basic protein – and of one astrocyte marker, glial fibrillary acidic protein, was analysed on days 7, 14 and 18 *in vitro*.

The number of galactocerebroside-positive oligodendrocytes increases during development between the 7th and the 14th days in a similar manner in both normal and *Jimpy* cultures. In normal cultures, a small percentage of galactocerebroside-positive oligodendrocytes undergoes a further dif-ferentiation, characterized by the appearance of myelin basic protein; in *Jimpy* cultures, the number of cells showing this second step of differentiation is only 5 % of the normal value. No apparent changes were observed in the expression of glial fibrillary acidic protein. These data suggest that in the *Jimpy* mutant the differentiation of oligodendrocytes which are both galactocerebroside- and myelin basic protein-positive is defective.

Acknowledgements

This work was supported by the Swiss National Research Foundation (No. 3.419.78). We thank Dr. Doris Dahl (Boston, USA) for the generous gift of the anti-GFAP serum, Miss Margrit Stoller for typing the manuscript and Mr. S. Stettler from Wild Leitz Ltd, Zürich, for photographic assistance.

References

1. Meier, C. Herschowitz, N. and Bischoff, A. (1974). Morphological and biochemical observations in the Jimpy spinal cord. *Acta Neuropathol. (Berl.)*, **27**, 349
2. Sidman, R. L., Dickie, M. M. and Appel, St. H. (1964). Mutant mice (Quaking and Jimpy) with deficient myelination in the central nervous system. *Science*, **144**, 309
3. Privat, A. Robain, O. and Mandel, P. (1972). Aspects ultrastructuraux du corps calleux chez la souris Jimpy. *Acta neuropathol.* (Berl.), **21**, 282
4. Meier, C., and Bischoff, A. (1974). Dysmyelination in 'Jimpy' mouse. Electron microscopic study. *J. Neuropathol. Exp. Neurol.*, **33**, 343
5. Meier, C. and Bischoff, A. (1975). Oligodendroglial cell development in Jimpy mice and controls. An electron microscopic study in the optic nerve. *J. Neurol. Sci.*, **26**, 517
6. Druse, M. J. and Hogan, E. L. (1972). Metabolism *in vivo* of brain galactolipids: the Jimpy mutant. *J. Neurochem.*, **19**, 2435
7. Matthieu, J.-M., Widmer, S. and Herschkowitz, N. (1973). Jimpy, an anomaly of myelin maturation; biochemical studies of myelination phases. *Brain Res.*, **55**, 403
8. Campagnoni, A. T. and Roberts, J. L. (1976). Isolation of myelin basic proteins from Jimpy mice. *Brain Res.*, **115**, 352
9. Jutzi, H., Siergrist, H. P., Burkart, T., Wiesmann, U. and Herschkowitz, N. (1979). Diminished cerebroside-sulfotransferase activity in the Jimpy mouse mutant due to altered lipid composition in microsomal membranes. *Biochim. Biophys. Acta*, **552**, 413
10. Wolf, M. K. and Holden, A. B. (1969). Tissue culture analysis of the inherited defect of central nervous system myelination in Jimpy mice. *J. Neuropathol. Exp. Neurol.*, **28**, 195
11. Meier, C., and Bischoff, A. (1977). Dysmyelination in Jimpy mouse due to astroglial hyperplasia? *Nature* **268**, 177

12. Skoff, R. (1977). Dysmyelination in Jimpy mouse due to astroglial hyperplasia? *Nature (London)*, **268**, 177

13. Skoff, R. P. (1976). Myelin deficit in the Jimpy mouse may be due to cellular abnormalities in astroglia. *Nature (London)*, **264**, 560

14. Raff, M. C., Mirsky, R., Fields, K. L., Lisak, R. P., Dorfman, S. H., Silberberg, D. H., Gregson, N. A., Leibowitz, S. and Kennedy, M. C. (1978). Galactocerebroside is a specific cell surface antigenic marker for oligodendrocytes in culture. *Nature (London)*, **274**, 813

15. Sternberger, N. H., Itoyama, Y., Kies, M. W., and de F. Webster, H. (1978). Myelinic basic protein demonstrated immunocytochemically in oligodendroglia prior to myelin sheaths formation. *Proc. Natl. Acad. Sci. USA*, **75**, 2521

16. Bignami, A., Eng., L. F., Dahl, D. and Uyeda, C. T. (1972). Localization of the glial fibrillary acidic protein in astrocytes by immunofluorescence. *Brain Res.*, **43**, 429

17. Bologa-Sandru, L., Siegrist, H. P., Z'graggen, A., Hofmann, K., Wiesmann, U., Dahl, D. and Herschkowitz, N. (1981). Expression of antigenic markers during the development of oligodendrocytes in mouse brain cell cultures. *Brain Res.*, **210**, 217

18. Johnson, G. D., Holborow, E. J. and Dorling, J. (1978). Immunofluorescence and immunoenzyme techniques. In Weir, D. M. (ed), *Handbook of experimental immunology*, Chap. 15. (London, Edinburgh, Melbourne: Blackwell Scientific Publications Oxford)

19. Barbarese, E., Carson, J. H. and Braun, P. E. (1979). Subcellular distribution and structural polymorphism of myelin basic protein in normal and Jimpy mouse brain. *J. Neurochem.*, **32**, 1437

SECTION FOUR

Consequences of Inborn Errors of Metabolism for the Individual, the Family and Society

16

Inborn errors of metabolism – consequences of long-term treatment for the individual, as derived from observations in phenylketonuria

H. Bickel and S. Grubel-Kaiser

For some 20 of the more than 100 well-defined inborn errors of metabolism, long-term treatment is now available or on trial. Therapy may be causal or symptomatic, and its effectiveness may be excellent, as in phenylketonuria (PKU) and galactosaemia, or still doubtful, as in histidinaemia and homocystinuria. In cystinosis and cystic fibrosis, treatment is certainly still purely symptomatic and therefore of limited value.

There are very few inborn errors of metabolism which are suited to answer the question concerning the consequences of long-term treatment for the individual. If such observations are to have any significance and reliability, treatment should be of proven value over a long period of time in a reasonably large group of individuals. In addition and in the context of this symposium, it should be complex enough to possibly interfere with the normal life and development of the individual patient, beyond its basic beneficial effect. The aim of this chapter is not so much to collect current evidence for the basic value of the therapy, but to consider how far this treatment, though of proven value in the management of the inborn error, may have unwanted side effects on the individual's psychosocial development.

Of the 16 inborn errors listed in Table 16.1, very few fulfil the conditions mentioned above. Effective therapy either has not been established for long enough or the number of patients is still too small to permit a valid statement concerning the consequences of long-term treatment. Ideally, the study should be conducted in a single centre in order to avoid any bias due to different modes of treatment or of testing its results. Our own clinical experience permits some first tentative statements only in the case of phenylketonuria, though similar observations at other centres seem feasible in patient groups suffering from galactosaemia, nephrogenic diabetes insipidus, or from some other relatively common inborn errors with a complex, effective therapy.

TABLE 16.1   Inborn errors of metabolism with long-term treatment

Amino acid metabolism	Carbohydrate and metal metabolism	Transport disorders
Phenylketonuria	Diabetes mellitus	Di- Monosacch. malabsorption
Maple-syrup urine disease	Galactosaemia	Renal tubular acidosis
Homocystinuria	Fructose intolerance	Nephrogenic diabetes insipidus
Histidinaemia	Wilson's disease	Vit D-resistant rickets
Methylmalonic acidaemia		Cystinuria
Cystinosis		Cystic fibrosis

In the last 20 years we have treated some 200 phenylketonuric patients[1,2] with a phenylalanine-restricted diet and have observed their development. This kind of therapy is very complex indeed. Ideally, it starts in the first two months of life and continues up to the age of 10 years and more. The diet is half-synthetic and must be rigidly controlled to avoid any biochemical imbalance with consequent brain damage. This means that for many years patients lead a rather unnatural life, being continually confronted with an unusual, partly unpalatable menu which differs fundamentally from that of their family, play- and schoolmates. Being different from their friends and always tempted to break the rules and to disobey their parents and doctors, they must soon be confronted with problems which may have consequences for their psychosocial development. Fortunately, their physical growth and other health parameters remain undisturbed by this therapy.

We have started a retrospective study of the psychosocial consequences which may develop during long-term dietary treatment in phenylketonuric children and adolescents. We consider their intellectual development, success at school, social contact and their situation within the family. To try to answer these questions, we gathered from the Heidelberg PKU group 26 early- and late-discovered patients who are now 13–20 years old, have had treatment over many years and are available and suitable for the tests. Some of them have finished their schooling, and are pursuing further professional training. Two of the 26 patients are still on a strictly reduced phenylalanine intake, whilst the others have received, since the age of 8 or later, a protein-restricted but otherwise normal diet, with a protein intake of 0.8—1 g/kg per day, resulting in phenylalanine blood levels of 15–20 mg %. In none of the patients has the diet been completely terminated.

The aim of this study is to recognize psychosocial problems occurring during school life and adolescence under this long-term treatment, and to measure any deviation from normal by standardized psychological test methods. In addition, individual statements of parents and patients have been evaluated.

RESULTS AND DISCUSSION

Of the 26 patients shown on Table 16.2, 19 were detected early, during the first three months of life, the other seven belatedly, between the 11th and 52nd months. The present age of the early treated group is 12–20 years, of the late treated group 13–19 years. Sex distribution is equal, 13 being boys and 13 girls. Intellectual development was measured with the Wechsler Intelligence Scale for Children[3], giving in the early-treated group an average IQ of 109, with a range of 72–137, and in the late-treated group an average IQ of 92, with a range of 57–107. The low IQ of 72 in one patient of the early-treated group is exceptional and is probably due to a complicating birth trauma, all other IQs of this group being above 90.

TABLE 16.2 IQ of 26 early and late-treated PKU patients
on strict or relaxed low-phenylalanine diet

No of patients	Age at start of diet (months)	Mean IQ of patients	Present age (years)
19	1–3 (early)	109 (72–137)	12–20
7	11–52 (late)	92 (57–107)	13–19

Eighteen further late-detected patients have not been included in the study because they were mentally unable to perform the psychological tests, having been damaged too badly before therapy could be started.

Education

For their schooling, the 26 patients attended the types of schools listed in Table 16.3; 13 of them were able to attend a higher (secondary) school, whilst special school care was necessary for four patients, three of them belonging to the late-treated group.

Twelve of the 26 early- and late-treated patients have finished school; seven attended an intermediate school and five attended secondary school. Now, at of 16–20 years of age they are undertaking further professional training as tax adviser, bank clerk, commercial employee, car mechanic, precision mechanic, sales woman, policeman, and are attending schools for agriculture, housekeeping and for nursing.

The results of school and professional training of this group of patients are satisfactory. Half of the 26 have been able to attend higher schools, three of them being late-detected patients. The transition of the school leavers to a broadly distributed professional training illustrates further the success of their school education.

Anxiety feelings at school

Additional psychological evaluation of the 26 patients deals with their anxiety feelings at school. They were examined with the "Questionnaire on Anxiety for Pupils"[4]. This questionnaire ascertains the anxious and unpleasant experiences of pupils at school and is applicable for children age of 9–17 years. It deals with the following four aspects:

(1) Anxiety on examination.
    Records are made of feelings of incapacity and helplessness during examination, fear of unsuccessful performance combined with slow reactions.

(2) General anxiety symptoms
    Symptoms such as 'heart throbbing', nervousness, disturbed sleep and concentration, timidity and lack of self-confidence.

(3) Aversion to school.

TABLE 16.3 School success of 26-early and late-treated PKU patients (present age 12–20 yrs)

Type of school	Start of diet			Total		School terminated
	1–3 m	11–52 m	n	per cent		Further trade education
Elementary + intermediate school	8	1	9	35		7
Secondary school (Realschule)	5	3	8	31	⎫ 50%	5
Grammar school (Gymnasium)	5	—	5	19	⎬	—
Special school (Sonderschule)	1	3	4	15	⎭	—
Total	19	7	26	100		12

Unpleasant experiences at school, reduced motivation towards lessons and subject matters are recorded.

(4) Desire to be socially accepted.
   This item includes fear of deviating from the desired standard of social behaviour and an increased tendency to impersonate normal behaviour.

The results of the test are shown in Table 16.4. Pronounced anxiety on examination, general anxiety and aversion against school were no more frequently encountered in our patients than in normal school children. None of the eight patients of 9–11 years of age expressed an increased desire to be socially acknowledged, whilst this desire was definitely above normal in patients aged 12–17. This suggests that from the twelfth year on, three times as many patients treated with the diet over a long time exhibit increased anxiety and a greater desire to be socially acknowledged than than normal children of the same age. However, before a general rule can be derived from this behaviour, a larger group of patients must be examined.

Neuroticism and extroversion

A psychological evaluation on neuroticism and extroversion was carried out with the "Junior Eysenck Personality Inventory"[5] in 16 of the 26 long-term treated PKU patients. The questionnaire ascertains certain further aspects of individual reactions, namely neuroticism or emotional lability as well as extroversion or introversion in children and adolescents aged 8–18. It consists of the following two aspects:

(1) Neuroticism.
   This includes feelings of inadequacy combined with oversensitivity and vulnerability, a tendency to dream and meditate, to exhibit fluctuating moods, especially depression, to worry about health, hypochondriacal behaviour, anxiety concerning the future, restlessness and nervousness, excitability, disturbed sleep, frequent weariness, fatigue and headaches.

(2) Extroversion.
   This is expressed as interest in the company of others, to enjoy cheerful contact (sociability), to exhibit liveliness, a drive to adventure and carefree behaviour (activity).

The results are shown in Table 16.5. Of the 16 patients tested for

TABLE 16.4   Psychological evaluation of "Anxiety of Pupils" questionnaire in PKU patients

Age at test (yrs)	Aspects of questionnaire	No of patients involved	Results Symptoms
9–17	Anxiety on examination General anxiety symptoms Aversion to school	3 of 26 (= 12%)	Increased anxiety. Frequency similar to normal pop. (= 15%)
9–11	Desire to be socially acknowledged	0 of 8 (= 0%)	With increased desire for social contact
12–17	Desire to be socially acknowledged	9 of 18 (= 50%)	With increased desire for social contact. Frequency threefold normal (= 15%)

TABLE 16.5 Results of psychological evaluation in PKU patients. "Junior Eysenck Personality Inventory", newly constructed by Buggle and Baumgärtel[5]

Age at test (yrs)	No of patients involved	Main symptoms according to questionnaire
10–17	6 of 16 (= 38%)	Increased emotional lability. ≐ Double normal frequency (= 22%)
10–17	9 of 15 (= 60%)	Increased striving for social contact (= extroversion) ≐ Threefold normal frequency (= 22%)
10–17	5 of 15 (= 33%)	Increased activity (= extroversion). Slightly higher frequency than normal (= 22%)

neuroticism, six (38 %) exhibited increased emotional lability, which is found in only 22 % of healthy children of this age group. As regards extroversion, nine of 15 patients (60 %) exhibited a strongly pronounced strive for social contact, which is three times as frequent as in normal youngsters of this age. Five of 15 patients (33 %) showed a definitely increased level of activity which is again somewhat more frequent than in normal children of this age.

Social contact

These observations suggest that PKU children and adolescents who have undergone long-term dietary treatment, miss social contact because of their special therapeutic situation. They make special efforts to achieve this contact and to have their own activities approved.

In addition to the above psychometric tests concerned with success at school and during professional training, school anxiety, and neuroticism and extroversion, we sought further insight into the consequences of long-term treatment by asking our patients and their families for written or oral statements concerning their own experiences. So far we have received such statements from 15 patients, their parents and one brother. They confirmed the results of the psychological tests and added some further points of interest.

On starting school, many patients develop feelings of inadequacy, increased social sensitivity and vulnerability in connection with their special diet, especially during school breaks, at invitations and parties, during school excursions, but also in their own family. They complain of the continuing dependence on the mother concerning dietary management, resulting in resentment of overprotection up to the age of 18 and beyond.

There is also the worrying question of how far patients and parents should reveal the disease and its consequences to friends, school-mates, teachers and other authorities, or how far their illness should be kept secret or trivialized. One 16-year-old boy writes: "At school I have rarely spoken about my disease and the diet, and I disliked this topic". An 18-year-old girl describes how difficult it was for her to defend her position in her class, having been overprotected and isolated for too long by her family. She was teased a lot by her schoolmates and now feels suspicious and insecure in circles of young people she does not know. Still another 13-year-old girl, now fully established socially as class speaker and treasurer, suffered from being made fun of until the teacher explained her special situation to her class-mates. It is not surprising that in some patients such experiences provoke moodiness, sadness, shame, anger and worry concerning health and the future, especially during the years of puberty and adolescence.

Whilst realizing the problems of these patients, it is gratifying that many families, especially of course the mothers, but also fathers, grandparents and even siblings do their best to help. In our group of patients the parents are generally described as very strict and consistent in conducting the diet, especially if there is a predamaged untreated child in the family. Some parents confess that, as a kind of compensation, they tend to spoil their child in other respects. Some mothers strive to ease their child's social contacts, for instance by preparing protein-free cakes for birthday celebrations and other parties. They occasionally even accompany their children on longer school excursions to supervise their diet. Other parents are less skilful, isolating themselves and their children by abstaining from parties, other activities and even from holidays. One nice exception: a girl patient whose parents are passionate weekend hikers has covered, over the last $2\frac{1}{2}$ years, a walking distance of 5000 km.

Fortunately, serious family problems arising between the parents and patients on the long-term therapy, have very rarely been encountered in our patients. Some siblings complain that the patient occupies too much of a central position in the family, the healthy siblings sometimes being included in a common protein-restricted Sunday meal. One healthy brother confessed that he had to eat sausage clandestinely and "with somewhat bad conscience". He once answered his parents furiously: "After all, it is not my fault that I was born healthy".

Patients repeatedly criticize their parents and doctors for not being informed early enough, before starting school, about their disease, their treatment and how to integrate this into school life. Older teenagers, especially, resent the fact that laboratory results and diet adjustments are brought to the attention of their parents, not to themselves. Every one of the older patients would like to stop dietary restrictions as soon as possible, especially the bad-tasting amino-acid preparations. One 18-year-old girl describes the flavour of one of the older preparations as "disgusting", "goose-flesh producing", another more recent preparation as "resembling a soup made of sawdust". She would be "very grateful to all research workers if they could find a preparation which does not taste so peculiar and could perhaps be taken on alternate days. That would really be terrific".

In this and other patients' letters there are not only complaints but also interesting positive remarks about the diet. Some patients feel that they are not only less spoilt concerning their eating habits than healthy children, but also less egotistic, more ready to take over responsibilities, representing their classmates in various activities which do not stand in high esteem, such as running competitions on a Sunday morning.

Summing up our patients' statements, there is no great interindividual difference in attitude to disease and diet. All complain of difficulty in eating bad tasting preparations, but they also realize the necessity of treatment and accept it in order to be successful at school. Some patients lack self-esteem, feel insecure and not established in their social surrounding. They have interests different to those of their peers and take life more seriously. They consider their parents to be very strict but also helpful, although they resent the over-protection, especially by the mother. All long for an unrestricted diet in the near future. They are upset not to be fully healthy, and they worry about their professional future. When applying for a job, they try to keep their disease secret.

The parents' approach in coping with the long-term treatment of their children is somewhat different. For some, the management of the diet means a load for the whole family, hard to bear and with serious restriction of their free-time activities, holidays and so on. For other parents, dietary management becomes a natural habit, an accepted responsibility for the entire family, although sometimes with considerable restrictions in their dietary habits and range of foods. As managers of the diet, parents become more closely attached to their children and experience satisfaction through their successes, whilst the affected child is clearly the suffering party in this symbiosis.

CONCLUSIONS

We would like to summarize the results of this study. The effectiveness of long-term treatment on the patients' intellectual development – as measured by psychological tests – is obviously good. The latest mean IQ of the early treated patient group is within the normal range, of the late treated group low normal. It should be noted that this late-treated group is selected, as previously defined.

The long-term results of treatment on school success in the various types of schools again show no important deviations from normal, especially in the early-treated patients. Late-treated patients do not do so well because of the delayed onset of therapy, not because of its long duration. The patients' further professional training confirms their school behaviour and also follows a normal pattern.

In this context it seems important that, despite long-term treatment, no increased anxiety on examination, aversion against school or general anxiety symptoms have been encountered in these patients. However, from about the age of 12, patients often experience an increased desire to conform as far as possible to their school mates, to be socially acknowledged by them and to be in no way inferior. This trend is also shown in the psychological tests on neuroticism and extroversion, which reveal a pronounced striving for social contact, for an active life in the community, and increased emotional lability derived from the fear that the aim to compete with and emulate the others successfully may not be achieved. Many patients are worried because they do not understand their disease and its implications sufficiently well, especially the contrast of feeling quite healthy but nevertheless needing treatment of a more or less incisive nature.

The results of this pilot study are certainly still preliminary and incomplete. So far they seem somewhat trivial and not unexpected. One would expect similar psychosocial reactions in other chronic diseases with a complex treatment, such as in diabetes mellitus. In fact, a recent study of this disease by Steinhausen and Börner has shown comparable reactions in diabetic children and adolescents[6]. It is of course necessary to differentiate clearly the consequences of the treatment *per se* from any late manifestation of the disease itself, arising perhaps from insufficient treatment or its delayed start. This differentiation may sometimes be difficult or impossible. To us, the consequences of long-term treatment of metabolic disease are neither trivial nor banal. Doctors, parents and patients should be familiar with them. They should do their best to avoid them at an early stage, starting to combat them before school age and especially before puberty. Although most of the psychosocial problems arise from therapy prolonged beyond the age of ten, it is our opinion that the continuation of treatment beyond this age – usually in a somewhat relaxed form – is necessary if permanent damage to the brain is to be avoided. If unavoidable, certain psychosocial consequences of this prolonged treatment must be accepted rather than prevented by cutting short an essential treatment.

References

1. Bickel, H. and Grubel-Kaiser, S. (1971). Ueber die Phenylketonurie. Psychometrische Erfolgsbeurteilung der phenylalaninarmen Diät bei phenylketonurischen Kindern. *Dtsch. Med. Wochenschr.*, **96,** 1415
2. Grubel-Kaiser, S. and Schmid-Rüter, E. (1978). Phenylketonurie: Schulerfolg bei Früherfassung. *Mschr. Kinderheilk.* **126,** 379
3. Wechsler, D. (1966). Bondy, C. (ed.), *Hamburg–Wechsler–Intelligenztest für*

Kinder (HAWIK). (Deutsche Bearbeitung der Wechsler-Intelligence Scale for Children – WISC). (Bern and Stuttgart: Huber)

4. Wieczerkowski, W., Nickel, H., Janowski, A., Fittkau, B. and Rauer, W. (1974). *Angstfragebogen für Schüler (AFS)*. (Braunschweig: Westermann)

5. Buggle, F. and Baumgärtel, F. (1975). Hanes, K. J. (ed.) *Hamburger Neurotizismus- und Extraversionsskala für Kinder und Jugendliche*. (Göttingen Hogrefe)

6. Steinhausen, H. Chr. and Börner, S. (1978). *Kinder und Jugendliche mit Diabetes*. Psychologie einer chronischen Krankheit. Beiheft No. 20 Praxis f. Kinderpsychologie u. Kinderpsychiatrie. (Göttingen: Verlag Med. Psychologie, Vandenhoeck & Ruprecht)

17

Social aspects of the handicapped person

Y. Posternak

INTRODUCTION

To say that I feel greatly honoured to have been asked to participate at this symposium is only half of the truth. The other half is that I have experienced a growing sense of awe at the prospect of imparting to biochemists and biologists this set of socio-educational issues. We have already heard of the great extent to which biological and medical research is intimately intertwined in problems of inborn metabolic errors in humans and how many future advances in the prevention and treatment of handicapping conditions will be based on applications of fundamental information.

However our optimism is still restrained as the World Health Organization (WHO), the International Labour Office (ILO) and UNESCO, in 1980, stressed that 12–15 % of children and adults in a given population are physically or mentally handicapped. The mere existence of these handicapped persons reveals the extent of the task that lies ahead; we cannot think in terms of a society without handicap. Although prevention is clearly the ultimate goal, the amelioration of existing handicap must also receive a high priority and intensification and enlargement of applied research on education, social and economic problems is an urgent necessity.

I thank you for this opportunity to share my interest in the welfare of handicapped children and adults, and for following me into a socio-educational field. One more introductory word. In my work I have been most directly concerned with mentally handicapped people, including the most severely handicapped; hence my examples tend to fall in that category, although I shall try to make reference to other conditions.

WHO ARE THE MENTALLY HANDICAPPED CHILDREN AND ADULTS? WHAT ARE THEIR NEEDS? WHAT CAN THEY DO?

Mentally retarded children are those who mature at a slower than average rate and experience unusual difficulty in learning, social adjustment and economic activity. The mentally retarded are children and adults who have feelings of love and loneliness, a need for affection, comradeship and a sense of belonging. Above all they are human beings just like the rest of us; the remarkable thing is that this simple fact has to be emphasized time and time again.

Mental retardation can be caused by any condition which impairs development of the brain before birth, during birth or early childhood. Well over 250 causes have already been discovered, but they account for only some 25% of all known cases of mental retardation. In 75% of the cases, therefore, the specific cause remains unknown.

In general, the rates found up to now in all parts of the world indicate that 1–3 per cent of the population are mentally retarded to some greater or lesser degree. Mental retardation can be prevented and cannot be cured in the customary sense of the word, but almost all mentally retarded individuals have the capacity to learn, to develop, and are susceptible to improvement.

WHAT HAPPENS TO MENTALLY HANDICAPPED PERSONS IN DIFFERENT PARTS OF THE WORLD?

It is generally assumed that mentally handicapped people fare better in our affluent western societies than in developing countries. The reality is quite different, for we find that luckily, interest in the welfare of the handicapped represents a social phenomenon of considerable consequence in many developing countries and in many deprived areas of the world. Let us not forget that love and feelings of parents toward their children are the same all over the world.

Excellent programmes exist for the handicapped in all parts of the world. For instance, there are several agricultural and craft schools in central Java, in the north of Thailand and in India. Countries so politically opposed as Israel and Libya are involved in setting up good facilities for the handicapped. The argument, therefore, about priorities which finds its expression in such statements as "Emerging countries have more important things to do than provide services for handicapped and non-productive persons", contrary to expectation, is not advanced by the majority of emerging countries. Today, it is in the industrialized countries that we are more likely to hear that investment in services for the handicapped must be curtailed or even stopped until economic conditions improve. We forget that some expenditures will reduce other costs. This is especially true of rehabilitation. Legislators are presently crying "we have to allocate funds according to priorities". Indeed this is true. But we must be alert and ever sensitive as to how priorities are established. Indubitably, what will happen is that an increasing number of people will try to impose their own personal values of human worth.

In new or developing countries where governments or local authorities do not yet provide for the disabled, parents' associations play an important role. Indeed, they exist in 64 countries, showing drive and determination in starting simple, but very often excellent, services adapted to their own culture and resources. One can only have the greatest respect for the way children are accepted in other cultures. Just one example which is well known to me comes from the Pacific region. There, services for the handicapped exist even in the small nation islands of the South Seas, so well described by Robert Louis Stevenson, who himself was physically handicapped. In search of a better climate, he settled down in Samoa and wrote his classic *Treasure Island*. In the South Seas, one finds that the life style and future of handicapped people are becoming more meaningful and less depressing than in many western countries, despite a limited, almost precarious economy and high unemployment. In the *Fiji Islands*, hundreds of severely mentally handicapped children are integrated into excellent schools, attended by non-disabled Fijian, Hindu, Chinese and white children. In *Tonga* and in *Western Samoa* as in *New Caledonia*, you will meet active parents' and friends' associations of the handicapped; in the *Cook Islands*, special teaching material and wheelchairs have been shipped recently from New Zealand and handicapped young people are employed in the crafts and skills of village life, planting, weaving, and fishing. There is an increasing acceptance of the handicapped in the traditional way of life.

Progress in providing for the handicapped in the fields of care, education and law, although very slow, has nevertheless been considerable in many countries, including those represented here. Today many handicapped children have access to education; many disabled adults live in suitable accommodation with their families and not in horrible asylums of the past; many lead an active social and working life.

But much more needs to be done. For example, we must make it known that even mental retardation is not a stable life-long condition but can become dynamic in its nature. This means that it is susceptible to improvement, provided that we do not adopt a passive attitude toward the handicapped. Out of every hundred mentally handicapped individuals, 95 have the capacity to learn, to become partially or even fully economically productive or to lead a more or less independent life. They can be developed to the same degree as other persons, namely to the optimum of their capacity. The small minority of the very profoundly handicapped has as much right to a dignified life and respect as any other human being.

It is obvious that no one will ever be able to convert a deux-chevaux car into a speeding Ferrari and there are limits to everything; the point is: what goals should we help handicapped persons achieve? Let me illustrate this last point and consider the differences in the development of children and adults suffering from Down's syndrome. These retarded people form a clear-cut group; they look like each other and, as a rule, are sharply different physically from both normal and other retarded people. In view of the frequency of this syndrome, there are ample opportunities for comparative studies. Some of these handicapped persons can function at a relatively high level (I am not speaking here of the exceptional mosaicism cases). As adults, they can carry out useful tasks in working situations but their potential is still underestimated. Perhaps I have a great advantage in that I am personally acquainted with many young people with Down's syndrome who live a good and useful life because they were given the opportunity to learn and develop. For example, François earns his life as a clerk in an International Organization in Brussels; Michael works skilfully in the orange groves outside Jerusalem, while Renata in Geneva is employed by a pharmaceutical concern and prepares surgical packs. But to other young people with the same Down's syndrome, the world still appears a rather grim and forbidding place. What does it mean for them to be mentally retarded? A rigid and unimaginative classification has resulted in an unjustifiable denial of assistance. They live a secluded life in institutions or with ageing parents; it means loneliness; it means social neglect; it means focus on pathology to the detriment of their developmental potential; it means deprivation of affection and of close emotional bonds.

The question therefore remains: why is it that certain persons with

mental disabilities become totally dependent and resigned to an unproductive and custodial life, while others achieve an unusual degree of development? Why are there such striking differences between the handicapped? It
would appear that, up to a point, the same defects do not produce similar
types of maladjustment and degrees of dependency, and it may be
hypothesized that the difficulties do not stem from mental causes alone.

One of the answers may be that the handicapping effects of retardation
have been exaggerated by policies of neglect, isolation and abuse. The
prevailing idea has been – once a mongol, always a mongol – and that
hardly provides for a programme aimed at respect and rehabilitation. It is
important to emphasize that, even in such a genetically determined
condition due to a chromosome anomaly, the role of the environment in
developing individual potential may be considerable. Such differences are
partly the outcome of (1) educational and social policies, (2) attitudes
towards a faceless mythical group called 'the handicapped', and
(3) obsolete legislation.

CHANGES IN EDUCATIONAL AND SOCIAL POLICIES

I will now consider, instead of mental retardation, a sensory deficiency –
blindness. In most European countries the approach is to send blind
children to segregated institutions for the blind or to special schools for the
blind. Few countries have a policy of sending blind children to the regular
schools, with the necessary special supporting services at the classroom
level. The results of these two types of education, in integrated or
segregated premises, will not be the same.

Let us first consider a blind child attending an institution for the blind.
He will be taught via techniques for the blind; he will also be taught to
'behave' as a blind person and later he will find it difficult to achieve an
integrated social life in the sighted community. Meanwhile, we tend to sit
back and appreciate how much is done for the blind in such special
surroundings, instead of questioning more closely in a critical, scientific
way how well such segregated educational arrangements prepare the
handicapped child for the harsh realities of the everyday world of work and
life which he must face on leaving school.

Italy[1], *Norway* and *Sweden*[2] provide stimulating examples of European
countries which have developed forward-looking policies for the education
of handicapped children, no matter what the nature (sensory, physical or
mental) and severity of the handicap. The majority of disabled children in
these three countries are integrated in regular classrooms and it is in the

regular classroom where the needed special help is provided.

Let me give you in a little more detail what I have seen in *Italy*, both in the more affluent industrialized northern areas as well as the predominantly rural and sparsely settled regions of the south.

> In one elementary school, a nine year old girl, blind, sits with her normal peers in the regular classroom. She needed special instruction in Braille; instead of taking the child out of the school, an itinerant teacher introduced Braille to the class and by now all the other children know how to use this alphabet. For them, it is just a game. Braille is now a normal educational experience for a whole class of 25 children who will not only be able to help their handicapped companion during the basic compulsory schooling years, but equally important, it will help ensure that they themselves will grow up to understand and appreciate human problems. As for the little blind girl, she will be raised in normal surroundings, in her own family, not hidden away in a remote institution.

I feel sure you will agree that few aspects in a child's life are more important than the sharing of normal educational and social experiences with children of his own age. So you may feel too that the stress, bitterness, and frustration encountered in families with children with severe handicaps can be considerably diminished when the support provided respects family ties. As I travelled through Italy and visited other schools, I met children with severe cerebral palsy, children with Down's syndrome and other handicapping conditions. The ordinary school was the natural setting for all handicapped children. None was isolated or obviously disabled in a group which accepted them naturally.

As this point we should ask ourselves what is happening to the normal children caught up in this new policy of sharing daily life with a severely handicapped comrade. Will they suffer unusual stress? Will they be intellectually neglected? What of their academic attainment? In Norway and Italy, one finds a certain similarity in programme development and results.

(1) A well-prepared system of enrolment of handicapped children has forced the schools to make basic changes resulting in better schooling for everyone.

(2) Teaching for all children has become more individualized; consequently, inside the classroom there is a general increase of self-confidence and self-direction.

(3) The presence of the handicapped child has not lowered the standard of school; cognitive growth has not been endangered.

(4) It has been recognized that the various barriers between handicap-

ped and non-handicapped children are also detrimental to the normal child.

The normal child may leave school unacquainted with some of the fundamental areas of human understanding and without the tolerant view of human nature that is so essential both for a well balanced personality and for social behaviour. In both countries, there is a clear determination to go on with the reshaping of schools and educational programmes so that more handicapped children can be admitted in future.

CHANGES IN ATTITUDES

Now that we have seen some of the beneficial innovative changes in education, let us consider another problem: the need for changes in attitudes. We all need around us a climate of understanding and acceptance; but handicapped people still suffer from rejection and negative attitudes. What are the reasons for these difficulties and what stands in the way of removing them? In part, as we have just seen, we promote them ourselves by *segregating* disabled individuals from their community. It is only in recent years that rigid segregation policies against the weaker and less privileged members of modern society have been re-examined and relaxed. We tend to *denigrate and reject those who fail to reach the 'norms'* that we have manufactured for ourselves and our society. The sharp distinction between 'the handicapped' and 'the normal' is no longer tenable. What kind of norms are these, that demand our allegiance and that shape our attitudes towards those who are handicapped? They are what you would expect of an industrialized society. They are norms in which fast is good and slow is bad. They are norms of competition, and not always of healthy competition: we compete in school, at play, at love and at work. Where do the handicapped fit in, those who can go to school, can play, can love, can work, but cannot excel in competition?

Identifying without labelling

Too frequently, we stigmatize children and adults by *labels and categories* that make them easy to count but difficult to help. Nicholas Hobbs, from Vanderbilt University, USA, has weighed up the effects of labelling and of experiences that come to children as a consequence of being classified[3]. He has made recommendations for diminishing the harmful effects of classification, yet preserving the benefits in planning and providing services. The model proposed by Hobbs overcomes a number of difficulties. By describing the services a person needs and indicating who is to deliver them an overall classification system is no longer necessary. Once a child is classified as handicapped, the label will stick, even if later he is able to work and look for a job. It is not a label which is needed but a profile of the child's functioning from different perspectives. Recently, I had the pleasure of listening to the opera *La Tosca* by Puccini in La Scala, Milan. One of the characters in the opera is Sciarrone, a jailor. The singer had a warm, impressive bass voice; he was also a severely handicapped dwarf. This artist must have had clever, devoted and loving parents, as well as encouragement from kind teachers. They offered him the same musical training and opportunities that he would have received had he been a normal child. Now, La Scala has gained a great singer, and the category of 'dwarf' is short of one of its number!

We have become more and more obsessed with abbreviating categories: the CP (cerebral palsied); the NI (neurologically impaired). This is then followed by stereotyped programmes. We are in fact addicted to packaged programmes -- programmes for the retarded as a group, for the elderly, for the gifted, all of which take them further and further away from everyday reality and human contact. I suggest we begin resisting these obsessions and lay greater stress on individuality. Another major difficulty, of our own making, is a tendency to discriminate because of prejudice and to concentrate on the handicaps, disregarding any qualities that a person may have.

A low expectation of the handicapped is part of the traditional approach to the care of disabled persons. When a person is perceived as deviant, he is cast for a role that carries with it powerful negative expectancies. On the other hand, Rosenthal and Jacobsen in a well-known experiment demonstrated that a child's intelligence may rise when the teacher in his classroom is led to believe that the child is brighter than he is. In the course of this experiment, 20 % of children in a public elementary school were reported to their teachers as showing unusual potential for intellectual growth. The names of these children were drawn at random by numbers. Eight months later, these unusual or 'gifted' children showed significantly greater intellectual gains than did the remaining children who had not been singled out for teacher attention. The change in the teachers' expectations regarding the intellectual performance of these allegedly 'special' and randomly selected children had led to an actual change in their intellectual performance. The results of this experiment have been published in a book entitled *Pygmalion in the Classroom*. Why Pygmalion? You may all recall

G. B. Shaw's play *Pygmalion*, a satirical study of English society, in which Professor Higgins, alias Pygmalion Higgins, decides to teach a flower girl, Eliza Doolittle, to forget her Cockney accent and to make her a lady. Listen now to Eliza:

> You see, really and truly, apart from the things anyone can pick up (how to dress and the proper way of speaking, and so on) the difference between a lady and a flower girl is not how she behaves, but how she is *treated*. I shall always be a flower girl to Professor Higgins, because he always treats me as a flower girl, and always will; but I know I can be a lady to you, because you always treat me as a lady, and always will.

So let us treat the handicapped person as someone who can learn and progress and who can give and not only receive. Let us accept that a handicap is not something which is solely due to factors within the individual, but is also the result of shortcomings in the interaction between the individual and the environment.

CHANGING LEGISLATION

Following the Second World War, and as a result of the widespread revulsion at the massive deprivation of human rights, there was strong pressure for international guarantees of human rights. Yet no one worried in particular about the rights of mentally handicapped people. The subsequent revolt came from parents, not only with great similarity from country to country, but as a spontaneous phenomenon. The year 1971 marked an important step forward for the mentally handicapped of the world. In that year the United Nations adopted the '*Declaration on the Rights of Mentally Retarded Persons*'. It enumerates in seven articles aspects of care, security, and protection to which the mentally retarded person is entitled. It stresses the word 'person'. Was this necessary? Yes. because the names which have been applied to the mentally handicapped are themselves a fascinating subject for study. Terms like idiot, imbecile, and subnormal reflect the fears, the prejudices, the ignorance and arrogance, that mentally handicapped persons have evoked over the years: that he was first *a person* was readily forgotten. The Declaration had been drafted by a Swede, Richard Sterner, an economist, a jurist and a parent with a strong personality. Once Sterner, when listening to a psychiatrist who declared "I give my patients their rights", jumped to his feet and said coldly: "You don't give anybody his rights; you can only take them away. You are not speaking about privileges which are given or withheld, but about rights, which are inherent in the human estate."

The Declaration is not a request for pity but a demand for respect; it is not a plea for charity but a cry for justice. It is interesting to note that most of the people who fought for the rights of the handicapped in the past, as well as in more recent periods, held liberal and advanced views in many other social fields. Among the early pioneers, we find in the USA Gridley Howe, who in 1848 opened the first Institution for the Disabled in Massachusetts. This excellent Institution was described in glowing terms by Charles Dickens during his first visit to the USA. Gridley Howe, a surgeon who had graduated from Harvard Medical School, was not only a strong upholder of the rights of handicapped children. He believed in freedom and went to Greece as a volunteer surgeon during the war of liberation; back in the USA he acted as a public advocate of negro emancipation. Another great pioneer in the USA, Edouard Seguin, greatly contributed in around 1850 to the special education field. Seguin, a French citizen by origin, had a strong philosophical and political concept of liberty and it was as an exile that he left France for the USA, having opposed the reactionary politics of the then King of France, Charles X. Nearer our own time (after World War II), in Norway and in Denmark, for example, the people who spoke out most strongly against the segregation of the handicapped were those who had actively participated in the Resistance movements in their own countries. All these people felt that with the rights and freedom of the handicapped under attack, the rights of all citizens were also in danger.

The question of segregation

Since 1971, new legislation has positively affected the status of the handicapped in many countries. In the field of education, I have already mentioned new practices in Norway and in Italy. Let us turn towards the USA where, up to 1974, the situation was generally characterized by the fact that the regular school system had disclaimed responsibility for handicapped children[5]. Children were excluded under various pretexts, for example, not enough teachers; the child cannot walk; the child has behavioural problems. Since 1974, *Public Law 93–380* requires that handicapped children be educated with children who are not handicapped. This Law also states that segregation of the handicapped child is anti-educational and anti-social. The Law compares segregation of handicapped children with racial segregation of negro children; it is based on a decision made in 1954 by the Supreme Court of the USA (Brown *v*. Education) which opened schools, hitherto segregated, to all negro children. In its conclusion, the Supreme Court stated that in the field of education 'separate' has no place and that separate educational facilities are inherently unequal.

New legislation also affects adults. We now see an increasing number of handicapped young people coming forward for training and employment. Once again, it is clear that in the past underestimation of the capabilities of the mentally handicapped has influenced the methods of management that have been adopted. We need sound vocational training of the handicapped and a more imaginative approach to finding suitable work for them. When you travel by air, just reflect that many of the pillowcases of major European and American companies have been made by handicapped workers. If you travel by car in *New Zealand*, you will find several motels run by handicapped persons: they do most of the work, the laundry, the house-cleaning, wash your car and they feel productive and worthwhile. In *Oregon*, as in the *Netherlands* or here in *Switzerland*, they are able to put together from 10 to 50 elements in a switch, with a quality equal to that of industry. The key to this result is that the assembly process has been broken down into easy steps and simple operations.

Some handicapped people are better at crafts; for the small minority for whom work is impossible, it is the awareness of their surroundings, enjoyment of life, interest in happenings that should be offered and developed. What is still so tragic is that the same person could easily be a hopeless, unresponding hospital patient instead of the young person embarking on a programme of vocational training. Where he was born, the kind of advice parents were given, the attitude and acceptance of society can make such a difference to his life.

A FINAL WORD

(1) Undoubtedly there is a great need for more research and for the biomedical sciences to disseminate their knowledge for prevention, treatment and care. By all means let us pursue prevention as fully as possible, but we should not use this as a screen to obscure the needs of the handicapped who are with us today and will be for many years to come. Scientific progress would be an ironic mockery if the elementary needs of the handicapped remain unmet.

(2) Let us not set the quality of 'humanness' as entirely dependent upon the degree of measured intelligence. Handicapped persons have to be enabled not merely to exist, but to live in the full sense of the word.

For the majority of them there has been a considerable underestimation of what they could achieve: perhaps the most dramatic findings relate to the severely handicapped for whom possibilities of amelioration were scarcely considered until ten years ago.

(3) Maximum integration into the community rather than segregation must be sought. Handicapped people, like old people, have to live in the social context to which they belong and should not be removed to far-away 'magic' Institutions or Hospitals. What is needed is to acknowledge the real array of support that is ready to be activated in the community. It is therefore up to us to help people to obtain an existence as close to the normal as possible. Do we try to meet handicapped people? Do we know how they live, where they are? Have we ever encouraged our own children to play with a handicapped child, or rather do we consider the handicapped child as a potential threat to our normal child?

(4) Do we accept the philosophy that people differ in need and are equal in human rights?

(5) A last point; handicapped children, to be sure, are not the kind of children we would choose to have in our traditional societies. It is, of course, true that they destroy our hopes and fantasies about what we wish our children to be. But as parents, we should perhaps be reminded less seldom by the specialists that even these children will bring us, as all other children, sorrow *and* happiness, if we as parents, and you, as members of society (*their society*) will share responsibilities.

References

1. Organization for Economic Co-operation and Development (OECD) (1979). *Integration of Handicapped Children and Adolescents in Italy.* CERI/HA/79. 12. (Paris: Chateau de la Muette, OECD)
2. Söder, M. (1980). Research and development concerning integration of handicapped pupils into the ordinary school system. *School integration of the Mentally Retarded.* (Stockholm: National Swedish Board of Education)
3. Hobbs, N. (1975). *Issues in the Classification of Children.* (San Francisco: Jossey-Bass)
4. Rosenthal, R. and Jacobson L. (1968). *Pygmalion in the Classroom. Teacher expectation and Pupils' Intellectual Development*, p. 240. (Holt, Rinehart and Winston)
5. The President's Committee on Mental Retardation. (1976). *The Mentally Retarded Citizen and the Law*, p. 738. (New York: Macmillan)

18

Psychological and educational aspects of handicap
C. C. Cunningham

INTRODUCTION

It is now generally accepted that because a child is intellectually handicapped as a result of biomedical or genetic damage, this does not necessarily mean that he is unable to benefit from educational methods or that his treatment and care must be predominantly medical. Indeed, much optimism is being expressed at present regarding the effects of educational approaches for such children and this is nowhere more evident than in the area of early intervention. It is my intention to examine this area and to question whether our optimism is justified. I will begin with a brief overview of the theoretical changes that have influenced practice and then draw upon our own research concerning early intervention with Down's syndrome infants to illustrate the main points.

MAJOR CHANGES

Up to the 1940s and 1950s intelligence was assumed to be a relatively unitary trait, fixed at conception, stable over time and having generalized control of mental behaviours[1]. In the field of developmental psychology, maturationalists, such as McGraw[2] and Gesell and Amatruda[3], had produced well documented descriptions of hierarchically ordered behavioural sequences of development. These sequences showed strong common patterns and regularity of growth and were used to argue for the dominance of intrinsic stabilizing factors which preserve the balance and direction of the child's development. Whilst it was accepted that environmental factors might support this growth, they did not engender it. Because of this regularity in growth, it was possible to produce standardized scales of development which described the normal age range and the approximate order in which one could expect to see the emergence of behaviours in infants and young children. By comparing an individual child's level of achievement on such tests (i.e. his mental age, MA) with that expected from the standardization samples for his chronological age, it is possible to quantify the rate of development of the child. This is expressed as a developmental or intelligence quotient (DQ or IQ). If this measure falls below two standard deviations from the norm the child is considered to be mentally handicapped. Thus a child with a mental age of eight months but a chronological age of 16 months would have a quotient of 50 and be considered mentally handicapped.

This quantification of the rate of mental growth led to the equating of developmental delay with mental handicap. Unfortunately, it also led to the expectation that the child with a mental age of eight months would be equivalent to an eight-month-old child. This expectation reflects the unitary notions of intelligence and development and rests upon the assumption that the handicapped child develops normally but more slowly —and also that he will be equally slow in all areas of development. Consequently, the major differences between handicapped and non-handicapped children were often seen as quantitative rather than qualitative. It is worth noting that Binet, who pioneered the development of mental tests, rejected this assumption from the beginning, arguing that the specific characteristics of retarded children are their unequal and imperfect development[4].

Two implications of such thinking were important for mental handicap. The first implied that if there was a failure in learning or development then one looked for a defect in the ability of the learner. Consequently there was little impetus to seek out influences from the environment or to seek out qualitative defects in specific learning processes. This further restricted the search for special educational approaches which might be necessary to counter the effects of such deficits.

Secondly, such a viewpoint implied that no special measures were necessary for mentally handicapped children and that all that was required was to provide the same experiences and learning opportunities available to normal children of comparable levels of development. In the 1960s many teachers working with mentally handicapped children appeared to accept this viewpoint, and adopted the current infant and nursery education methods. This emphasized the provision of a rich and stimulating environment in which a child was encouraged to take advantage of a wide range of materials and opportunities. Thus it is still not uncommon to find mentally handicapped adolescents being provided with materials developed for the 2–5-year-old non-handicapped child.

By the 1950s these notions of intelligence and development were under attack from a wide range of sources, including the egalitarian philosophies of western societies. In psychology, major influences came from the appraisal of the results of intelligence tests and the rise of behavioural learning theories.

It was argued that if intelligence is a constant predetermined trait, then one must predict high correlations between measures of intelligence (IQs) or development (DQs) at different ages. Further, if it is a unitary all-embracing trait, one must predict correlations within tests and between different aspects of mental functioning. Such correlations have not generally been found and so the assumptions have been seriously questioned[5]. Intelligence and development are now increasingly seen as being made up of discrete but interrelated domains of abilities and skills strongly influenced by environmental conditions. Developmental psychology has become more concerned with understanding the organization of the developmental process rather than merely charting the appearance of developmental milestones. Consequently the learning processes and sensory channelling systems which may mediate between the environment and the biological base have become key areas for consideration.

For example, in contrast to the findings in non-handicapped children, high correlations and good predictions have been found between early developmental test scores and later IQ measures in mentally handicapped children. One explanation is to assume low inherited mental capacity or slow maturation. However, it is also necessary to consider the possibility of specific sensory or cognitive deficits distorting or complicating the developmental process. A third viewpoint would emphasize the possibility that development is affected by lack of experience or a whole range of environmental deprivations, as well as positively by active teaching.

These factors are not mutually exclusive. Indeed, because elements of all three will inevitably be present the clinician or educator has to estimate their relative contribution in explaining the delay in an individual child's development. These considerations will also determine the choice and optimism in selecting possible treatments. In this, two further factors must be recognized. Firstly, are there periods or areas of development when the

organization is most susceptible to definite types of stimulation and likely to
have long-term consequences? One can infer that this notion is, implicitly
at least, accepted by many workers, judging by the enthusiasm for early
intervention and the emphasis on the importance of the first years of life.
Secondly, to what extent can teaching overcome these deprivations or
compensate for specific disorders in learning? We can begin to answer this
question by considering the influence of those behavioural learning
theories which have emphasized an environmental position.

Primarily these theories focussed attention on the immediate environmental conditions controlling the behaviour of the child. If one found a
failure in learning or development, one began to look for an explanation in
the actual teaching and social interactions taking place. This viewpoint
freed many workers from a preoccupation with defects in hereditary or
environment (e.g. early social deprivation) and gave an optimistic impetus
to search for therapeutic techniques which might improve the achievement
and skills of handicapped individuals.

The techniques that eventually proved most useful emphasized the need
to carry out a detailed assessment of the individuals' strengths, weaknesses
and interests using standardized instruments, and observation under free
or controlled conditions. From this one selects a task which is within the
attainment of the learner in the near future and which is considered to be
desirable for him. This is carefully analysed in a series of small steps of
learning with the aim of eliminating failure. The learner is then taught step
by step, with each successful response being immediately rewarded.
Records of the progress are kept, particularly where errors occur, so that
one can re-examine the teaching programme in the case of failure and not
assume learner disability[6].

Using these systematic teaching techniques many workers demonstrated
that mentally handicapped children and adults could attain far higher
levels of skill than previously thought possible. Further, it was also shown
that the level of final performance reached on such tasks was largely
independent both of IQ and of initial performance[7].

The relative success of these individualized systematic teaching techniques can be interpreted in the light of evidence relating to specific defects
in learning processes in the mentally handicapped. Clarke and Clarke have
succinctly encapsulated these in their notion of spontaneous deficit[8]. They
argue that there is an obvious constitutional deficit which imposes severe
limits upon the severely mentally handicapped person's development and
which includes a relative inability to spontaneously structure ordinary life
experiences. Specifically, they are unable to organize and encode incoming
stimuli, build up schemata, respond selectively, perceive relationships and

make deductions without the intervention of a human agent. This produces a high frequency of failure and a corresponding loss of motivation.

Structured teaching techniques appear to partially compensate for these difficulties in attention and information processing. By breaking down complex tasks into a series of small steps and using cues or prompts, they focus attention on the relevant elements. By frequent repetition and over-learning and mastery of each step, they may compensate for difficulties in memory and retrieval. Once learned, these steps are carefully chained together which assists synthesis. Incidental learning, often seen as deficient in mental handicap, is not expected or required as all the information needed by the learner is taught directly. Finally, each small step is rewarded and the whole system reduces the chances of failure, thus aiding motivation. Seen from this perspective, the application of systematic behavioural techniques has again focussed attention on the importance of specific constitutional disorders in mental handicap.

It is highly plausible that both environmental defects and constitutional disorders may prevent or distort the child's interactions with his environment from birth and thus affect the process of development. If development is hierarchical, with each stage building on the previous ones, then such early distortions are likely to have a cumulative effect. Thus, early intervention which reduces environmental deprivations and applies systematic teaching procedures may well prevent or reduce distortion and delay in development and the consequential handicap.

The evidence from early intervention programmes with socially and economically deprived children provides some support for these notions. Relatively large and lasting gains in achievement have been found, provided that the child is enrolled in the programme from an early age; that parents are used as co-educators and the home is recognized as a major variable; that the programme has specific and developmentally appropriate objectives and uses systematic teaching approaches rather than mere enrichment; and that it is maintained over long periods of time and attempts to generalize the learning to the wider environment[9]. Recently Lazar and Darlington selected 12 such programmes which were considered to be properly designed with well recorded data[10]. With great care they evaluated the long-term effects and found that the children involved were less likely to be assigned to special education classes, less likely to be retained within year grades or drop out of school early. Achievement in mathematics at age ten was significantly improved and there was a trend toward better reading test scores than the controls. The children had more 'achievement orientation' and their mothers indicated higher vocational aspirations.

The children involved in these studies are primarily 'at risk' for mental retardation as a result of social/economic deprivations. Thus one cannot readily assume that results of intervention found with them will be found in severely handicapped children where constitutional impairments are paramount. This distinction between the two groups is often overlooked in both the discussions of early intervention and the development and application of programmes. A further distinction worth noting is that organically impaired children are distributed across all socio-economic categories and do not cluster particularly in the deprived classifications.

In considering the outcome of early intervention for children with severe handicap associated with biological disorder, one must accept that the disorder will set limits to what can be achieved. But we do not really know what these limits are because we have only just begun to test them by means of structured teaching programmes applied from birth. Further, if one accepts the model that development is made up of discrete domains, reacting to and requiring different types of stimulation at different times in the sequence, it will follow that we need to know considerably more about how to phase our intervention into the developmental process. Until we have an efficient and effective system which can do this, we will not be able to draw conclusions on possible outcomes. Since the history of this field has indicated that theories emphasizing limitations have largely discouraged attempts to seek solutions, it seems better to err on the side of optimism at the present time.

I will now consider some of the evidence on early development and intervention with Down's syndrome infants to illustrate these points.

EARLY INTERVENTION WITH DOWN'S SYNDROME INFANTS

Table 18.1 provides a summary of the mean developmental and intelligence test results of samples of Down's syndrome children taken from longitudinal studies encompassing the first years of life. The striking feature of the table is that despite the use of different tests, year of publication and country of origin, the results are highly similar across ages and care conditions. Children raised in institutions have lower scores than those raised at home. This finding has been supported by other studies[20-22]. The effect of institutional placement is apparently manifested within the first year of life and not only in quantitative measures of development. Francis for example, reports that home-reared infants showed more initiative and exploration in play than those in institutions[23]. The studies also suggest

TABLE 18.1   Mean DQs and IQs for young children with Down's syndrome – from longitudinal studies

Reference	1 y	2 y	3 y	4 y	5 y	n	Test
Reared at home/no intervention							
Share et al.[11]	68.0	58.0	51.0	46.0	49.0	45	Gesell/Binet
Loeffler and							
Smith[12]	65.0	51.0	46.0	43.0	43.0	47–34	Cattell
Carr[13]	66.7	56.0*	48.0	48.0	—	45	Bayley*
Dicks-Mireaux[14]	67.0	57.0†	—	—	—	21	Gesell
de Coriat et al.[15]	66.4	54.5	48.2	44.1	42.6	9–189	Gesell
Ludlow and							
Allen[16]	69.0	61.0	53.0	48.8	44.0	23–71	Griffiths/Binet
Institution reared							
Dameron[17]	59.0	46.0†	—	—	—	12	California‡
Carr[13] §	56.0	44.6*	37.1	35.2	—	7	Bayley
Ludlow and							
Allen[16]	68.0	44.0	42.0	40.0	38	8–22	Griffiths/Binet
Intervention given							
de Coriat et al.[15]	87.7	69.6	65.6	61.0	61.4	9–189	Gesell
Ludlow and							
Allen[16]	79.8	70.0	62.7	57.8	56.4	9–63	Griffiths/Binet
Brinkworth[18]	—	66.8	—	—	—		Griffiths
Cunningham[19]	75.4	66.4*	—	—	—	59–68	Bayley*

* The BSID provide developmental indices whilst the other infant tests quote DQs based on the simple ratio formula MA/CA × 100. Thus the Mental Ages obtained in the studies using BSID have been converted to DQs using the formula for the purpose of comparability
† Assessed at mean age of 18 months
‡ Original version of Bayley Scale
§ These infants were 'boarded out' in family group homes, not in large institutions

that children reared at home for the first years of life are not only in advance of those placed in the institution but that the benefit is maintained for several subsequent years of institutional care[22]. It is important to note that it is not institutions *per se* that retard development but the lack of stimulation provided, and that not all institutions necessarily depress performance[24].

Comparisons of home- and institution-reared samples indicate that infants with Down's syndrome are vulnerable to lack of stimulation from the first months of life and hence variation in environmental conditions can be seen as contributing to the degree of handicap. However, it would be wrong to infer from such findings that early intervention which uses systematic stimulation programmes necessarily have added benefit. The institution–home comparison studies merely show the effects of stimulus deprivation on development. The contention that such programmes would be beneficial is given support from the higher developmental scores found in samples where some form of early intervention was given. In the de Coriat *et al.*[15] and Ludlow and Allen[16] studies the scores of the intervention groups were reported as being significantly greater at all ages than the group not receiving intervention. Unfortunately de Coriat *et al.*[15] give no details on how the two groups were selected and in Ludlow and Allen's study[16] the non-intervention group were those parents unable (possibly unwilling) to attend a clinic regularly. This reliance on parents willing to attend a centre may well cause a bias in sampling.

Our own study was based on regular home-visiting and we finally estimated that 85–90 % of all Down's syndrome infants born in the Greater Manchester area since October 1973 have been included. Thirty-nine per cent of our families felt that they would not or could not attend a central, University based clinic at the two or six-weekly intervals required. The majority of these included working mothers, mothers with other young children and families in the lower economic groups. Consequently, the faster rates of development reported by clinic-based studies may be based on favourably biased samples. Even if this is the case, the difference between the mean developmental scores at one and two years of our sample and de Coriat's and Ludlow and Allen's is only in the order of three to four points lower[15, 16]. A second methodological issue in these early intervention studies is the lack of assessment by independent observers who were unaware of the experimental groupings. In the majority of studies the intervener is also the assessor.

Several other studies have also reported positive findings of early intervention in the first years of life with Down's syndrome children[25-30], though again they frequently have methodological difficulties such as lack of controls and representative samples and lack of independent assessment. Despite these criticisms the present evidence generally supports the notion that early intervention can partially prevent delay in development.

The results presented in Table 18.1 also reflect the decline in developmental and intelligence test scores which have been found in a large number of studies. Many workers have argued that this decline reflects a progressive deterioration in mental abilities related to continuing neurological change[14, 31, 32]. Others have suggested that this decline is an artefact of the computation of DQ or IQs using the simple ratio formula (MA/CA × 100) because mental age continues to rise at a slower rate than chronological age.

Kirman[33] has put forward an alternative explanation, suggesting that the anomalies in Down's syndrome do not become fully manifest until the relevant stages of development are reached. He also notes that if there is a progressive deterioration in the brain, then attempts at birth to restore the physiology to normal may help to minimize the process. If progressive global deterioration is the case, then the developmental curves should show relatively steady declines with little relation to specific areas of development. On the other hand, one would predict from Kirman's suggestion that declines should be observed which correspond to the areas of development related to those parts of the nervous system likely to be impaired. Provided that developmental assessment has been sufficiently detailed and frequent, longitudinal curves should reflect these impairments.

Carr tentatively suggested that the pattern of development for Down's syndrome infants is one of rapid decline in DQ scores between six and ten months, and periods of prolonged plateaux when little development appears[13]. We attempted to explore this possibility by assessing a group of Down's syndrome infants at six-weekly intervals from six weeks of age using the Bayley Scales of Infant Development[34] in their own homes.

The 32 families of these infants were also given support and advice on ways of stimulating their infant[35] and we compared the effects of this with a delayed treatment group of 13 families included in the intervention programme when the child was between six and twelve months of age. Approximately 40% of assessments were carried out by one assessor who was unaware of the grouping. The groups were equated for social class, sex, maternal age, number of siblings, karyotype and added congenital difficulties such as heart disease. (We have now replicated this study on 50 more infants – 34 in an early treatment group and 16 in a delayed treatment group – using a nurse as the home visitor and found similar results.)

In Figure 18.1 we have compared our results with those of a similar sample reported by Carr[13,36]. There is little difference between our early-treatment group and Carr's group for the first six months, although a slight decline in mean DQs is apparent. At 24 and 30 weeks this decline is quite marked. The infants in Carr's 'boarded out' group showed the greatest decline. Those in Carr's home-reared group and our delayed-treatment group showed the next largest decline and have comparable levels of development up to 60 weeks of age. The group given intervention from birth have the least decline and have significantly higher scores at 24–54 weeks than the delayed treatment group.

By 60–66 weeks the delayed-treatment group had apparently caught up to the early treatment group. At this age, inspection of individual profiles revealed that the majority of the infants obtained the same raw score (± 1 point) on several test occasions giving the impression of a plateau. This period corresponds to the development from simple manipulatory play

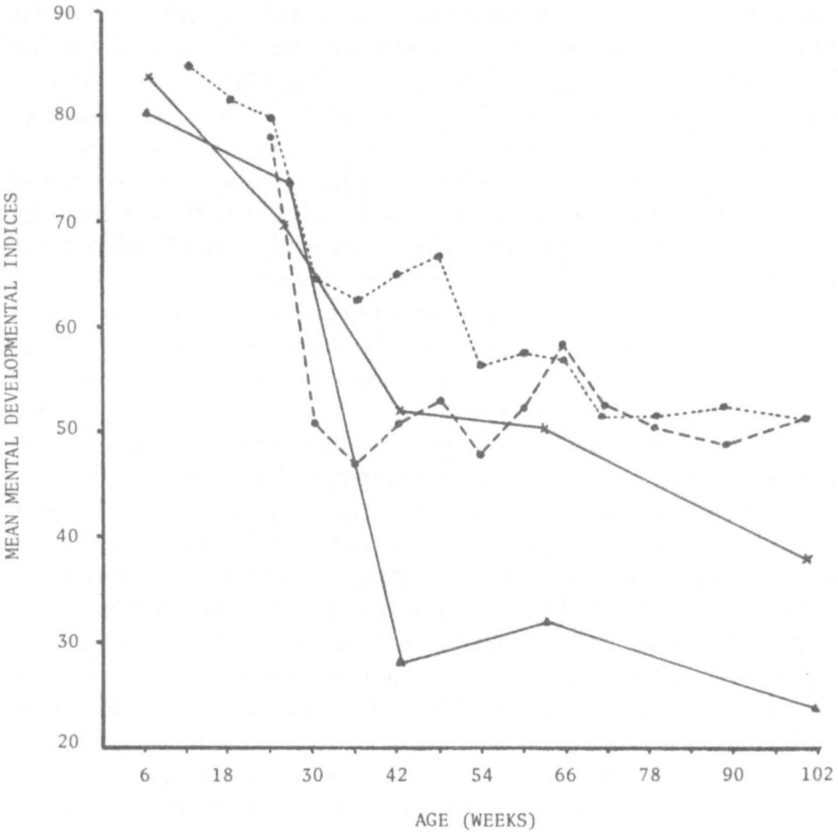

Figure 18.1 Comparison of Bayley mental developmental indices for early and delayed treatment Down's syndrome infants and those of Carr[13]

▲———▲ boarded out } Carr
×———× home reared } Carr
●- - - - -● delayed treatment } present study
●·········● early treatment and teaching } present study

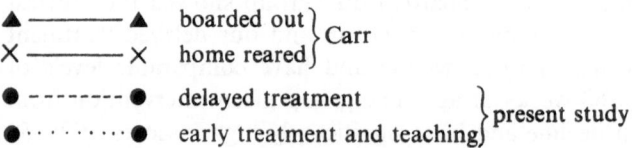

with single objects to relational play involving several objects, functional use of objects and increased span of attention. However it is not yet clear whether this reflects a maturational factor, i.e. the infants are not 'ready' to progress, or whether they need more time to consolidate the manipulative skills which have just emerged. Certainly, when compared to normal patterns of development these children appear to have exaggerated profiles of plateaux and relatively rapid periods of attainment. This observation is commonly reported by parents and researchers[36]. Similar results were found for gross motor development with plateaux occurring prior to independent sitting and walking.

These observations are not merely of academic interest. Once parents accept that systematic stimulation can aid their infant's development they also accept that lack of stimulation can add to the handicap. Thus we find the majority of parents in our sample express anxiety and sometimes guilt about "not doing enough". Equally common is the question "how much do we need to do?" This reflects the need for professionals advocating intervention programmes to consider the needs of the whole family and to ensure that an acceptable balance is maintained.

We have found that parents express great relief when we have been able to explain that the apparent lack of development at certain times in their infant is common to the majority and consequently is probably related to intrinsic developmental factors rather than their lack of effort or in-adequacy in applying stimulation programmes. Indeed, we are convinced that a major contribution of early intervention programmes lies in providing parents with a detailed explanation of developmental processes and the interactional model of specific deficits, maturation and environmental factors.

Unfortunately this knowledge is scarcely sufficient at present. In particular we do not know enough about the nature of timing of teaching programmes to allow accurate phasing of treatment with the development process. Nor do we know enough about the intensity (i.e. how often and how much) with which to apply specific training to ensure reasonably optimal outcomes.

For example, the data presented in Figure 18.1 would suggest that intervention in the first six to nine months was effective but lack of it did not appear to have long-term detrimental consequences – the delayed group caught up. However, it could be that the nature or the intensity of the stimulation programmes advised were not accurate or sufficient. The mean age for attainment of sitting unsupported for one minute in our sample was 10.2 months – which is in advance of the 12 month mean found by Carr[13], 11.3 months mean reported by Share et al.[11] and similar to that reported by Share and Veale[37]. However, both Connolly and Russell[29] and Hanson and Schwarz[28] report means of between seven and eight months for small samples of intensively trained Down's syndrome infants. If we assume that the differences are not due to sampling problems, then we must consider whether the treatments varied.

To test this, we began by examining the nature of the behaviours being assessed in the development scale at the time of the first major 'drop-off' in DQ scores at 30–36 weeks. On the mental-scale items this corresponded to the expected emergence of visually directed reaching and on the motor scale to the attainment of independent sitting. A detailed longitudinal study comparing the development of visually directed reaching and manipulatory skills of normal and Down's syndrome infants using video-tape recordings, revealed a lack of utilization and integration of visual feedback on prehensory behaviour in the handicapped sample[19]. Our observations of sitting development also suggested that the main delay was associated with those aspects involving balance rather than strength. This suggested impaired integration between balance and motor elements.

Consequently, we devised training programmes which emphasized balance (e.g. rocking from side to side) as well as strength (e.g. pulling to sitting) and visual attention to objects during reaching. We then matched two groups of 12 Down's syndrome infants and from the age of 12 weeks visited the home every two weeks. One group was shown how to carry out intensive training whilst the other was given advice similar to our previous intervention[38]. Parents in the intensive group were given written instructions and demonstrations for training and asked to carry out the exercises five times every day and to record results. Three parents could not cope with the intensive training programme and were dropped from the group.

Both groups attained higher development test scores than our previous samples, with the intensively trained group being significantly more advanced. The mean age for sitting independently was 8.4 months for the intensive group and 9.8 months for the control group. More significantly, the effect of training became increasingly apparent as the behaviour increasingly demanded the use of balance. This is illustrated in Figure 18.2 which compares the mean age of attainment of the two groups on the six items of the Bayley scales of infant development (BSID) which assess sitting and including the mean ages reported for the non-handicapped standardization sample of the test.

There is little difference between the means for the first two items, 'sits with support' and 'sits with slight support'. However, the control group are significantly slower to attain the next four items which involved independent sitting and the intensive training group show significant delay in attaining 'sits alone for 30 seconds or more' compared to the test norms. Comparable results were found for reaching behaviours. The intensively trained group appear to be maintaining their superiority after the intensive training has ceased at ten months up to 18 months, but data is not yet available beyond this age.

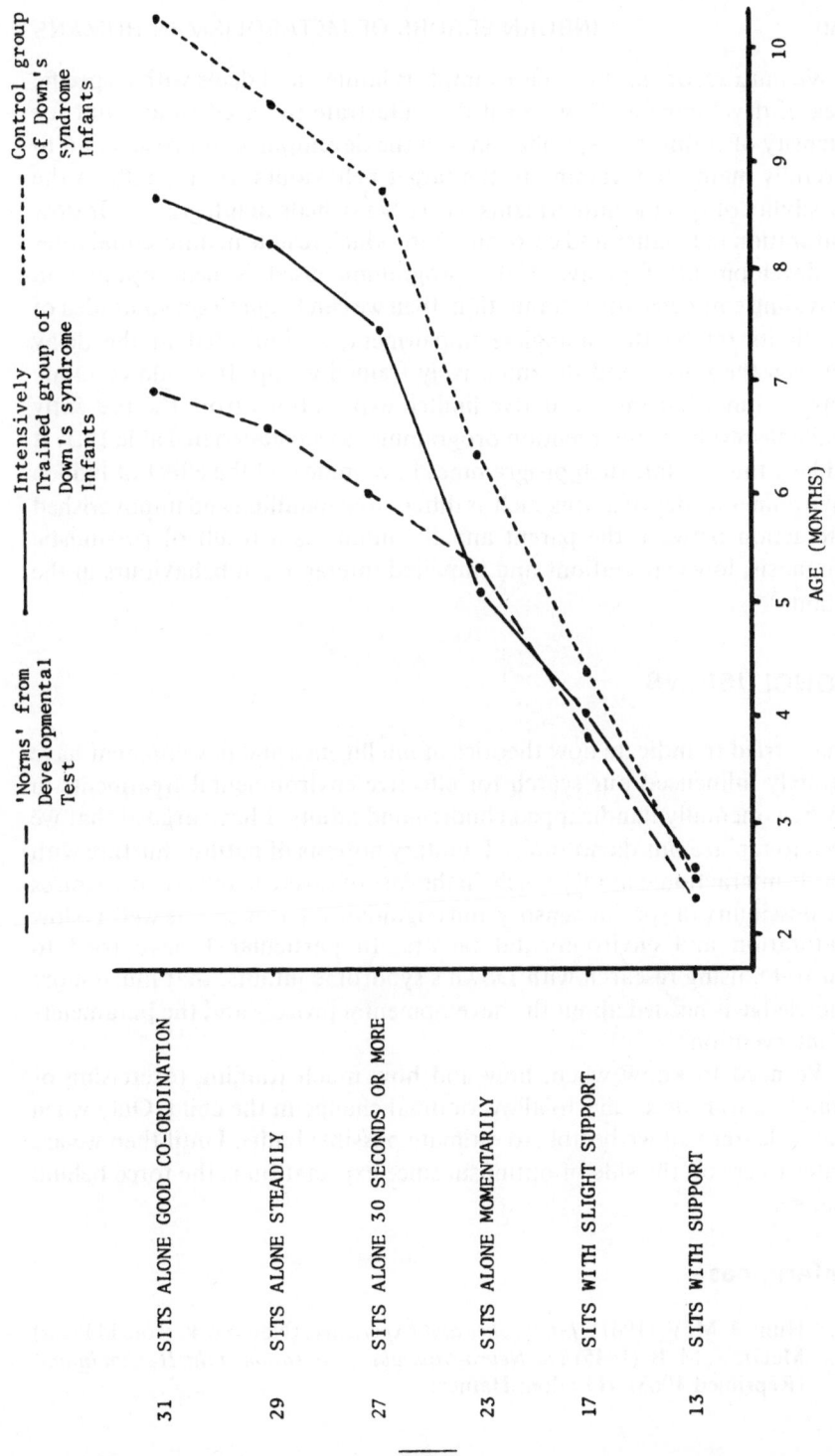

Figure 18.2 Mean age of attaining Bayley items assessing sitting (From Arnljotsdottir[38])

We must recognize that this example is limited and deals with a specific area of development. However it does illustrate the need to account for intensity of training at specific times in the developmental process and to carefully match the training to the target behaviours. It also reflects the possibility of specific impairments, i.e. either deficits in integration or slow maturation in balance and co-ordination, which results in differential rates of development. Equally, if the programme used is near optimal in providing compensatory stimulation, then we can begin to get some idea of the limits set by the biological impairment, as indicated in the delay between the norms and the intensively trained group. It would certainly appear somewhat rash to derive limited expectations from the presently available results of intervention programmes as suggested in Table 18.1. It is likely that, so far, such programmes have indicated the effect of hidden environmental deprivations such as differential handling and impoverished interaction between the parent and the infant as a result of pessimistic prognosis, low expectations and impaired interactional behaviours in the infants[39].

CONCLUSIONS

I have tried to indicate how theories of intelligence and development have strongly influenced our search for effective environmental treatments in severely mentally handicapped children and adults. I have argued that we need to replace our dichotomized, unitary notions of nature–nurture with a truly interactional model which, in the case of severe handicap, recognizes the possibility of specific sensory and cognitive impairments as well as slow maturation and environmental factors. In particular I have tried to illustrate, using research with Down's syndrome infants, that much more knowledge is needed about the developmental process and the parameters of intervention.

We need to know when, how and how much training (exercising or stimulation) is necessary to allow optimal change in the child. Only when this is clearer will we be able to estimate possible limits. Until then we are better to err on the side of optimism since expectation is the force behind change.

References

1. Hunt, J. McV. (1961). *Intelligence and Experience*. (New York: Ronald Press)
2. McGraw, M. B. (1945) *The Neuro-Muscular Maturation of the Human Infant*. (Reprinted 1963). (London: Hafner)

3. Gesell, A. and Amatruda, C. S. (1941). *Developmental Diagnosis*, 2nd Edn. (New .York: Hoeber)
4. Binet, A. and Simon, T. H. (1914). *Mentally Defective Children.* (translated by B. Drummond). (London: Arnold)
5. McCall, R. B. (1976). Toward an epigenetic conception of mental development in the first three years of life. In Lewis, M. (ed.) *Origins of Intelligence.* (New York, London: Plenum Publishing)
6. Cunningham, C. C. (1979). Early stimulation of the mentally handicapped child. In Craft, M. (ed.) *Tredgold's Mental Retardation,* 12th Edn. (Bailliere-Tindale)
7. Clarke, A. D. B. and Cookson, M. (1962). Perceptual motor transfer in imbeciles: a second series of experiments. *Br. J. Psychol.,* **53,** 321
8. Clarke, A. M. and Clarke, A. D. B. (1973). What are the problems? An evaluation of recent research relating to theory and practice. In Clarke, A. D. B. and Clarke A. M. (eds.) *Mental Retardation and Behavioural Research.* IRMR Study Group 4. (London: Churchill Livingstone)
9. Stedman, D. J. (1977). Important considerations in the review and evaluation intervention programme. In Mittler, P. J. (ed.) *Research to Practice in Mental Retardation,* Vol. 1, *Care and Intervention.* 4th Congress of I. A. S. S. M. D. (Baltimore, London, Washington: University Park Press)
10. Lazar, I. and Darlington, R. B. (1978). The Lasting Effects after Preschool. Pub. No. (OHDS) 79–30178 (Washington DC: W. S. Dept. of Health, Education and Welfare)
11. Share, J., Koch, R., Webb, A. and Graliker, B. (1964). The longitudinal development of infants and young children with Down's syndrome (Mongolism). *Am. J. Ment. Defic.,* **68,** 685
12. Loeffler, F. and Smith, G. F. (1964). Data quoted in Penrose, L. S. and Smith, G. F. (1966). *Down's Anomaly.* (London: Churchill)
13. Carr, J. (1970). Mental and motor development in young mongol children. *J. Ment. Defic. Res.,* **14,** 205
14. Dicks-Mireaux, M. J. (1972). Mental development of infants with Down's syndrome. *Am. J. Ment. Defic.,* **77,** 26
15. de Coriat, L. F., Theslenco, Z. and Waxsman, J. (1968). The effects of psychomotor stimulation on the IQ of young children with Trisomy 21. In Richards, B. W. (ed.) *Proceedings of the 1st Congress of the International Association for the Scientific Study of Mental Deficiency.* (Reigate: Jackson)
16. Ludlow, J. R. and Allen, L. M. (1979). The effect of early intervention and pre-school stimulus on the development of the Down's syndrome child. *J. Ment. Defic. Res.,* **23,** 29
17. Dameron, L. E. (1963). Development of intelligence of infants with mongolism. *Child Devel.,* **34,** 733
18. Brinkworth, R. (1973). The unfinished child: effects of early home training on the mongol infant. In Clarke, A. D. B. and Clarke, A. M. (eds.) *Mental Retardation and Behavioural Research.* Study Group 4, IRMR. (Edinburgh and London: Churchill Livingstone)
19. Cunningham, C. C. (1979). Aspects of early development in Down's syndrome infants. *Ph.D. Thesis,* University of Manchester
20. Centerwall, S. A. and Centerwall, W. R. (1960). A study of children with

mongolism reared in the home compared to those reared away from the home. *Pediatrics*, **25**, 678

21. Stedman, D. J. and Eichorn, D. H. (1964). A comparison of the growth and development of institutionalised and home-reared mongoloids during infancy and childhood. *Am. J. Ment. Defic.*, **69**, 391

22. Shipe, D. and Shotwell, A. M. (1965). Effect of out-of-home care on mongoloid children: a continuation study. *Am. J. Ment. Defic.*, **69**, 649

23. Francis, S. M. (1971). The effects of own home and institutional rearing on the behavioural development of normal and mongol children. *J. Child Psychol. Psychiat.*, **12**, 173

24. Tizard, J. and Tizard, B. (1974). The institution as an environment for development. In Richards, M. P. (ed.) *The Integration of a Child into a Social World*. (Cambridge: Cambridge University Press)

25. Hayden, A. H. and Haring, N. G. (1977). The acceleration and maintenance of development gains in Down's syndrome school-age children. In Mittler, P. J. (ed.) *Research to Practice in Mental Retardation*, Vol. 1, *Care and Intervention*. 4th Congress of I.A.S.S.M.D. (Washington, Baltimore, London: University Park Press)

26. Rynders, J. E. and Horrobin, J. M. (1975). Project EDGE: The University of Minnesota's communication stimulation program for Down's syndrome infants. In Friedlander, B. Z. et al. (eds.) *Exceptional Infant*, Vol. 3, *Assessment and Intervention*. (New York: Brunner/Mazel)

27. Aronson, M. and Fallstrom, K. (1977). Immediate and long-term effects of developmental training in children with Down's syndrome. *Devel. Med. Child Neurol.*, **19**, 489

28. Hanson, M. J. and Schwarz, R. H. (1978). Results of a longitudinal intervention program for Down's syndrome infants and their families. *Educ. Train. Ment. Retard.*, **13**, 403

29. Connolly, B. and Russell, F. (1976). Interdisciplinary early intervention program. *Physical Ther.*, **56**, 155

30. Clunies-Ross, G. G. (1979). Accelerating the development of Down's syndrome infants and young children. *J. Spec. Educ.*, **13**, 169

31. Masland, R. L., Sarason, S. B. and Gladwin, T. (1958). *Mental Subnormality*. (New York: Basic Books)

32. Gesell, A. (1940). *The First Five Years of Life: A Guide to the Study of the Pre-school Child*. (London: Methuen)

33. Kirman, B. (1975). Genetic errors: chromosome anomalies. In Kirman, B. and Bicknell, J. (eds.) *Mental Handicap*. (London: Churchill Livingstone)

34. Bayley, N. (1969). *Bayley Scales of Infant Development*. (New York: Psychological Corporation)

35. Cunningham, C. C. and Sloper, P. (1978). *Helping Your Handicapped Baby* (London: Souvenir Press) In USA – *Helping Your Exceptional Baby*. (New York: Pantheon Books)

36. Carr, J. (1975). *Young Children With Down's Syndrome*. IRMMH Monograph No. 4. (London: Butterworths)

37. Share, J. and Veale, A. M. D. (1974). *Developmental Landmarks for Children with Down's Syndrome (Mongolism)*. (Dunedin, New Zealand: University of Otago Press)

38.   Arnljotsdottir, M. (1980). Psycho-motor intervention with Down's syndrome infants. *M.Sc. Thesis*, University of Manchester
39.   Cunningham, C. C. and Mittler, P. J. (1981). Maturation, development and mental handicap. In Connolly, K. J. and Prechtl, H. R. (eds.) *Maturation and Development: Biological and Psychological Perspectives.* (London: Heinemann Medical)

19

Repercussions of screening

B. E. Clayton

Screening may apply to a whole or the major part of a community, it may involve a limited section of the population or perhaps be concerned only with extended family groups known to be at risk for some disorder. The present discussion is concerned with screening apparently healthy subjects in whom disease may be diagnosed as a consequence. This is very different from the conventional diagnosis of disease in an individual who is ill and seeking medical help.

Amongst healthy people of any age, screening programmes of a service nature should be clearly differentiated from those which are research projects[1]. The programme will set in motion a chain-reaction which is likely to involve the wider family circle and a whole variety of health workers. In particular it is likely to cause anxiety – not only in the mother of a newly born infant but also in adults who may be screened for such disorders as carcinoma of the cervix or diabetes mellitus. When the programme is of a research nature, the support which must be given to subjects having a positive screening-test result is even more important. This is an aspect of screening which may be seriously neglected when the project is too laboratory-orientated and insufficient thought and support have been given to the subjects being tested.

The technique which is used to screen for one particular disorder may, in fact, detect other conditions at the same time. For example, a Guthrie test for hyperphenylalaninaemia will only detect that biochemical abnormality, but a screening test employing chromatography will show other amino-acid disorders in addition. In the latter situation there has frequently been no clear plan for dealing with the unsolicited information. As a result infants have been placed on low proline or low histidine diets, for example, without any definitive co-ordinated therapeutic trial being undertaken. The expertise for doing this was not always available, and conclusive results on the outcome could not be obtained.

Over the years, experience gained in screening for inborn errors has affected society's attitudes to screening in general, and has helped to clarify the criteria which must be fulfilled for a successful screening programme[2,3]. These include:

(1) as much as possible should be known about the natural history of the disease;

(2) the condition must be an important health problem;

(3) there should be treatment for the condition;

(4) there must be facilities for diagnosis and treatment, including genetic counselling;

(5) the screening test must be acceptable to the subject and must satisfy criteria of sensitivity, precision and specificity;

(6) the whole process must be economically justifiable in the context of the rest of the claims on limited finance available for health care.

It is no longer sufficient to think of neonatal screening programmes as only embracing inherited metabolic disorders. Already many infants are screened for hypothyroidism. Although this is a metabolic disorder it is not an inherited condition in the majority of affected infants. In the future, therefore, programmes will be extended to include perhaps additional inherited disorders, other metabolic disorders which are not inherited, chromosome abnormalities, HLA typing and so on. In the organization of such a wide-ranging programme, co-ordination of all the different people who will be involved is vital and the number of individuals who are actually in direct contact with the mother, infant and family must be kept to a minimum. The screening tests themselves and certainly requests for repeat tests or additional specimens make the mother of a newly born infant very anxious and she should be supported by only two or three individuals whom she knows and trusts. In the United Kingdom this is generally the midwife or health visitor, and the general practitioner. These individuals should understand the programme and the need for repeat samples, but in order that they may not be confused and that their goodwill may be retained, the laboratory workers should coordinate the results of the different screening tests. Only one or two individuals in the laboratories should approach the health care workers who deal directly with the mother.

How far a pregnant woman or the mother of a newly born infant should be asked for informed consent before a screening test is performed is a debatable point. Pregnancy and the puerperium are not times when a woman should be worried if it is avoidable. The education of older schoolchildren should include such matters in the teaching of human biology. Certainly in the United Kingdom, and perhaps elsewhere, insufficient use is made of the high circulation of women's magazines and the press in disseminating information. It is, of course, essential for such information to be accurate and presented in a non-sensational way, but unfortunately this is not always the case.

Results arising from screening programmes have emphasized deficiencies in our knowledge of the natural history of many disorders[4]. They have also demonstrated the heterogeneous nature of what seemed in years gone by to be relatively straightforward diseases. Studies on the inborn errors have stimulated, too, the search for new methods of treatment. The problems posed by all these considerations are not, in fact, limited to inherited disorders of infancy.

Early screening programmes for phenylketonuria depended on the detection of abnormal metabolites in urine, but many cases were missed[5]. In the 1960s, tests based on the finding of raised phenylalanine in blood began to be widely used. Over the years there has been gradual recognition that 'phenylketonuria' is not a single disease entity but encompasses a number of disorders of differing clinical and biochemical severity and the term 'hyperphenylalaninaemia' embraces this heterogeneous collection more appropriately. Most patients with persistent hyperphenylalaninaemia have one of several defects of phenylalanine hydroxylase activity[6], but a few rare patients have abnormalities of biopterin metabolism[7, 8].

Amongst 51 infants with persistently elevated blood phenylalanine levels [greater than 240 µmol/l (4 mg/100 ml)] detected in a screening programme in North London[9] there were considerable variations in the amount of natural protein which they could tolerate in their diets. Some persistently tolerated 10 g or more daily, whilst others could tolerate only between 3 and 6 g daily. The North London programme has shown also how environmental changes may affect the findings in a screening programme. Amongst the three quarters of a million infants tested between October 1969 and December 1978 there was a significant fall in the incidence of uncomplicated transient hyperphenylalaninaemia with and without tyrosinaemia. The decrease coincided with, and is likely to be due to, the change in infant feeding practice which led to lower intakes of protein and hence of phenylalanine intake in infants born after 1974 in the United Kingdom[10].

A similar explanation has been proposed to account for the decreased incidence of transient hypermethioninaemia and homocystinuria detected in recent years in the same North London screening area[11]. It has thus become essential for every infant who has a screening test giving a value of 240 µmol phenylalanine/l blood (4 mg phenylalanine/100 ml) or more to be followed up carefully.

Screening of neonates for congenital hypothyroidism is proving rewarding and in a programme in North London, for example, the incidence was one in 3363 births[12] compared with one in 15 000 for hyperphenyl-alaninaemia[9]. A programme was first introduced in Quebec in 1974[13] and since then others have been developed elsewhere. Although absolutely firm evidence that early diagnosis and treatment improves prognosis is lacking, all the experience which is accumulating indicates that this is so[14].

For ethical reasons double blind clinical trials are impossible, but in a retrospective survey of patients with congenital hypothyroidism in North London, it was found that diagnosis of the condition had often been delayed, only 40 % of cases being recognized before 3 months of age. In addition, one third of the children required special schooling and one quarter had IQs of less than- 70[12].

In the North London screening programme only two of the 26 infants detected had been diagnosed by conventional methods by the time the results of screening became available, one because of functional intestinal obstruction and the other because of pronounced clinical signs of hypothyroidism. After the screening test was reported it was found that nine babies had feeding problems, three were still jaundiced after 10 days and other symptoms included constipation in seven and a hoarse cry in five. Six infants were considered to be asymptomatic by their mothers, although two had fairly pronounced signs of hypothyroidism. Eleven infants had an ectopic thyroid, there were seven with large thyroids and four with only remnants of thyroid tissue. Two were athyrotic and three had goitres, which were probably familial in two of them. In seven babies, the thyroid was in the normal position; one had a hemithyroid, three had apparently hypoplastic glands and two may have been transient cases. Only now, are we able to follow such infants in considerable numbers from early life. In particular, it will be necessary to determine how many infants have a transient form of the condition.

A consideration of cystic fibrosis, which is the commonest serious genetic disease in Caucasian children, demonstrates the moral dilemma of whether or not to screen. The hallmarks of a patient who clearly has the condition include chronic suppurative staphylococcal or pseudomonas lung disease, exocrine pancreatic insufficiency and an abnormally increased concentration of sodium in sweat. Cystic fibrosis as at present recognized is still life-threatening, carries a poor prognosis and requires life-long treatment which usually necessitates a number of hospital admissions. It is a serious matter when the diagnosis is made and if the diagnosis should be wrong, much distress will have been caused.

The natural history of cystic fibrosis appears to have changed over the years so that there has been some improvement in survival and the quality of life. The biochemical basis of the condition is unknown and whether or not it is heterogeneous in its nature as with so many inborn errors, remains to be elucidated. Recent screening tests in the newborn have included those based on raised albumin in meconium[15], diminished trypsin activity in stools employing benzoyl-arginine-p-nitroanilide as a substrate[16] and the demonstration of raised immunoreactive trypsin in dried blood spots[17, 18]. None of them are perfect and with such a dreadful condition false negatives and positives are of serious concern. Confirmation of the diagnosis requires a sweat test. This is frequently performed badly and should be carried out only in centres with considerable and on-going experience of its use[19]. In young infants, sweating is sometimes inadequate and repeat sweat tests and waiting for the infant to become a little older before retesting cause the parents much anxiety. Although heterozygote detection is to some extent possible in research studies, its unreliable nature renders it inappropriate for use in a service situation at present.

Duchenne muscular dystrophy leads to an inability to walk by the age of 12 and death in the late teens or early twenties. It probably has an incidence approaching one in 3000 male births[20], but the new mutation rate is high and accounts for about a third of patients[21]. Antenatal fetal sexing with selective abortion of a male fetus may be carried out, but there are serious doubts about the reliability of tests for fetal serum creatine kinase activity in the prenatal diagnosis of the condition in infant boys[20].

The condition can be detected in the affected newborn male infant since the creatine kinase activity will be very high. Screening is feasible as the enzyme is stable in dried blood spots and several screening projects have been performed. For example in France amongst 109 100 infants screened[22], nine cases of the condition were confirmed. Screening is not excessively expensive and is effective. However, there is much debate about the ethics of screening an infant for an untreatable disease, although parents of affected children often appear to be in favour. The worry is the reaction of parents faced with an apparently normal male infant who has a lethal condition. Since it is the mother who is the carrier the problems are much greater than with a disorder with an autosomal recessive inheritance where the parents cannot blame each other. The period after childbirth is not a good time for a mother to learn about such a dreadful disease in her infant and for her to appreciate that she is responsible. The sensible suggestion has been made[23] that it would be better to screen all boys who are not walking by the age of 18 months.

Carrier detection should be pursued vigorously in the extended family whenever Duchenne muscular dystrophy is diagnosed in one of its members. In this context, the girls in such families should be tested at the time of leaving school. There are those who would screen for carrier status amongst all female neonates. Assessment of carrier status is not perfect and the significance of a positive result in the screening test may remain in doubt. A positive test is a burden which would be with the parents throughout childhood. Ethical views on this differ, but I have no doubt that we are wrong to inflict such a worry on the parents of a child, particularly whilst we do not know the cause of the condition.

There are inherited conditions with definite biochemical abnormalities, the clinical significance of which is not understood. Histidinaemia provides a good example. The biochemical abnormalities found in this condition include increased histidine in plasma and urine, increased urinary excretion of metabolites of histidine, marked reduction in histidine ammonia lyase (histidase) activity and urocanic acid content in the skin, and an abnormal histidine tolerance curve. Originally the biochemical changes were discovered during the investigation of mentally subnormal patients. Further studies raised doubts as to whether or not these biochemical findings were in fact related to the patient's condition[24]. When 'biochemical histidinaemia' is detected during the screening of newborns an ethical problem arises, some clinicians considering that the infant should be treated and others that it is unnecessary to do so. It must be remembered that any diet in childhood imposes strains on the child and family, and in any case no synthetic diet can be better than present knowledge allows. No untoward findings have been observed in prospective studies of untreated infants with biochemical histidinaemia detected by screening, some for more than 15 years (Neville, B. G. R. and Clayton, B. E., unpublished). It is still too soon to state unequivocally that histidinaemia may not produce some abnormalities in later life. It has been suggested[25] that histidinaemia may be genetically heterogeneous like so many other inherited metabolic disorders. If this is the case, all the evidence points to the form(s) detected by screening being benign. Parents of infants in such prospective studies require much support and intelligent, educated parents are particularly anxious about the outcome.

All the problems, dilemmas and ethical considerations faced in screening programmes for the neonate have occurred too when screening adults. A good example is screening women for carcinoma of the cervix. This has been carried out with varying degrees of enthusiasm in different parts of the world for about 30 years, but much of this has occurred in a haphazard manner at the behest of pressure groups. The lack of well-designed trials has made it difficult to assess its efficacy[26, 27]. This is an important point because if it is really useful, then many women must have been deprived of a beneficial screening service. Only in recent years has firm scientific evidence accumulated so that more rational decisions based on facts rather than dogma can be made. There are now well-designed studies such as that from Iceland[28], indicating that screening results had reduced mortality in women aged 25–59 years and that deaths and advanced tumours will be confined largely to women who have not been screened and treated. The Icelandic authors considered alternative explanations for their findings before concluding that screening was the cause of the improvement. The natural history of the disease as detected by screening was unknown and one of the problems has been the significance of positive smears. In an important paper, Kinlen and Spriggs[29] described 101 women with unsuspected positive smears who had had no biopsy by at least two years later for a variety of reasons. Seventy of them were traced; seven had clinically diagnosed carcinoma of the cervix and of these five died. Fifty-three were studied after a mean interval of 5.2 years without any follow-up. The important observation was made that 19 of these showed no lesion at this time, regression being confined to women under 40 years of age. The other subjects had evidence of malignancy. It is still impossible to say whether those smears which regress represent a separate and harmless condition, or whether in the long-term the positive smear will have indicated a truly pre-cancerous lesion. Smears which fall short of malignancy certainly generate anxiety in the women concerned and such studies as that of Kinlen and Spriggs are very helpful for the health care workers who have to support them.

Certain abnormalities in the fetus may be detected by screening the mother. At present maternal screening for raised serum α-fetoprotein (AFP) is being introduced in many places. At the eighteenth week of gestation the concentration of AFP correlates with the frequency of anencephaly and open neural-tube defects[30]. The prevalence of these defects varies from one to almost 10 per 1000 births, depending on the geographical region and the ethnic group from which the population comes. Although it is much higher where there is a family history and for a pregnancy in a woman who has had two previously affected children, in the United Kingdom 90 % of all affected children result from pregnancies not known to be at risk for this group of conditions. In order to obtain maximum benefit from the screening programme three aspects are important: the precision of the AFP measurement, the reliability of the estimated stage of gestation and careful assessment including a further measurement before undertaking amniocentesis. Quality control of AFP reagents and of the assay itself has been considered recently[31] and it was recommended that there should be national maternal serum and amniotic fluid reference materials against which producers and users of reagents would be able to calibrate their own working standards, and that national materials should be calibrated against the World Health Authority AFP reference material.

Although screening for AFP has benefits, it also has undesirable side effects. It has been estimated that the increased risk to a normal fetus arising from amniocentesis which has resulted in accidental abortion or perinatal morbidity will possibly occur about four times in 10 000 women screened[32]. For this reason it has been advised that adequate monitoring both nationally and locally is necessary in order to assess the efficacy of the programme and to identify side-effects. Maybe experience will show that it should be applied only to limited populations of pregnant women. Information on the test should be available, preferably so that the woman has knowledge of it before she is pregnant. Some consultants would question the extent to which a detailed explanation of AFP and the need to obtain formal consent for the first test is necessary. Nevertheless, the test, if positive, will raise the issue of amniocentesis with the risks (albeit minimal) which that entails and the moral issues which it raises.

Fetal lymphocytes pass actively into the mother's blood relatively early in pregnancy[33] and many remain there for long periods. There is also passage of erythrocytes from fetus to mother. The lymphocytes, particularly, will surely be used for prenatal diagnosis at some time in the future and may be employed in a programme which screens the fetus without invading its environment.

HLA typing is likely to be incorporated into screening programmes one day, to aid in the detection of disorders with familial clustering[34], e.g. ankylosing spondylitis, diabetes mellitus[35], coeliac disease[36] and perhaps in relation to potential malignancy. Such a programme might relate to fetal cells in the maternal circulation or to the infant after birth. Already HLA typing of amniotic-fluid cells can be used in the prenatal diagnosis of congenital adrenal hyperplasia due to C21-hydroxylase deficiency[37, 38]. This is highly specific and there is no linkage between HLA group and congenital adrenal hyperplasia due to C11-β-hydroxylase deficiency[39].

In conclusion, the team participating in a screening programme must always remember that the subjects concerned are apparently healthy. This raises many problems: ethical, medical, social and economic. The possible impact on a community should be beneficial, but without careful thought and support of the subjects with positive tests a programme may create distress.

References

1. Larsson, A. (1980). Screening of newborn infants in Sweden for congenital metabolic diseases. In *Skandia International Symposia Congenital Diseases in Childhood*, pp. 176–192. (Stockholm: Almqvist and Wicksell)
2. Whitby, L. G. (1974). Screening for disease. Definitions and criteria. *Lancet*, **2**, 819
3. Clayton, B. E. (1976). Principles in the management of inherited metabolic disorders. In T. E. Oppé and F. P. Woodford (eds.) *Early Management of Handicapping Disorders*, pp. 3–10. (Elsevier, Excerpta Medica, North-Holland)
4. Smith, I. and Wolff, O. H. (1974). Natural history of phenylketonuria and influence of early treatment. *Lancet*, **2**, 540
5. Stephenson, J. B. P. and McBean, M. S. (1967). Phenylketonuria: a reassessment of mass infant screening by napkin test. *Br. Med. J.*, **3**, 582
6. Kaufman, S. (1978). The enzymes of the hepatic phenylalanine hydroxylating system. *J. Inher. Metab. Dis.*, **1**, 63
7. Kaufman, S. (1980). Differential diagnosis of variant forms of hyper-phenylalaninaemia. *Pediatrics*, **65**, 840
8. O'Brien, D., Berlow, S., Donnell, G., Justice, P., Kaufman, S., Levy, H. L., McCabe, E. R. B. and Snyderman, S. (1980). New developments in hyperphenylalaninaemia. *Pediatrics*, **65**, 844
9. Walker, V., Clayton, B. E., Ersser, R. S., Francis, D. E. M., Lilly, P., Seakins, H. W. T., Smith, I. and Whiteman, P. D. (1980). Hyperphenylalaninaemia of various types amongst three quarters of a million neonates tested in a screening programme. *Arch. Dis. Child.*, **56**, 759
10. Department of Health and Social Security (1974). Present Day Practice in Infant Feeding. Reports on Health and Social Subjects. No. 9. (London: HMSO)
11. Whiteman, P. D., Clayton, B. E., Ersser, R. S., Lilly, P. and Seakins, J. W. T. (1979). Changing incidence of neonatal hypermethioninaemia: implications for the detection of homocystinuria. *Arch. Dis. Child.*, **54**, 593
12. Hulse, J. A., Grant, D. B., Clayton, B. E., Lilly, P., Jackson, D., Spracklan, A., Edwards, R. W. H. and Nurse, D. (1980). Population screening for congenital hypothyroidism. *Br. Med. J.*, **1**, 675
13. Dussault, J. H., Coulombe, P., Laberge, C., Letarte, J., Guyda, H. and Khoury, K. (1975). Preliminary report on a mass screening program for neonatal hypothyroidism. *J. Pediatr.*, **86**, 670
14. Smith, P. and Morris, A. (1979). Assessment of a programme to screen the newborn for congenital hypothyroidism. *Community Med.*, **1**, 14
15. Ryley, H. C., Neale, L. M., Brogan, T. D. and Bray, P. T. (1979). Screening for cystic fibrosis in the newborn by meconium analysis. *Arch. Dis. Child.*, **54**, 92

16. Crossley, J. R., Berryman, C. C. and Elliott, R. B. (1977). Cystic-fibrosis screening in the newborn. *Lancet*, **2,** 1093
17. Applegarth, D. A., Davidson, A. G. F., Kirby, L. T., Bridges, M., Sorensen, P., Wong, L. T. T. and Hardwick, D. F. (1979). Dried blood spot screening for cystic fibrosis. *Lancet*, **2,** 1236
18. King, D. N., Heeley, A. F., Walsh, M. P. and Kuzemko, J. A. (1979). Sensitive trypsin assay for dried-blood specimens as a screening procedure for early detection of cystic fibrosis. *Lancet*, **2,** 1217
19. Schwachman, H. and Mohmoodian, A. (1979). Quality of sweat test performance in the diagnosis of cystic fibrosis. *Clin. Chem.*, **25,** 158
20. Emery, A. E. H. (1980). Duchenne muscular dystrophy. *Br. Med. Bull.*, **36,** 117
21. Davie, A. M. and Emery, A. E. H. (1978). Estimation of proportion of new mutants among cases of Duchenne muscular dystrophy. *J. Med. Genet.*, **15,** 339
22. Dellamonica, C., Robert, J. M., Cotte, J., Plauchu, H. and Dorche, C. (1979). Dépistage néonatal systématique de la myopathie de Duchenne de Boulogne. *Nour. Pressé Méd.*, **8,** 1491
23. Gardner-Medwin, D. (1979). Controversies about Duchenne muscular dystrophy. (1) Neonatal screening. *Devel. Med. Child Neurol.*, **21,** 390
24. Neville, B. G. R., Bentovim, A., Clayton, B. E. and Shepherd, J. (1972). Histidinaemia. Study of relation between clinical and biological findings in seven subjects. *Arch. Dis. Child.* **47,** 190
25. Levy, H. L., Smith, V. E. and Madigan, P. M. (1974). Routine newborn screening for histidinaemia. *N. Engl. J. Med.*, **291,** 1214
26. Task Force appointed by the Conference of Deputy Ministers of Health (1976). Cervical Cancer Screening programs. *Can. Med. Assoc. J.*, **114,** 1003
27. Foltz, A. and Kelsey, J. L. (1978). The annual Pap test: a dubious policy success. *Millbank Memor. Fund Q./Health Soc.*, **56,** 426
28. Johannesson, G., Geirsson, G. and Day, N. (1978). The effect of mass screening in Iceland, 1965–74, on the incidence and mortality of cervical carcinoma. *Int. J. Cancer*, **21,** 418
29. Kinlen, L. J. and Spriggs, A. I. (1978). Women with positive cervical smears but without surgical intervention. A follow-up study. *Lancet*, **2,** 463
30. Report of UK Collaborative Study on alpha-fetoprotein in relation to neural tube defects (1977). *Lancet*, **1,** 1323
31. Report of a Workshop sponsored by the National Institute of Child Health and Human Development (NICHD), Bethesda, Md, USA (1980). *Clin. Chim. Acta*, **105,** 9
32. Report by the Working Group on Screening for Neural Tube Defects (1979), set up by the Standing Medical Advisory Committee to advise the Health Authorities. (This refers to the United Kingdom)
33. Zilliacus, R., Chapelle, A. de La, Schröder, J., Tiilikainen, A., Kohne, E. and Kleihauer, E. (1975). Transplacental passage of foetàl blood cells. *Scand. J. Haematol.*, **15,** 333
34. Dick, H. M. (1978). HLA and disease. *Br. Med. Bul.*, **34,** 271
35. Cudworth, A. G. and Festenstein, H. (1978). HLA Genetic heterogeneity in diabetes mellitus. *Br. Med. Bull.*, **34,** 285

36. Mackintosh, P. and Asquith, P. (1978). HLA and coeliac disease. *Br. Med. Bull.*, **34**, 291

37. Couillin, P., Nicolas, H., Boué, A. and Boué, J. (1979). HLA typing and amniotic fluid cells applied to prenatal diagnosis of congenital adrenal hyperplasia. *Lancet*, **1**, 1076

38. Levine, L. S., Zachmann, M., New, M. I., Prader, A., Pollack, M. S., O'Neill, G. J., Yang, S. Y., Oberfield, S. E. and Dupont, B. (1978). Genetic mapping of the 21-hydroxylase-deficiency gene within the HLA group. *N. Engl. J. Med.*, **299**, 911

39. Brautbar, C., Rösler, A. and 12 others (1979). No linkage between HLA and congenital adrenal hyperplasia due to 11-β-hydroxylase deficiency. *N. Engl. J. Med.*, **300**, 205

20

Some principles in the management of inherited metabolic disease

D. N. Raine

As Watchman on the King's ship you must be cautious and circumspect. Gales of earthliness are whistling violently, waves of this world are surging up, headlands of secular power threaten danger and death, and hypocrites lie in ambush like pirates. Amidst all these you must hold your course for the harbour.

Fulbert of Chartres, 1008

With Sir Archibald Garrod's Croonian lectures in 1908[1], inherited metabolic disease, as an entity, became recognizable; the discovery of an effective treatment for phenylketonuria in 1953 by Bickel, Gerrard and Hickmans[2], made it important. Even so, 10 years later, those pioneering a wider approach to the early detection of similar disorders were repeatedly challenged with the question "Why detect them when you can't treat them?" and in Birmingham two medical colleagues took active steps to prevent the introduction of the neonatal screening programme subsequently reported by Raine and co-workers[3], one argument being that the risk of a road accident to the midwife driving to collect the blood specimen would probably exceed any benefits to an infant as a result of the survey! Happily this phase passed, but there emerged a more real and overwhelming problem as the true magnitude of inherited metabolic disease became apparent and the wider implications beyond the care of the propositus were appreciated. It became clear that few specialists were likely to devote the necessary time to the subject to be able to recognize and treat individuals suffering from such a wide range of disorders.

Fortunately, the number of patients requiring this service is small, and it has been suggested that there would be enough specialist centres if each country provided one for each five[4] or ten[5] million of population. The annual number of new cases has been estimated in three different ways: those detected in screening surveys can be counted and provide a minimum number; a further assessment can be made from the proportion of paediatric deaths due to recessive and X-linked genetic disease; and a third assessment can be made from the proportion of paediatric hospital admissions due to these same disorders. These give an annual rate of not less than 20 per million population, more realistically 40 per million, ultimately rising to perhaps 50–60 per million as the appropriate diagnostic facilities become more widely available[6]. These figures are not just intelligent guesses, but are derived from reliable data detailed in the source cited.

Thus, having defined the problem it became possible by February 1974 to detail the components of a health-care system necessary to deal with it. Since then a number of countries (for example Canada, Denmark and the Netherlands) have established, and their governments have formally recognized, such systems, and it gives no satisfaction to report that the United Kingdom, from which the proposals were first made, is still not among them. However, world-wide there is now sufficient experience to allow, in the present discussion, a re-examination of this health-care system to see how well it is fulfilling its expectations. This leads to the enunciation of a number of principles which need to be borne in mind in discussing the international aspect of management of inherited metabolic disease, namely:

    P1.   The health care system for inherited metabolic disease
           will benefit too few people for it to command spontaneous
           consideration from national administrators.

Apart from their superficial relevance, the quotations from *The Letters and Poems of Fulbert of Chartres*[7] which punctuate this discussion, have a further purpose which will be explained at the conclusion.

INFORMATION

To be sure, truth will always out, but coming from an ignorant and unlearned man it cannot be proclaimed so as to be pleasing.

Hugh of Tours to Hubert of Angers, 1023

In 1978 McKusick[8] listed 1322 recessive and X-linked human genetic diseases, all of which can be expected, sometime, to be revealed to be specific metabolic disorders; indeed in 158 the precise enzyme deficiency is already known. None but the most dedicated specialist could expect to be sufficiently familiar with this corpus of knowledge to be able to recognize most conditions when cases present and, should he try, at the end of his working life he may well consider that he had failed to make practical use of as much as three quarters of the knowledge he had so painstakingly acquired.

It is not uncommon to find that the less dedicated specialist spends the time he can spare an individual patient in rationalizing away the need to investigate him for a rare metabolic disorder rather than consulting reference works or a distant specialist to discover the differential diagnosis, the appropriate diagnostic tests and the reference laboratories where these can be performed. In fact, in normal hospital circumstances, the task is quite hopeless and can only realistically be attempted if it is mechanized, preferably by electronic means. Several categories of information are required and these should be available at the touch of a key. Rapid retrieval of published data on the diseases is possible and a system tailored to this need has been designed to give literature citations under several headings (clinical, diagnosis, treatment, pathology, carrier detection, prenatal detection, enzyme data) for each disorder[9]. A team of informed workers would be required to form the initial data bank, but thereafter keeping it updated would call for no more time than is normally given by individual specialists to keeping abreast of recently published work. Microfiche copies of citations from a central store can be transmitted to remote centres by telephone line to supplement local library facilities.

Similar files of patients and their physicians would enable, without delay, those encountering a particular disorder for the first time to consult clinicians able to advise from practical experience. This would supplement statements of preferred treatments, prepared and updated at leisure, which would also be available with minimal delay and effort when a new diagnosis is made. Only if the abstruse information necessary for any aspect of the management of an inherited metabolic disease can be obtained at the touch of a key, can there be any assurance that it will be applied to most of the patients for whom it is relevant, and for this the information must be predigested, prepackaged and stored in a computer. Thus a second general principle can be enunciated:

P2.   The number and diversity of inherited metabolic disorders requires electronic aid for adequate retrieval of published data.

DIAGNOSIS

But the proper remedy for each disorder cannot be known unless their origins and, as it were, the roots are examined with care and discernment.

Hugh of Tours to Hubert of Angers, 1023

The number of inherited metabolic diseases and the relative rarity of each makes it impossible for most clinicians to know even their names, much less their diagnostic criteria, and in practice most patients who suffer from one will find themselves so remote from a specialist that their diagnosis will be made later rather than sooner or, more probably, not at all. Several very useful check lists of symptoms and signs are now available[10-12], but still quite an astonishing number of clinicians barely know about, and cannot easily turn to, the most basic reference works such as the McKusick catalogue. It is quite clear that something more is required.

An early attempt to provide an approach to diagnosis, based on four clinical features and an assessment of severity[5] proved, in practice, to be too crude. A similar approach, in which 22 clinical observations are compared with a comprehensive data bank comprising the answers to these questions for 157 disorders has been much more successful[13]. For each patient this system gives possible diagnoses in a preferential order and in a trial of 36 patients, representing 21 diseases, the correct diagnosis of 24 occurred within the first five listed by the computer[14]. In the next phase, each disorder will be accompanied by the special investigations required to establish the diagnosis, but at present this information is only conveniently available for about 300 disorders published in a table[15].

The combination of this computer facility with the computerized information retrieval system makes it so easy for the clinician to begin to seek an unusual diagnosis that, having got so far, he is unlikely to withdraw before bringing it to a successful conclusion: at present these opening gambits are so inhibiting that, in many instances, he makes only a gesture towards the task. This can be expressed as a general principle:

P3.   The diversity of diagnostic criteria and laboratory technique requires mechanical or electronic assistance and shared analytical resources.

This lead into the diagnostic problem, however, soon reveals the weakness in the next stage of the operation. Even when the computer-aided diagnostic print-out includes the crucial investigations that will confirm or exclude the clinical entities (in some no specific investigation is known and the diagnosis is made on a summation of criteria), finding a laboratory to perform these can be very difficult indeed. Even countries with established reference laboratories will soon need to refer some investigations beyond their national boundaries and, not infrequently, halfway across the world. One or two lists of reference laboratories have been published[16-18] but these provide false security to the unwary: often no quality control of the analyses exists, certainly none is published and rarely is any information available, such as the extent of the experience with a particular diagnostic test from which the referring clinician, or local laboratory, can assess the reliability of a centre or compare that of competing centres. Moreover:

P4.   New knowledge of inherited metabolic disease is progressing so rapidly that both present techniques and previous diagnoses require periodic review.

It is our practice to have the details of each patient in a folder under the heading of the disease and in the past 15 years we have taken certain diseases in which advances have been made perhaps in the previous five years, e.g. glycogen storage disease, and reviewed every case to see whether the statements made at the time of initial diagnosis were still valid.

I believe this is a most important aspect of management that we will have to attend to continuously in the future. Diseases that were once not well understood and were imprecisely diagnosed need to be clarified. Some diseases such as the Sanfilippo syndrome have been split, first of all into two, then into three and recently into four separate entities. Remember that if we make a wrong diagnosis and fail to confirm the precise enzyme deficiency underlying the disease in a given patient there is every possibility that a mistake in prenatal detection will occur in the future and the consequences of that both on ethical and medico-legal grounds may be very substantial indeed.

EARLY DETECTION (TOTAL POPULATION SCREENING)

I thank you for your vigilance in sending me forewarning, simple-minded as I am, for I truly need to be forewarned on many counts because of my tendency to be imprudent and negligent.

Fulbert of Chartres, 1021

Although methods, sufficiently simple to be applied to large populations, are available for the analysis of small samples of blood or urine in order to detect infants suffering from one of several inherited metabolic diseases, it is interesting that still the only one to find universal acceptance is that for phenylketonuria using the Guthrie microbiological procedure or, less commonly, the Scriver chromatographic method. A detection method that seems most likely to be accorded similar approval, that for congenital thyroid deficiency by assaying thyroxine or thyroid stimulating hormone or both, is the most recent. Thus the exciting prospects of detecting galactosaemia, histidinaemia, cystic fibrosis and Duchenne muscular dystrophy remain unrealized in most quarters. Since the early detection of some of these diseases could be of considerable practical importance, it is of interest to examine the reasons why some programmes are implemented and others not.

Centres where the neonatal screening programme for phenylketonuria was extended, either by further investigation of the Guthrie blood spot by a chromatographic method[19] or by the initial use of the Scriver one-dimensional chromatography of plasma separated from blood collected in a capillary tube[3, 20], have the potential to detect about 20 amino-acid disorders. Indeed, apart from transient abnormalities, the Birmingham study showed that from 1 million of population (20 000 births each year), in addition to the two phenylketonuric patients expected, five more patients with a metabolic disorder were recognized. After this scheme had been in operation for about five years, a selection of participants were asked to write freely, to an independent person, of their experience of all aspects of the screen and its consequences. The selection of correspondents covered the whole range of experience, from those whose initial test was normal and were not seen again, to those whose test revealed phenylketonuria requiring continued hospital attendance. It was recognized that the screen would generate anxiety in the parents and where it was necessary to repeat tests or follow up for longer periods, a metabolic clinic was established to give parents the opportunity for full explanation and discussion. In spite of this, the results of the survey were startling[21] and since by this time it was apparent that, apart from phenylketonuria, the other disorders detected either did not require treatment (prolinaemia type I and probably histidinaemia) or could not be treated very satisfactorily (tyrosinosis, lipidaemia type I), it was considered that the anxiety generated by this extended form of amino-acid screen far outweighed the advantages of being able to detect more than one disorder. Although the same technical processes are still used to screen for phenylketonuria, only tests showing increased phenylalanine are followed up and almost all other abnormalities are ignored. It was this experience that led Raine[22], after summarizing the strict criteria that McKeown[23] required to be met before embarking upon any new screening programme, to state "Perhaps the lesson to be learned from the experience with PKU screening is that while strict criteria must be met before embarking upon a mass screening programme there is almost certainly a need for limited pilot surveys, which do not pay too much heed to these restrictions. For a rare inherited metabolic disease, such surveys will require the co-operation of very large populations (at least 1 million). The investigator should give as careful consideration as he can to the need for, the benefits expected from, and the extent of the interference with the population: he should be able to persuade his professional colleagues who protect the interests of the public health on these matters: and his mind should remain sufficiently open so that, *should his expectations not be fulfilled, he will be prepared to modify or even discontinue the pilot study.*" Stated as a general principle:

P5. Unless the McKeown criteria for the total population screening can be satisfied, national programmes should be preceded by pilot studies of appropriate size and duration.

TREATMENT

It is a physician's duty to offer those who are suffering from depression, insanity, or any other illness, what he has learned in the exercise of his art, and to apply himself with all diligence to the task of curing them even if they are ungrateful and insult his skill.

Hugh of Tours to Hubert of Angers, 1023

If satisfactory treatment of these rare disorders is to be achieved reasonably quickly, it is important that the relatively few opportunities that occur are concentrated in a few hands. As with diagnosis, it is also helpful if the current state of the art and the next most promising proposal are formulated ready for immediate implementation, when the next patient is recognized. Previous patients and their attendent clinicians should be listed and the collective experience in treating a particular disorder should be reviewed continuously by a respected authority who would provide help where it is needed. In practice, local clinicians readily sacrifice their natural possessiveness towards their patients – an attitude which stems only from an overriding desire to do the best by them – once it is seen that the reference centre is more able than themselves to initiate an effective or hopeful regimen. Thus:

> P6. Clinical experience must be centralized rapidly and shared. Individually rare disorders are too diluted for effective consolidation within a working life-time.

It is a simple fact stemming from the rarity of these diseases that if all the cases in a region of, say five million, were sent to the main Children's Hospital and all were seen by one paediatrician, he may, even so, only see one or two cases of the more common metabolic diseases a year and it is entirely possible that within his working life-time very little progress can be made in the management of any particular disorder. We therefore need a different kind of system and I would recommend that in the network of referral centres there is included a structure for lodging the details of each case as it arises and the clinician caring for the particular patient so that progress can be reviewed almost continuously.

Apart from the best advice, it is necessary to have immediate access to any special food, drugs or other preparations required for the treatment and the reference centre should also provide rapid means of delivering these to the patient. The principle being:

> P7. Appropriate and prompt treatment of individually rare disorders requires a central bank of unusual therapeutic agents with detailed guidance on their use.

It is well established that the successful management of some of these patients depends very much on prompt implementation. Unless these reagents are delivered to the site where they are required within 24 hours, it may be that successful treatment is not possible.

Professor Scriver has been noteworthy in establishing a food-bank in Canada. I know well that this food-bank has supplied materials that would not have been otherwise available, except after several weeks or months, to patients in countries well outside of Canada as well as to many patients within that country.

A special problem in the treatment of these (and indeed other) rare diseases arises, ironically, from the protective measures designed to safeguard the public from adverse side-effects of drugs. It is now so costly for pharamaceutical manufacturers to introduce a new drug that this can only be justified where there is a very considerable market potential. Sales for a chelating agent to remove toxic deposits of copper from patients with Wilson's disease will, mercifully, always be small, but there can be few diseases more worth treating by the most effective and least noxious agent than this. The cost of the legally required tests prior to marketing such a substance, for which there will be so little demand, has prevented manufacturers from producing it, and supplies in the United Kingdom[24] and apparently also in Sweden[25] are only available from physicians who make it in their own laboratories[26,27]. Some means must be found whereby such drugs can be produced, perhaps for restricted use, when they are required.

Treatment of a patient with an inherited metabolic disease, including satisfactory management of his parents and family, calls for contributions from several members of a team. Apart from the family practitioner and the local paediatrician, those at the reference centre – clinician, dietitian, biochemist and social worker – all need to work closely together and it is commonly found that this is most effectively achieved by the attendance of this latter group, at the reference centre out-patient clinic, followed by case conferences on all patients every two or three weeks. Between visits to the centre, the dietitian or biochemist often gives further help by telephone.

Apart from the acute and the more esoteric aspects of their treatment, patients with life-long disorders call for other forms of support. Few can survive long without it being known that they are 'different' and anecdotes illustrating the effects on patient and family during early childhood are related with enormous impact by Clothier[28]; the problem, indicated by the sub-title 'notes on the management of spoiled identity' to his book on *Stigma* is analysed in a more general way, for all ages, by Goffman[29]. Nor should it be forgotten that, in the early stages of establishing treatment of a new genetic disorder, support will be required by patients and their families in the face of trials that fail, while effort is given to devising and supervising measures expected to be more successful. The care of the child or adolescent whose death is inevitable calls for deep understanding and any inclined to dismiss lightly the effect of recurring stillbirths or neonatal death in a family at risk for a known genetic disorder will find something to reflect upon in the publication for parents issued by the National Stillbirth Study Group[30] (see also Lancet editorial 1977)[31]. Thus as a general principle:

P8.   Management of inherited metabolic disease calls for
               eight forms of service. Patients should have access
               to all of these and none should be offered in
               isolation.

HETEROZYGOTE DETECTION

This discovery gave rise to conjecture.

Fulbert of Chartres, 1019

When this component of the management of inherited metabolic disease
was discussed five years ago[6], it seemed to be an area in which growth was
certain. Although all that was said at that time still stands – assessment of
carrier status is required by siblings of a propositus, laboratories should
standardize conditions for testing, there is still general scope for improving
the methods of testing, and the role of genetic counselling clinics requires
evaluation – little progress has been made since then.

The recommendations by Westwood and Raine[32,33] to replace the
traditional binary (yes–no) approach to tests of heterozygotes for these
biochemical disorders by one based on probability – as used for less
precisely understood genetic disease – have been adopted by some[34] but
others still try for an absolute statement by increasing the number of
parameters used for each assessment[35,36]. Analysis of the problem[32] still
suggests that, in the majority of cases, reliable absolute determination of
heterozygous status cannot be achieved by any of the methods used
hitherto, although the gene dissection methods seem likely to provide this
for some diseases soon[37] and, perhaps, ultimately for most.

PRENATAL DIAGNOSIS

*So if you are satisfied that the offer is sincere (and I emphasize sincere – that no
attempt is being made to bring your soul into jeopardy) I advise you not to reject
it.*

Fulbert of Chartres, 1008

Of all the components of a health-care system for inherited metabolic
disease, this has seen the greatest growth in the last five years. The potential
for prenatal recognition by enzymic analysis of cultured amniotic cells and
by a few supplementary techniques has been shown to be no less wide than

was anticipated, and a number of centres have now significant, although not yet substantial, experience with several disorders. It is still too soon to regard prenatal diagnosis as an established service and there are many problems, both technical and social, still to be evaluated. It would be safer for the immediate future to continue to regard each consultation as an experiment embarked upon jointly by both parents and their clinical adviser.

There is no doubt, however, that as techniques improve and confidence grows, prenatal examination, with the implied abortion of an affected fetus, will be an important component in the management of inherited metabolic disease. Initially amniocentesis was regarded only as a pre-liminary to abortion of an affected fetus and, because facilities are restricted, some centres would only undertake the investigation if parents consented to this second stage. Such a precondition is now wholly unacceptable and even if parents intend to proceed to abortion, they should be absolutely free to change their minds at any stage prior to the abortion itself. The ethical guidelines formulated by the Hastings Centre[38] seem likely to be acceptable to practitioners in most parts of the world. It is essential that such a service should grow slowly enough to accommodate public opinion, however, in this respect, it is interesting to read paragraph 15 of the Russian Soviet Federative Socialist Republic's 1936 statement[39] of the 'Medical Indications for the Artificial Interruption of Pregnancy (Abortion)':

Abortion is permitted if mother, father or one of the children have suffered or are suffering from one of the following hereditary diseases: haemophilia, idiocy, genuine epilepsy, severe forms of schizophrenia or manic depressive psychosis, which have been treated in hospitals; serious hereditary diseases of the eye leading to blindness; hereditary deaf and dumbness; hereditary progressive diseases of the nervous system (progressive muscular atrophy, hereditary ataxia).

The final principle to be considered:

P9.   Management of inherited metabolic disease in-volves more healthy relatives than sick propositi, calling for greater accuracy and precision than traditional medicine, and I have in fact touched on this point also.

We must never forget that the implications of making a genetic diagnosis in a child who may well die within days or weeks of making that diagnosis are then lodged in that family and will affect all of their futures. If we were wrong in the initial diagnosis, a great deal of harm can ensue and we must take every precaution to ensure that that initial diagnosis is correct and founded on sound scientific data. This may well require the establishment of routine skin biopsies and cultures from all propositi or as many as it is possible to achieve.

NATURAL HISTORY

So that the way we are reasoning may not seem to savour too much of the severity of the old law, let us also set forth the new.

Fulbert of Chartres, 1019

Such a new and promising field as inherited metabolic disease is undergoing constant change and the discovery of new principles requires existing knowledge to be reviewed. Several inherited biochemically unusual conditions are known which were first described in patients with clinical features later discovered to be accidental associations. Examples include Joseph's syndrome of iminoglycinuria and hiatus hernia, hydroxy-prolinaemia, prolinaemia type 1, and very probably histidinaemia. So, too, the clinical presentation of a disorder in different patients or at different ages may be sufficiently distinct as to be described as different diseases, only later to be shown to have a common underlying cause (for example metachromatic leukodystrophy and amaurotic idiocy, combined features of, McKusick 24980, and sulphatidosis, juvenile, Austin type, McKusick 27220). In the latest edition of his catalogue McKusick (1978)[8] has made a valuable contribution in distinguishing by an asterisk those diseases for which there is unequivocal evidence for the stated mode of inheritance in contrast to the rest, where the evidence is less certain, with the possibility that, in some, the underlying cause may not be genetic at all.

The study of all such rare disorders must continue purely at the descriptive level and those caring for new patients with apparently established disorders should, as far as possible, repeat and, where appropriate, publish observations already reported. The reluctance of some editors of medical and scientific journals to publish single case reports was an important factor in leading the Society for the Study of Inborn Errors of Metabolism to establish in 1978 the *Journal of Inherited Metabolic Disease*.

CO-ORDINATION

The judges will see whether the effect is matched to cause. If not, we shall rest content with having admonished you as to what we think you ought to correct.

Fulbert of Chartres, 1019.

In such a multi-component health-care system, the need for some co-ordination was never more amply demonstrated than by a recent incident. A paediatrician caring for a patient with an apparent mucopolysaccharidosis had this diagnosis confirmed by his nearest biochemical reference laboratory, which, at the same time, established a skin fibroblast culture from both the propositus and one parent. When the mother became pregnant again, amniotic fluid obtained by her obstetrician was handled by three laboratories in sequence. Only then was it learned that cultures from members of this family, with which the amniotic cells could be compared, were already available. (There are few enough ways of increasing the precision of prenatal diagnosis by enzyme analysis and it would have been a pity to have missed the opportunity to compare findings within the same genetic pool.) Only at this late stage did the one person most able to co-ordinate the whole exercise, the paediatrician caring for the propositus, learn of this new pregnancy. In this case the fetal diagnosis was achieved within an appropriate time, but only after considerable urgent activity by several enterprising people.

The risk of failure in such circumstances would be minimized by following the recommendation to have a central list of patients, their clinicians, and of known heterozygotes, which can be scanned electronically[6]. Those who object that such files risk infringing privacy can easily be satisfied, since the information can be kept entirely within the medical profession by using a dedicated computer of minimal size and cost (say £20 000). Moreover, the same computer could provide the basis for the literature information retrieval system referred to earlier. Other aspects of this health-care system also require co-ordination: the quality of analyses from different laboratories should be monitored and it would be an advantage to include some of the functions of the DHSS–MRC Phenylketonuria Register initially established in Liverpool[40] and since transferred to London.

GENERAL COMMENTS AND CONCLUSIONS

The eight headings, under which the management of inherited metabolic disease has been discussed, constitute the components of an administrative structure. There are, however, some more general considerations which have emerged from the experience of recent years.

Legislation and litigation

In traditional medicine, on which almost all medical practice is still based – to the point where many clinicians are unable to think beyond this – the initiating act is a complaint from the client, combined with a request for help. In a substantial part of genetic medicine, and especially in total population screening, the first encounter by an unsuspecting and apparently completely healthy subject is an unsolicited visit from an unknown 'specialist' or nursing officer sent by 'them' to virtually impose investigations, at first of simple but sometimes of increasing complexity. In the first context the doctor can expect acquiescence to almost anything he suggests and even his mistakes, if not too serious, are likely to be overlooked; in the second context there can only be concealed (sometimes overt) resentment and any suspicion of defect or error arising from the encounter is likely to be pursued with vigour. Clearly, if those concerned with these more public forms of medical care are aware of this difference, their approach can be modified to minimize conflict. However, there is ample scope for further discovery and improved guidance in dealing with such matters as the carrier status of individuals outside, or even inside, the immediate sibship at risk for an unpleasant disorder; the discussion of abortion of an affected fetus; the prospective discussion of prenatal investigation, with all its implied consequences, before the parents can know whether they will have to take an onerous decision or not. There is always the more familiar problem of the guilt often felt by parents who have given rise to an affected child and the discussion, none-the-less painful for being irrelevant, of with which side of the family it all started.

Equally serious is the emergence of considerable legislation in preventive medicine – laws imposing neonatal screening programmes sometimes before techniques are generally considered satisfactory; sometimes for disorders for which some would consider screening inappropriate. In this respect, the variations between different National (and in the United States of America, State) Legislatures suggests that the most appropriate contribution of the law, at best a cumbersome tool in health-care, has yet to emerge[41,42].

In a more personal way, the courts are being invoked to determine practice as the result of test cases in various areas[43], a traumatic experience for the practitioner who advises sincerely and who has never claimed infallibility. Nothing can stop these developments, but they should be watched carefully by the medical profession, who should be ready to help their legal colleagues to construct a framework of case law that is just to all concerned – patients, parents, doctors and, in a Welfare State, to Society itself[44].

Accommodation of ethnic differences

Few can doubt the well-meaning intentions of those who initiate, often at considerable effort and expense, measures contributing to the management of some aspect of genetic disease. It must therefore have come as something of a shock when the United States screening programme for sickle cell disease was seen as yet another form of discrimination, if not persecution, of the blacks[45]! However, when a similar screening programme was established in Birmingham, which has a substantial Asian and African immigrant population, it was decided to select those to be treated entirely on the colour of their skin. This seemed to be the most logical and economical method of selection and, having thought out the arguments carefully, and detailed them to the medical officers involved, the programme has proceeded without incident for several years[46,47].

Programmes to detect, in the Jewish population, those at risk for GM_2 gangliosidosis have had notable success in North America[48,49]. It, therefore, came as a surprise to find that there was almost no response to a similar programme in Britain[50]. There appears to be no single factor to explain this convincingly; differing degrees of Rabbinical orthodoxy are not the cause and there is little evidence from genetic markers that British Jews, thought to have come via Spain, differ from American Jews believed to have migrated from Eastern Europe. Nor, for that matter, does this type of evidence support the view that one or both groups are Khazar converts and not from Askenazi stock[51]. These different attitudes towards screening for Tay–Sachs disease, however, are real – and as yet unexplained.

Again, contrast the contribution abortion might make to the management of inherited metabolic disease in northern and eastern European countries with that in South and West. Many more such differences will emerge as the management of genetic disease progresses throughout the world and in such public forms of medical care it behoves all who initiate these programmes to enter into close and continued dialogue with the communities concerned, regardless of whether or not there are obvious cultural differences. This dialogue will present problems of cross-cultural communication both between and within nations, and there will also be problems arising from the different levels of social stratification that exist within any ethnic group. Some ground has been broken, albeit in different fields, by anthropologists[52] and those concerned with the integration of immigrant communities[53]. Indeed the whole of medicine would benefit from a greater awareness of these problems when, as in the management of many inherited metabolic diseases, instructions must be given and unfamiliar concepts and serious consequences need to be explained.

Finally, the promised explanation of the quotations. What has been attempted here, starting with *The Need for a National Policy for the Management of Inherited Metabolic Disease*[6], is the definition and refinement of an administrative system, in this case for an aspect of health care. It seemed that if the components that have emerged are valid, they will be reflected in other administrative systems. None was so well established or so successful as that governing the mediaeval church and fewer practised this as ably as Fulbert, Bishop of Chartres. Some surprisingly close parallels emerge; so perhaps the last word should come from that quarter –

> *In sending you this warning, brother, I am not being haughty and lording my teaching office over you, but rather carrying out in all trepidation my duty as your archbishop. If you agree to do as I have said, you will, I think, be taking thought for your salvation; but if (heaven forbid) you should be of a different opinion, the fault will not be mine, for I have warned you.*

Hugh of Tours to Hubert of Angers, 1023

References

1. Garrod, A. E. (1908). The Croonian lectures on inborn errors of metabolism. *Lancet*, **2**, 1, 73, 142 and 2114
2. Bickel, H., Gerrard, J. and Hickmans, E. M. (1953). Influence of phenylalanine intake on phenylketonuria. *Lancet*, **2**, 812
3. Raine, D. N., Cook, J. R., Andrews, W. A. and Mahon, D. F. (1972). Screening for inherited metabolic disease by plasma chromatography (Scriver) in a large city. *Br. Med. J.*, **3**, 7
4. Komrower, G. M. (1975). Screening for phenylketonuria. *Lancet*, **1**, 331
5. Raine, D. N. (1972). Management of inherited metabolic disease. *Br. Med. J.*, **2**, 329
6. Raine, D. N. (1974). The need for a national policy for the management of inherited metabolic disease. In Raine, D. N. (ed.) *Molecular Variants in Disease. J. Clin. Pathol.*, **27**, Suppl., R. Coll. Pathol., **8**, 156–163. Reprinted with amendments in Raine, D. N. (ed.) (1977). *Medico-Social Management of Inherited Metabolic Disease*, pp. 3–20. (Lancaster: MTP)
7. Behrends, F. (1976). *The Letters and Poems of Fulbert of Chartres*, (London: Oxford University Press)

8. McKusick, V. A. (1978). *Mendelian Inheritance in Man*, 4th Ed. (Baltimore: Johns Hopkins University)
9. Emmerson, J. S. and Raine, D. N. (1977). Mechanised storage and retrieval of information. In Raine, D. N. (ed.) *Medico-Social Management of Inherited Metabolic Disease*, pp. 247–258 (Lancaster: MTP)
10. Gellis, S. S. and Feingold, M. (1968). *Atlas of Mental Retardation Syndromes*, pp. 168–186. (Washington: U.S. Dept. Health, Education, and Welfare)
11. Smith, D. W. (1970). *Recognizable Patterns of Human Malformation*, pp. 278–294. (Philadelphia: Saunders)
12. Harley, R. D. (1975). *Pediatric Ophthalmology*, pp. 598–606. (Philadelphia: Saunders)
13. Raine, D. N., Rees, N. G. and Terry, S. H. (1977). Computer-aided diagnosis of inherited metabolic disease. In Raine, D. N. (ed.) *Medico-Social Management of Inherited Metabolic Disease*, pp. 259–271. (Lancaster: MTP)
14. Raine, D. N. (1977). Diagnosis of inherited metabolic disease using a computer-operated matrix matching system. *Arch. Dis. Child.*, **52**, 516
15. Raine, D. N. (1979). Inherited metabolic disease. In Brown, S. S., Mitchell, F. L. and Young, D. S. (eds.) *Chemical Diagnosis of Disease*, pp. 927–1008. (Amsterdam: Elsevier)
16. Clinical Chemistry (1977). Directory of rare analyses. *Clin. Chem.*, **23**, 323
17. Deutsche Gesellschaft fur Klinische Chemie (1977). Wer bestimmt was?. Laboratorien, in denen spezielle und seltenene Bestimmungen durchgefuhrt werden. *Dtsch. Ges. Klin. Chem. Mitteil.*, **8**, 25
18. Whalen, R. P. and Porter, I. H. (1978). Metabolic eye disease register: specialized laboratory services for birth defects and inherited genetic diseases, biochemical–cytogenetic, New York State. *Metabol. Ophthalmol.*, **2**, 77
19. Ireland, J. T. and Read, R. A. (1972). A thin-layer chromatographic method for use in neonatal screening to detect excess amino acidaemia. *Ann. Clin. Biochem.*, **9**, 129
20. Komrower, G. M., Fowler, B., Griffiths, M. J. and Lambert, A. M. (1968). A prospective community survey for aminoacidaemias. *Proc. R. Soc. Med.*, **61**, 294
21. May, E. C. (1977). Parent reaction to medical care and screening. In Raine, D. N. (ed.) *Medico-Social Management of Inherited Metabolic Disease*, pp. 81–91. (Lancaster: MTP)
22. Raine, D. N. (1974). Screening for disease: Inherited metabolic disease. *Lancet*, **2**, 996
23. McKeown, T. (1968). *Screening in Medical Care*. (London: Oxford University Press)
24. Walshe, J. M. (1975). Drugs for rare diseases. *Br. Med. J.*, **3**, 701
25. Bucer, I. and Hasselgren, K. H. (1975). Treatment of Wilson's disease. *Lancet*, **2**, 1218
26. Editorial (1976). Drugs for rare diseases. *Lancet*, **2**, 835
27. Hopley, P. J. (1976). Drugs for rare diseases. *Lancet*, **2**, 1021
28. Clothier, C. (1977). Management of dietary treatment in the home. In Raine, D. N., (ed.) *Medico-Social Management of Inherited Metabolic Disease*, pp. 51–61 (Lancaster: MTP)
29. Goffman, E. (1963). *Stigma: Notes on the Management of Spoiled Identity*.

(Englewood Cliffs: Prentice Hall) (Reprinted, 1979, Harmondsworth: Penguin Books)

30. National Stillbirth Study Group (*ca.* 1979). *The Loss of Your Baby*, 10pp. National Stillbirth Study Group, 24, Wimpole Street, London, WIM 7AD
31. Editorial (1977). The abhorrence of stillbirth. *Lancet*, **1**, 1188
32. Westwood, A. and Raine, D. N. (1973). Some problems of heterozygote recognition in inherited metabolic disease with special reference to phenylketonuria. In Seakins, J. W. T., Saunders, R. A. and Toothill C. (eds.) *Treatmenn of Inborn Errors of Metabolism*, pp. 63–76. (London: Churchill Livingstone)
33. Westwood, A. and Raine, D. N. (1975). Heterozygote detection in phenylketonuria. Measurements of discriminatory ability and interpretation of the phenylalanine loading test by determination of the heterozygote likelihood ratio. *J. Med. Gen.*, **12**, 327
34. Güttler, F. and Hansen, G. (1977). Heterozygote detection in phenylketonuria. *Clin. Genet.*, **11**, 137
35. Gold, R. J. M., Maag, U. R., Neal, J. L. and Scriver, C. R. (1973). The use of biochemical data in screening for mutant alleles and in genetic counselling. *Ann. Hum. Genet.*, **37**, 315
36. Delvin, E., Pottier, A., Scriver, C. R. and Gold. R. J. M. (1974). The application of an automated hexosaminidase assay to genetic screening. *Clin. Chim. Acta*, **53**, 135
37. Kan, Y. W. and Dozy, A. M. (1978). Antenatal diagnosis of sickle-cell anaemia by DNA analysis of amniotic-fluid cells. *Lancet*, **2**, 910
38. Powledge, T. M. and Fletcher, J. (1979). Guidelines for the ethical, social and legal issues in prenatal diagnosis. *N. Engl. J. Med.*, **300**, 168
39. Sigerist, H. E. (1937). *Socialised Medicine in the Soviet Union*, p. 370. (London: Gollancz)
40. Hudson, F. P. and Hawcroft, J. (1977). The phenylketonuria register for the United Kingdom. In Raine, D. N. (ed.) *Medico-Social Management of Inherited Metabolic Disease*, pp. 217–224
41. Committee for the Study of Inborn Errors of Metabolism (1975). The development of legislation and regulations for P.K.U. Screening. In *Genetic Screening, Programmes, Principles and Research*, pp. 44–87. (Washington: National Academy of Sciences)
42. Culliton, B. J. (1976). Genetic screening: States may be writing the wrong kinds of laws. *Science*, **191**, 926
43. Ratner, G. A. (1977). The coming of the second genetic code: eugenic abortion in the United Kingdom. In Raine, D. N. (ed.) *Medico-Social Management of Inherited Metabolic Disease*, pp. 119–139. (Lancaster: MTP)
44. Milunsky, A. and Annas, G. J. (1976). *Genetics and the Law*. (New York: Plenum Press)
45. Whitten, C. F. (1973). Sickle-cell programming – an imperiled promise. *N. Engl. J. Med*, **288**, 318
46. Stuart, J., Schwartz, F. C. M., Little, A. J. and Raine, D. N. (1973). Screening for abnormal haemoglobins: a pilot study. *Br. Med. J.*, **4**, 284
47. Raine, D. N. and Pepper, J. M. (1974). Screening for abnormal haemoglobins in the immigrant community. *Arch. Dis. Chiid.* **49**, 496
48. Kaback, M. M., Zieger, R. S., Reynolds, L. W. and Sonneborn, M. (1974).

Approaches to the control and prevention of Tay–Sachs disease. In Steinberg, A. G. and Bearn, A. (eds.) *Progress in Medical Genetics*, pp. 103–134. (New York: Grune and Stratton)

49. Lowden, J. A., Zuker, S., Wilensky, A. J. and Skomorowski, M. A. (1974). Screening for carriers of Tay–Sachs disease. *Can. Med. Assoc. J.*, **111**, 229

50. Evans, P. R. (1977). Screening for Tay–Sachs disease. In Raine, D. N. (ed.) *Medico-Social Management of Inherited Metabolic Disease*, pp. 93–101 (Lancaster: MTP)

51. Mourent, A. E., Kopec, A. C. and Domaniewska-Sobocak, K. (1978). *The Genetics of the Jews.* (Oxford: Clarendon Press)

52. Adler, L. L. (1977). Issues in cross cultural research. *Ann NY Acad. Sci.*, **285**, 753

53. Gumperz, J. J., Jupp, T. C. and Roberts, C. (1979). *Crosstalk: A Study of Cross-Cultural Communication,* p.59. National Centre for Industrial Language Training, Havelock Centre, Havelock Road, Southall, Middlesex, UK

Index

abortion, medical indications in USSR 277
acanthosis nigricans 82
acatalasia 159
  encapsulated catalase 133, 134
acid hydrolases
  causes of heterogeneity 108
  molecular weight of chains 106
  recognition marker 105
activated charcoal, microencapsulated
  adsorbent 132
  treatments 132, 134
adenine phosphoribosyl transferase 22
adenosylcobalamin 40, 45, 60
adrenal hyperplasia, lipoid 80
adrenal insufficiency 73
adrenal steroids
  biosynthesis 70–3
  defects and features 73–5
  synthesis sites 73
adrenogenital syndrome 69, 73
  acquired 76
  defects causing 73–5
  3β-dehydrogenase 80
  11β-hydroxylase 76, 77
  21-hydroxylase 75, 76
adrenoleukodystrophy 77
adsorbents, encapsulated 132
AFP see alphafetoprotein
albumin
  charcoal coated 132
  tryptophan bound and transport 93
alcaptonuria 111
alcoholism, severity 9
aldosterone
  biosynthesis 70, 72
  structure 71

allopurinol
  in Lesch–Nyhan syndrome 22
  and xanthine oxidase 18
alphafetoprotein (AFP) 261–3
  quality control of testing 262
amino acids
  brain availability 87–95
  neutral, pharmacology 94
  ratio and brain availability 96
  site competition in brain 87
amino acid transport 87–95; see also blood–
    brain barrier
  competition role 90, 91
  peripheral tissue, K_m values 91
amniocentesis, risk 262
anaemia, megaloblastic 48, 61
androstenediol biosynthesis 78, 79
androstenedione biosynthesis 78, 79
anencephaly
  genetic basis 162
  screening 261
animal models of inborn metabolic errors
    157–207
  brain development in mice 161–70
  defect level 158
  enzymes and proteins 159
  metabolites 159
  organ systems 158
  phenylketonuria 193–8
apoenzymes, mutants 41–4
aromatase
  defect effects 82
  steroid biosynthesis 78
artificial cell
  encapsulated enzymes 131–36
  metabolite removal 133–35

principle 131, 132
arylsulphatase A, enzyme replacement 142, 143
Ashkenazi Jews 6, 281
astrocyte development in *Jimpy* mice 202, 206
athetoid dysarthria 14
athetoid dysphagia 14
8-azaguanine 19, 21
azaribine and homocystinuria 62

Bayley scale of Infant Development 243, 245
    early treatment of Down's syndrome 245, 246
    and sitting 248, 249
behaviour
    Lesch–Nyhan syndrome 14–16
    modification 24
    partial HGPRT deficiency 26
    sequences of development 238
biopterin metabolism abnormalities 257
biotin
    activating enzymes 46
    cofactor 45, 46
    metabolism disorders 47–9
    mitochondrion role 46, 47
    responsive defects 48, 49
    transport 45
    see also propionyl CoA carboxylase
blacks and sickle cell disease 281
blood–brain barrier
    carrier modulation 89
    permeability and enzyme replacement 145
    tissue sampling–carotid injection technique 88
    transport systems 88, 89
    tryptophan–albumen competition 92, 93
blood–brain barrier amino acid transport 87–95
    basic 80
    competition and brain disease 95
    K_m values 90
    neonatal 93, 94
    neutral 90
    neutral and competition 91, 93
    phenylalanine affinity 90
    tryptophan competition 91, 93
Braille 230
brain development 157–9
    cerebellar 164, 166
    genetic disease 161
    mice 161–70

carbonic anhydrase 176

carcinoma of the cervix, value of screening 261
cathepsin D 97, 104
cells
    amniotic 276
    chinese hamster ovary 104
    Jimpy mouse brain cell 202
    see also fibroblast
ceramide galactosyltransferase localisation 176
ceramidetrihexosidase isolation 146
ceramide trihexoside
    accumulation in Fabry's disease 142
    effects of replacement 146, 147
    plasma derived 147
cerebellar atrophy, mouse model 166
cerebellum defects in mice 164, 166
cerebroside sulphotransferase, *trembler* mice 185
Charcot–Marie–Tooth neuropathy, mouse model 179, 185
p-chlorophenylalanine and experimental phenylketonuria 197
cholesterol
    biosynthesis 70–2, 78
    structure 71
chromatography 255, 256
chromosome, X 14, 20, 31, 82
cobalamin
    cofactors 45
    and homocysteine transferase 60, 61
    inherited defects 48
    metabolism disorders 47–9, 60
    -responsive defects 48, 49
    transport 45
    see also methylmalonyl CoA mutase
coma, hepatic 132
complementation analysis 7
congenital adrenal hyperplasia 69
    diagnosis 262
congenital metabolic disorders *see* inborn errors
cortisol
    biosynthesis 70–2
    production defects 73
    structure 71
creatine kinase in muscular dystrophy 259
cross reacting material (CRM) 41
culture media
    hypoxanthine–aminopterin–thymidine (HAT) 21, 22, 26
    minimal essential 27
cystathionine synthase
    apoenzyme and coenzyme 58

genetic heterogeneity 57
cystathionine synthase deficiency 55, 56
    biochemical findings 63
    clinical signs 64
    see also homocystinuria
cystic fibrosis
    dilemma of screening 258, 259
    natural history 259
    test 259

data of inherited metabolic disease 269, 270,
    279
deanol, choline precursor 89
3β-dehydrogenase
    defect symptoms 80
    steroid biosynthesis 72, 73
Dejerine–Sottas neuropathy, mouse model
    179, 185
17,20-desmolase 78
    defect 81
20,22-desmolase defect 80
    complex system 80
22,22-desmolase function 72, 73
developmental delay 238
developmental psychology 239
developmental quotient (DQ) 238
    Down's syndrome 242, 243
    drop-off in Down's syndrome and signifi-
        cance 248
diagnosis
    co-ordination 279
    early and screening 272, 273
    effect on family 277, 278
    and growth of knowledge 271
    metabolic disease 270, 271
    prenatal 20, 276–8
    success 270
diet
    food bank 274
    homocystinuria 58, 59
    modulation of brain disease 95
    palatability 220
    phenylalanine and body, brain weights
        195
    and therapeutic effects of amino acids 94
dihydrotestosterone biosynthesis 78, 79
DNA 4
L-DOPA effect in Parkinson's disease and
    diet 94
Down's syndrome 230
    appearance of anomalies 244, 245
    assessment times 245, 246
    delayed treatment effects 245–7
    early intervention 242–50

    Manchester study 244
    non-intervention 243, 244
    sitting, age of attaining 248, 249
    variable care 228
drugs, availability of unusual 275
dysraphic disorders
    man 162
    mice 162, 163

early detection 272, 273
ectopia lentis 54
education
    attitudes and handicap 231–34
    policy changes 229–31
    see also teaching
endocytosis, fibroblast 125
enzyme activity loss 5
enzyme replacement therapy 139–50
    blood–brain barrier permeability 145
    and function site 147
    further developments, 149, 150
    success 145
enzymes
    artificial cell encapsulated 132–36
    encapsulation materials 133
    erythrocyte entrapped 135
    extracellular enzyme removal 134, 135
    intracellular actions of introduced 135,
        136
    myelin specific 176
    replacement therapy 111, 139–50
    see also lysosomal
enzyme substitution by fibroblast transplan-
    tation 111–126
epilepsy
    centralopathic 168
    mice mutations 164, 167–9
erythrocyte, entrapped enzymes 135, 136
erythrocyte metabolism
    amino acid transport 91
    and haemolytic disease 7
ethnic differences and management 281

Fabry's disease 142
    ceramidetrihexoside use 146
    enzyme replacement 145–47
    renal transplantation 142
feto-placental unit
    lymphocyte passage 262
    oestrogen biosynthesis 82, 83
    steroid defects 82
fibroblasts 26, 30, 62, 104
    bio complementation group 49
    correction of defective 143

culture in Lesch–Nyhan diagnosis 21, 26
I cell enzymes 105
implantation uses 140
lysosomal enzyme release 125
fibroblast transplantation
  effectiveness 114–123
  enzyme substitution 111–126
  survival time 126
  and viability 125
Friedrich's ataxia, mouse model 167, 170

galactocerebroside 202
galactosylceramidase deficiency 187
gangliosidases GM$_2$ 281
Gaucher's disease, type I 159
  enzyme deficient 140
  enzyme replacement 145, 148, 149
  fibroblast implantation 140
  kidney transplantation 141
  liver transplantation 141
  spleen transplant 140, 141
gene action mechanism 4
genetic defects
  numbers in humans 269
  rodents 161
  see also inborn errors
genetic heterogeneity 3–10, 20, 53, 75, 77
  background 8, 9
  causes 4–10
  consequences 63, 64
  definition 3
  environmental interaction 9, 10
  therapeutic implications 8
genitalia
  correction 74
  development 74
globoid cell leukodystrophy (Krabbe's disease) 179
  mouse model 187
globoside in Tay–Sachs disease 143, 144
glucocerebrosidase 140
  clearance and catabolism 148
  clinical use 148, 149
  depot 140
  kidney 141
  mannose linking 149
  oligosaccharide and receptors 149
  origin 148
  replacement in Gaucher's disease 148, 149
  see also Gaucher's disease
glucocorticoids see steroids C-21
glucosamine N-sulphatase deficiency 114
glucose-6-phosphate dehydrogenase
  types in Lesch Nyhan syndrome 21

glycosaminoglycans
  accumulation of degraded 112
  analysis 113, 114
  catabolism 112, 113
  fibroblast accumulation 112
gout 13
  HGPRT variants 24, 25
gouty arthritis, onset 29
guanine metabolism 19
guanylic acid 19
Guthrie test 255, 272

haemolytic disease 7
haemoperfusion
  activated charcoal, uses 132
  encapsulated adsorbants 134
hair follicle, HGPRT assay 22
handicap
  blind care 229
  incidence 225
  labelling 232
  opera singer 232
  progress in care 227, 228
  psychological and educational aspects 237–50
  social aspects 225–236
  see also mental handicap
health-care systems 268
  small benefit 268
heterozygosity 6
  detection 276
hexosamidase A 7
  brain assay 143
  deficiency and replacement 143–45
  function 143
  metabolic effects of replacement 143
  neuronal receptors 145
  placental 144
  see also Tay–Sachs disease
hexosaminidase B 143
  deficiency and replacement 143–45
  see also Tay–Sachs disease
β-hexaminidase
  chain molecular weight 106
  isolation 103
  maturation process 104
  protease resistance 104
HGPRT see hypoxanthine guanine phosphoribosyl transferase
high pressure liquid chromatography, purines 27, 28
histidinaemia 260
HLA genotype
  21-hydroxylase deficiency 75

typing and screening 262
homocysteine methyl transferase 57
  cobalamin dependence 59
  defects 59, 60
homocysteine transferase
  and cobalamin 60, 61, 64
  deficiency, biochemical findings 63
homocystinuria 53–64, 258
  amino acid profile 56
  biochemical findings 63
  causes of death 59
  classical 53–57
  clinical features 54, 55
  cobalamin role 60, 61
  development 54
  diet 59
  drug-induced 62, 63
  enzyme deficiencies 56, 57, 59
  eye symptoms 54
  features distinguishing types 64
  heterogeneity 53, 57, 63, 64
  homocystine transferase 60, 61
  inheritance 57
  and Marfan's syndrome 55
  methyl cobalamin response 60
  5,10-methylene tetrahydrofolate reductase 61, 62
  pyridoxine response 57–9
  thrombosis 55
human chorionic gonadotrophin
  testosterone stimulation test 79, 80
human menopausal gonadotrophin and oestrogen production 82
Hunter syndrome (mucopolysaccharidosis type II) 7
  corrective factor and fibroblast transplant 122, 123
  enzyme deficiency 114
  fibroblast transplantation 113–126
  iduronate sulphatase activity 125
  oligosaccharide fractions 114, 117, 118
  sulphate : uronic acid ratios 121
  uronic acid excretion and fibroblast transplantation 114, 115, 117
Hurler syndrome 7
hydrocephalus
  genetic causes 164
  mouse mutants 164, 165
11 β-hydroxylase defect 75, 262
  genetic heterogeneity 61
  severity 60
11 β-hydroxylase function 72, 73
17-hydroxylase
  deficiency 75, 81

function 72, 73
21-hydroxylase
  deficiency 262
  and steroid biosynthesis 72, 73
  systems and adrenal zones 75
21-hydroxylase defect 75, 76, 262
  effects 75
  HLA linkage 75, 76
  prevalence 75
hydrolases, lysosomal 103
5-hydroxytryptophan 24
hyperaldosteronism 65
hyperaminoacidaemia, CNS sensitivity 94
hypermethioninaemia 258
hyperphenylalaninaemia
  Guthrie test 255
  induced in rats, effects 194, 195
  protein tolerance and children 257
  spectrum of causes 257
hyperprolinaemia 159
hypertension and steroid biosynthesis defects 74, 75
hyperuricaemia 14
  partial HGPRT deficiency 25–9
hypogonadism 79
hypothyroidism
  congenital 256, 258
  delayed and diagnosis 258
  screening of congenital 256, 258
hypoxanthine, solubility 23
hypoxanthine–guanine phosphoribosyl transferase (HGPRT)
  activity calculation 28
  brain concentrations 29
  cross reactivity 20
  electrophoresis 20
  erythrocyte measurement 19, 20, 21, 25
  hair follicle 22
  and purine metabolism inhibitors 19, 21
  reaction catalysed 19
  see also Lesch–Nyhan syndrome
hypoxanthine–guanine phosphoribosyl transferase deficiency
  clinical features 25
  gout 25
  neurological 25
  partial, electrophoresis 26
  variants and disorders 24–9
  see also Lesch–Nyhan syndrome

Iceland, cervical carcinoma screening 261
ichthyosis, X-linked 82, 83
α-L-iduronidase maturation 104

α-L-idurono-2-sulphate   sulphatase   deficiency 113, 114
   assay 113
   corrective factors 121
   fibroblast transplantation 121, 122
   in Hurler's syndrome, corrected 123, 125
immunosuppression 125
inborn errors of metabolism 267
   animal models 158, 159
   brain development 157
   causes 5
   diagnosis 270, 271, 276–8
   early detection 271, 272
   health-care system 268
   information sources 269, 270
   long-term treatment effects 211–22
   major groups 131
   management 267–82
   metabolites 159
   natural history 278
   numbers 111
   proteins 159
   screening 255–63
   treatment 272–5
   see also individual diseases
inbreeding and autosomal recessives 6
Institution for the Disabled, Massachusetts
   234
intelligence
   attitudes 237–42
   predetermined 239
Intelligence Quotient (IQ) 238
   and development tests 238, 239
   Down's syndrome 242, 243
International Labour Office 228
intersexuality 74
intestine, amino acid transport 91
Italy
   blind education 230
   education of handicapped 229–31

Jews 281; see also Ashkenazi
Jimpy mouse 168, 179, 180, 201–7
   brain cell culture 202
   brain cell enzymes 203, 204, 206
   discovery 201
   oligodendrocyte development 202
   reduced myelin 201
Junior Eysenck Personality Inventory and
   long-term treatment 216, 218

ketotic hyperglycinaemia syndrome 37
kidney, amino acid transport 91
kinky hair disease 159

lacrimal glands, congenital absence 29
de Lange syndrome 24
legislation 280, 281
   and health care 280, 281
   mental handicap 233–5
   vocational training 235
Lesch–Nyhan syndrome 14–24
   allelic mutants 5
   amine imbalance 24
   arthritis 16
   autopsy findings 17
   behaviour modification 24
   cerebral symptoms 14
   cerebrospinal fluid 19, 29
   chromosome site 14, 20, 21
   clinical characteristics 14–16
   diagnosis 20, 21
   enzyme defect 19, 20, 23
   genetic heterogeneity 20
   glycine metabolism 18
   HGPRT activity 28, 29
   hypoxanthine excretion and studies 18
   lip loss 15
   management 23, 24
   maternal mosaic 21
   pain sensation 15, 16
   pathogenesis of behaviour 16
   purine metabolism 17–24
   restraining 15, 16, 23, 24
   self-mutilation 14–16
   treatment 22
   uric acid accumulation 16
   uric acid excretion 17
lipid storage disorders
   organ transplantation 140–2
   therapeutic strategies 139
liposomes
   enzymes carried 135
   uses 135, 136
litigation 280
liver
   amino acid transport 91
   transplant in lipid storage diseases 141
lysosomal enzymes
   I cell 105
   inherited deficiencies 111
   maturation 103–108
   molecular weight of chains 106
   phosphorylation 107, 108
   pulse-chase 103, 104
   recognition marker 105
   T cell 105
   transfer and transplant 126
   types 103

McKeown criteria, total population screening 273
management of inherited metabolic disease 267–82
  abortion and prenatal diagnosis 276–8
  access to service 276
  data retrieval 270
  diagnosis 270, 271
  ethnic differences 281, 282
  information sources 269, 270, 274, 279
  need for national policy 282
  new knowledge 271
  see also treatment
mannose 6-phosphate 105
  residues and targeting 107
α-mannosidase, lymphocyte transfer 126
maple syrup urine disease 88
Marfan's syndrome, clinical features 55
Medical Indication for the Artificial Interruption of Pregnancy, USSR 277
Menkes steely hair syndrome, mouse model 179, 186
mental handicap
  capacity to learn 228
  care, world-wide 226–9
  causes 226
  changes in attitude 237–42
  definition 226
  developing world, care 227
  and developmental delay 238
  early intervention 241
  educational policy 229–31
  interaction, shortcomings 233
  IQ and developmental test 239
  labelling, adverse effects 231, 232
  legislation 233–5
  low expectation 232, 233
  progress in care 227, 228
  rights 233
  segregation 231, 234, 235
  social changes 229–31
  step-by-step teaching 240, 241
  stimulation 239
  teaching techniques 229–31, 240, 241
  UN declaration 233, 234
  western, lack of care 226, 227
mental retardation, amino acid disorders 54
metabolite removal methods, extracellular compartment 133–35
metachromic leukodystrophy 126, 159
  arylsulphatase A replacement 142, 143
methaemoglobinaemia, incidence of congenital 10
methionine transsulphuration and remethylation pathway 56, 57
methylcobalamin 45, 60
β-methylcrotonyl CoA carboxylase 46
5,10-methylene tetrahydrofolate reductase deficiency 61, 62, 64
  amino acid profile 62
  biochemical findings 63
  fibroblast culture 62
  folate medication 64
methylmalonic acidaemia 37–49
methylmalonic aciduria 7, 60, 61
  mutation 8
  vitamin B$_{12}$ response 8
methylmalonyl CoA mutase (MUT)
  apoenzyme mutants 41, 42
  and cobalamin 38, 39
  coenzyme mutants and disorders 44–9
  cross reacting material 41, 42
  deficiency 37, 60
  molecular weight 39, 40
  mutation and apoenzyme 8
  reaction catalysed 37, 38
  structural features 39, 40
methyltetrahydrofolate homocysteine methyltransferase 45
mice
  blotchy 186
  brindled 186
  cerebellar mutants 164, 166
  cribriform degeneration 187
  crinkled 186
  ducky 168, 170, 188
  dwarf 186
  dysraphic disorders 163
  dystrophic 184, 185
  epilepsy 164, 166, 168, 169
  genetic defects and brain development 161–70
  and human myelination disorders 179
  hydrocephalus 164, 175
  Jimpy 168, 179, 180, 201–7
  mld 169, 175, 178, 183, 184
  mottled 186
  msd 180, 181
  muscular dystrophy 184
  myelination mutations 173–89
  neurological mutants 170
  quaking 168, 176, 177
  shambling 188
  shiverer 169, 180, 181, 183, 184
  sprawling 188
  tabby 187
  trembler 181, 183, 184
  twitcher 187

wabbler lethal 169, 188
wobbler 170, 187
mineralocorticoids *see* steroids C-21
mitochondrion, biotin reactions 45–7
microencapsulated enzymes 134–36
 asparaginase 133
 catalase 133, 134
 transaminase 135
 tyrosinase 134, 135
 uricase 134
mucolipidosis III 107
mucopolysaccharidoses 112; *see also* Hunter's and Sanfilippo syndromes
multiple allelism in genetic heterogeneity 4–6
multiple loci and genetic heterogeneity 6–8
muscular dystrophy
 carrier detection 260
 Duchenne, screening 259
 incidence 259
MUT *see* methylmalonyl CoA mutase
mutation
 functional consequences 4
 and gene action 5
 mouse myelin 173–89
 mouse, neurological 161–70
myelin
 basic protein 175
 components, half-lives 196
 composition, central and peripheral 174, 175
 dystrophic mutants 184, 185
 half-lives and hyperphenylalaninaemia 196
 isolation 174
 Jimpy mutants 179–81
 lipid analysis of *trembler* 185
 localised enzymes 176
 metabolism and phenylalanine effects 193–8
 mld 169, 175, 182–4
 msd mutants 180, 181
 murine mutations 173–89
 mutants with secondary effects 185–8
 quaking proteins 168, 176, 177, 181
 sheath 173–5
 shiverer mutant 180–4
 synthesis in mutant rats 197
 trembler mutants 181, 183, 185
 turnover and age in rat mutants 194–7
 turnover and diet in rats 197
myelination
 hormone effects 186
 human disease models 179
 mouse 173

secondary effects of mutation 185–8
start of brain 173

National Stillbirth Study Group 275
neonates
 amino acid transport 93, 94
 parenteral nutrition 89
neural tube defects, screening 261, 262
Niemann–Pick disease 159
 liver transplant 141
noradrenaline and convulsions 167
Norway, handicapped education 229–31

17β-oestradiol
 biosynthesis 71, 72, 78
 structure 71
oestrogen biosynthesis, feto-placental unit 82, 83
oligodendrocyte
 abnormal differentiation in *Jimpy* mouse 201–7
 biochemical markers 202
 enzyme changes 203, 204, 206
 immunofluorescence 202, 203, 205
oligosaccharide fractionation 113
 elution profile, Hunter's syndrome 118
 elution profile, Sanfilippo syndrome 119
optic nerves, *mld* mutant mouse 182, 184
oxypurines 22, 23
 and allopurinol treatment 23

pancreas amino acid transport 75
parents association, world-wide for mental handicap 227
PCC *see* propionyl CoA carboxylase
Pelizaeus–Merzbacher syndrome, mouse model 179–81
phaeochromocytoma 94
phenylalanine
 dietary stimulation 194, 195
 and myelin metabolism 193–8
phenylalanine catabolism deficiency 167
phenylketonuria 88, 267
 anxiety at school 215–17
 brain amino acid uptake 94
 diet 95, 198, 212, 220
 diet start and psychosocial effects 213, 215
 family role 219, 220
 induced 193
 long term treatment effects 211–22
 mouse model 168
 neuroticism and extraversion 216, 219
 psychological evaluation 218
 rat model 198

screening 272, 273
social contact 218–20
symptoms 193
Phenylketonuria Register, DHSS–MRC 279
plasma transfusion 112
polymorphisms 8, 9
polyribosyl pyrophosphate (PRPP) syn-
    thetase
  abnormalities 29–31
  enzyme catalysis 30
  fibroblasts 30
  product role 30
  X-chromosome 31
positron emission tomography 95
prednisone and enzyme replacement 149
pregnenolone biosynthesis 78
probenecid 22
progesterone biosynthesis 78
propionate pathway 38
propionic acidaemia 37–49
propionyl CoA carboxylase (PCC)
  apoenzyme mutants 41–4
  and biotin 38, 39, 46
  coenzyme mutants and disorders 44–9
  cross reacting material 43
  deficiency 37
  immunotitration 43
  model, subunits 40
  molecular weight 39
  mutant antigenicity 43
  mutants, site of action 44
  reaction catalysed 37, 38
  structural features 39
  subunit abnormality 42
PRPP see polyribosyl pyrophosphate
pseudohermaphroditism 79–81
pseudo-Hurler polydystrophy see mucolipi-
    dosis III 107
Public Law 93-38, education of handicapped
    234
purine metabolism
  analogue inhibitors 19
  cell culture study 26
  genetic heterogeneity in disorders 27
  inborn errors 13–31
  interrelations 23
  Lesch–Nyhan syndrome 17–24
  overproduction 30
Pygmalion in the Classroom 232, 233
pyridoxine in homocystinuria 143–5
pyruvate kinase deficiency 6

rats, phenylalanine response of mutants 194,
    195

recognition markers 105
5α-reductase
  defect effects 81, 82
  sex steroid biosynthesis 78
17-reductase 78
  defect 81, 82
  effects of defect 81
renal failure, Lesch–Nyhan syndrome 17
renal transplantation
  Fabry's disease 142
  Gaucher's disease 141
renin hypotension in childhood 77
reticuloendothelial system in sphingolipid
    storage disease 149
RNA types and gene action 4

saltatory conduction 174
salt loss 73
Sandhoff disease 104
  protein 7
Sanfilippo syndromes (mucopolysacchari-
    dosis type III) 7, 271
  corrective factor excretion 125
  corrective factor and transplant 123, 124
  enzyme deficiency 113, 114
  fibroblast transplantation 113–126
  oligosaccharide fractions 114, 117, 119,
    120
  sulphamino : hexosamine ratio 120, 121
  uronic acid excretion and fibroblast trans-
    plantation 114, 116, 117
Scheie syndrome 7
school see also education
  anxiety 214, 216
  and long term treatment 214–16
Schwann cells in dystrophic mice 184, 185
screening 255–63
  alphafetoprotein 261, 262
  anxiety causes 273
  carrier detection 260
  centres 268
  cervix carcinoma 261
  consent and timing 257
  criteria for programme 256
  cystic fibrosis 258, 259
  and diagnosis 255, 272, 273
  and follow up 258
  HLA typing 262
  hyperphenylalaninaemia 257
  hypothyroidism 256, 258
  McKeown criteria 273
  muscular dystrophy 259, 260
Scriver chromatographic method 272
Seguin, Edouard 234

self-mutilation 14, 15
sex steroid defects 79, 80
sex steroids, biosynthesis 77–79
side-effects of long-term treatment, assessment 213
sitting, age of attaining and Down's syndrome 248, 249
South Sea Islands, mental handicap care 227
sphingomyelin 140, 141
spina bifida, genetics and mouse model 162, 163
spleen transplant, Gaucher's disease 140, 141
Stein–Leventhal syndrome 82
steroid biosynthesis
  biochemistry 70
  17-deoxy pathway 71
  known defects 70
  pathway 69
  see also adrenal, sex steroids
steroid biosynthesis defects 69–83
  feto-placental unit 82, 83
steroids, C-21 synthesis 72
Stigma 275
stones, xanthine 23
Strumpell–Lorrain paraplegia, mouse model 170
sudanophilic leukodystrophy, mouse model 179
sulphatase defect 82, 83
Sweden, education and handicapped 229

Tay–Sachs disease 104, 281
  Ashkenazi Jews 6
  enzyme replacement 143–45
  globosides 143, 144
  hexosaminidases 143
  proteins 7
  therapeutic strategy 145
teaching techniques 229–31
  handicap 229–31, 240, 241
  for sitting 248
  timing in Down's syndrome 247
testosterone
  biosynthesis 70–2
  biosynthesis defect 79
6-thioguanine 19, 21
transcobalamin 45
  II critical role 48
  deficiencies 47, 48

transketolase in alcoholism 9
transport systems and blood–brain barrier 88, 89
treatment 273–6
  and cooperation 274
  and information 274
  therapeutic agent bank 274
treatment, long-term 211–22
  anxiety assessment 215–17
  educational experiences 214–16
  IQ 213
  parents role 219, 220
  psychosocial side-effects 212
  and social contact 219–21
tryptophan, blood–brain barrier transport competition 91–3
tyrosinosis in Quebecois 6

UNESCO 225
United Nations Declaration on the Rights of Mentally Retarded Persons 233, 234
uric acid accumulation 13; see also gout
uronic acid excretion and mucopolysaccharidosis 114–116

vitamin A, teratogen 162
vitamin B_{12} deficiency 61
vitamin metabolism, enzyme mutant sites of action 44
vitamin-responsive inherited metabolic disorders 37–49
vocational training 235
vomiting 14, 16

Wallerian degeneration 185
Werdnig–Hoffman syndrome, animal model 167, 170, 179, 187
Wernicke–Korsakoff syndrome 9
  enzyme deficiency 9
  thiamine 9
  transketolase 9, 10
Wilson's disease, copper chelation 275
Wolfgram proteins, mld mice 178, 182, 183
World Health Organisation 225
  alphafetoprotein reference material 262

xanthine oxidase
  congenital defect 18
  inhibition 23